Cutaneous Disorders of the Lower Extremities

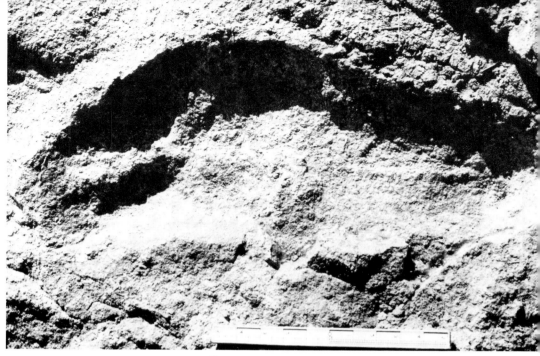

Footprint in 3.6-million-year-old volcanic rock in the Laetoli region
(Olduvai Gorge, Tanzania) (Photo courtesy of Dr. Mary D. Leakey;
Peter Jones, © National Geographic Society)

Some 3,600,000 years ago, the first certain ancestor of man walked with a foot that is almost indistinguishable from the foot of modern man.

During my stay in Tanzania in the spring of 1979 as Visiting Professor at the University of Dar es Salaam, I had the opportunity to visit the site in the Laetoli region (in Olduvai Gorge) where, in 1978, Dr. Mary D. Leakey discovered the hominid footprints that are remarkably similar to those of modern man.[1] Later, I visited The Louis Leakey Institute in Nairobi where Dr. John Harris showed me the fiberglass mold of these footprints. Excitedly, I viewed the remarkable detail and recalled Dr. Leakey's description: "the form of the foot was exactly the same as ours."[2] I had a question: Is it possible that plantar markings (dermatoglyphics) could have been visualized in the original footprints? Dr. Leakey was away, so I directed the question to her in a letter. She was most kind to respond as follows: "The sediment in which the prints are made is not sufficiently fine-grained to take impression of skin markings," and sent with her letter a photo of a hominid footprint and permission to publish the photo in our book.[3] (Photograph above.)

I am extremely grateful to Dr. Leakey.

Although the skin markings are not defined, the illustration is highly relevant to the concepts in our text. We can hypothesize that as man evolved into his present form, separate sets of anatomically specialized cells developed during embryonic life. We have noted a curious linkage between certain internal disease syndromes and skin changes on the lower extremities. The reason for these associations is obscure but in view of the frequent associations it is apparent that certain distinctive characteristic lesions on the lower extremities are "skin markers" of a corresponding internal disease.

1. Leakey MD: Footprints in the ashes of time, National Geographic, 155: 446–457, 1979
2. Ibid., p 453
3. Personal correspondence, August 4, 1979

Cutaneous Disorders of the Lower Extremities

M.H. SAMITZ, M.D., M.Sc. (Med.)

Emeritus Professor of Dermatology
School of Medicine
University of Pennsylvania;
Past Chairman and Consultant, Department of Dermatology
Graduate Hospital; and
Emeritus Professor and Consultant in Dermatology
Pennsylvania College of Podiatric Medicine
Philadelphia, Pennsylvania

second edition

6 CONTRIBUTORS

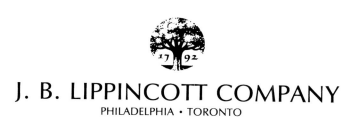

J. B. LIPPINCOTT COMPANY
PHILADELPHIA · TORONTO

The authors and publisher have exerted every effort to ensure that drug selection and dosage set forth in this text are in accord with current recommendations and practice at the time of publication. However, in view of ongoing research, changes in government regulations, and the constant flow of information relating to drug therapy and drug reactions, the reader is urged to check the package insert for each drug for any change in indications and dosage and for added warnings and precautions. This is particularly important when the recommended agent is a new or infrequently employed drug.

Library of Congress Cataloging in Publication Data

Samitz, MH,   DATE
  Cutaneous disorders of the lower extremities.

  First ed. published in 1971 under title: Cutaneous lesions of the lower extremities.
  Includes bibliographical references.
  1. Skin—Diseases. 2. Extremities, Lower—Diseases.
3. Cutaneous manifestations of general diseases.
I. Title. [DNLM: 1. Leg dermatoses. 2. Foot
dermatoses.
RL72.S33 1981   616.5'4   80-25266
ISBN 0-397-50427-6

To Doris

CONTENTS

CONTRIBUTORS

ORLANDO CANIZARES, M.D.
Professor of Clinical Dermatology
New York University College of Medicine
New York, New York

CHARLES L. HEATON, M.D.
Associate Professor of Dermatology
University of Cincinnati College of Medicine
Cincinnati, Ohio

SIDNEY HURWITZ, M.D.
Associate Clinical Professor of Pediatrics and Dermatology
Yale University School of Medicine
New Haven, Connecticut

JOHN N. LABOWS, JR., Ph.D.
Associate Member
Monell Chemical Senses Center
Philadelphia, Pennsylvania

JOHN E. LEWIS, M.D.
Sparks Regional Medical Center
Fort Smith, Arkansas

JOSEPH A. WITKOWSKI, M.D.
Clinical Associate Professor of Dermatology
University of Pennsylvania School of Medicine, and
Associate Professor of Dermatology
Pennsylvania College of Podiatric Medicine
Philadelphia, Pennsylvania

PREFACE

Many people have helped and encouraged us with the second edition, but none more than our students and colleagues.

The response to *Cutaneous Lesions of the Lower Extremities* showed that there was clearly a need for this particular text because its contents presented information previously unavailable. From comments received from colleagues and readers, it is apparent the book has succeeded in meeting the needs of not only the general practitioner but also of the internist, the surgeon, the dermatologist, and the podiatrist. It has been adopted by the schools of podiatric medicine as the basic text in dermatology.

Reviews of the first edition were highly favorable and such widespread acceptance confirmed our original motive for writing the book and was most gratifying. Some changes were recommended by several reviewers if another edition were contemplated. Some of these were relevant and they have been incorporated into the new text.

Our perspective has been expanded. The title of the second edition has been changed to *Cutaneous Disorders of the Lower Extremities* to accommodate a more balanced point of view for the reader wishing more information. We have taken the opportunity to add certain fresh facts and make some modifications in the light of knowledge gained since the first edition appeared. Several sections have been revised and updated. Recent information in immunodermatology, cutaneous physiology, and on microcirculation involved in pathogenetic mechanisms underlying many common disorders have been included. Eight new chapters have been added in which the syndromes described are of sufficient importance and distinction to accurately and clearly reveal the relation to disease locale, such as nutritional deficiencies, cutaneous manifestations of systemic diseases, pediatric-dermatologic problems on the lower extremities, the geriatric foot, the swollen leg, skin tumors of the lower extremities, toenail disorders, and skin foot problems in association with sports. The last chapter on miscellaneous disorders covers a wide range of subjects from corns and calluses to foot odor and unusual conditions that can affect the legs. We have arbitrarily chosen to emphasize subjects of current interest concerned with clinical problems found in many areas of everyday practice. These choices have been made because they provide a general perspective; the text is by no means a catalog of all diseases that can occur on the lower extremities.

Selected references follow each chapter and are grouped according to subject matter, which is a feature that should be helpful to both the student and the practitioner. Cross-references to chapters dealing with special subjects are used in order to avoid repetition.

The material is based on experience in our offices and in the dermatology clinics of the Hospital of the University of Pennsylvania and the Graduate Hospital of the University of Pennsylvania as well as on my experience as Consultant to the Pennsylvania College of Podiatric Medicine.

M.H. Samitz, M.D., M.Sc. (Med.)

PREFACE TO THE FIRST EDITION

Cutaneous disorders that show a predilection for the lower extremities are the subject of this text.

Lesions of the lower extremity are a significant diagnostic and therapeutic challenge not only to the general practitioner, but also to the internist, surgeon and dermatologist. It is hoped that this book will be useful in the teaching of dermatology in schools of podiatry, and practical information for the podiatric practitioner has also been emphasized.

Although the diagnostic importance of the regional localization of lesions can be exaggerated, there is often great significance in the specialized patterns of their distribution. This might involve cutaneous lesions that are the sole expression of disease—such as tinea pedis, which reflects purely local factors such as moisture, heat and maceration—or those cutaneous lesions that reflect a systemic disease affecting various organ systems, such as ulcers in hematopoietic disease or necrobiosis lipoidica seen with diabetes.

Topics have been selected on the basis of their importance in the clinical practice of the internist and dermatologist. New data on physiologic and biochemical properties that clarify skin function in health and disease are discussed, and clinical applications are emphasized.

The material is based on experience in our offices and in the dermatology clinics of the Hospital of the University of Pennsylvania and the Graduate Hospital of the University of Pennsylvania. Some ideas have been expressed by others; the selected bibliographies indicate the sources of this information.

ACKNOWLEDGMENTS

I am indebted to more people that I can possibly name, but I must especially thank the contributors and collaborators who were most kind to offer their expertise in their particular fields and were responsible for substantial contributions.

Joseph A. Witkowski, M.D., Clinical Associate Professor of Dermatology, University of Pennsylvania, School of Medicine, and Associate Professor of Dermatology, Pennsylvania College of Podiatric Medicine, collaborated in Chapters 1, 2, and 5 and permitted the use of the photographs of gout, necrobiosis lipoidica diabeticorum ulceration, "toasted skin" syndrome, and the figure on dermatoglyphics, and gave invaluable assistance.

John E. Lewis, M.D., collaborated in the chapters on Toenails, The Geriatric Foot, Genodermatoses, and Tumors, and was indefatigable in the search of pertinent literature. He also reviewed the entire manuscript and gave constructive criticism.

Sidney Hurwitz, M.D., Associate Clinical Professor of Pediatrics and Dermatology, Yale University School of Medicine, was solely responsible for Chapter 8, Pediatric-Dermatologic Problems on the Lower Extremities, and the accompanying illustrations.

Orlando Canizares, M.D., Professor of Clinical Dermatology, New York University, College of Medicine, was responsible for the section on Tropical Dermatology.

Charles L. Heaton, M.D., Associate Professor of Dermatology, University of Cincinnati College of Medicine, updated his previous section on syphilis.

G. T. Anderson, M.D., wrote the excellent sections in the chapter on Immersion Injuries in the first edition and these have been retained in this edition with some modifications.

John N. Labows, Jr., Ph.D., Associate Member, Monell Chemical Senses Center, contributed the section on Foot Odor.

Jack Weiner, M.D., Clinical Assistant Professor of Dermatology, University of Pennsylvania, re-read the first edition for errors and offered suggestions for corrections.

Approximately 90% of the illustrations and photographs are of patients I have treated over the past 40 years. I am extremely grateful for selected photographs from Dr. G. Ted Anderson, Dr. Jack Weiner, Dr. Stanton S. Lebouitz, Dr. Steven E. Gammer, Dr. Harvey Lemont, Dr. Tom Ross, Dr. Donald L. Baxter, Dr. Carrel and Podiatric Affiliates (Buffalo, N.Y.), Dr. R.I. Patel (Nairobi, Kenya), and Dr. Aaron E.J. Masawe (Dar es Salaam, Tanzania).

I am inexpressibly grateful to Schering Laboratories, Kenilworth, New Jersey, for a grant that made possible the placement of the color plates in proximity to related text.

I owe much gratitude to my secretary, Ms. Margaretta Hummel, for the patience and dedication in typing and retyping the many drafts of the manuscript—she was a tremendous support.

I am extremely grateful to J. Stuart Freeman, Jr., Editor-in-Chief, Medical Books, J.B. Lippincott Company, who was never too busy to advise and encourage me, and to Darlene Pedersen, Manuscript Editor.

And to my former students and residents who lent a hand on my journey of some 40 years to make the learning and teaching of dermatology an exciting experience, my gratitude is equal.

Cutaneous Disorders of the Lower Extremities

1 BASIC PRINCIPLES

LOCALIZATION OF LESIONS ON THE LOWER EXTREMITIES

FACTS AND HYPOTHESES FOR THE REGIONAL PREDILECTION

Certain skin disorders tend to occur exclusively in specific body areas or, at times, remain confined to them. Frequently, the reason for such topographical distribution can be readily explained; however, in some disorders the explanation is subject to question.

The lower leg and foot do indeed present special and important features. If we consider disorders such as corns, callosities, plantar warts, tinea pedis, erythema ab igne, "toasted skin" syndrome, sweaty feet, varicose ulcers, shoe dermatitis, or stasis dermatitis, the circumstances accounting for their localization are readily explained by physical factors.

Weight bearing, abnormal biomechanics, and anatomical abnormalities contribute to the development of corns and callosities; warts in areas of pressure are in part related to the excessive weight placed on a small skin area or to mechanical factors. The interdigital spaces of some toes, such as the third and fourth interspaces, are relatively narrowed, allowing the skin to become macerated and increasing the tendency to bacterial, dermatophyte, and monilial infections.

The feet and legs endure more insults than do any other part of the body. As a result of injuries, hematomas, traumatic ulcers, and foreign body granulomas, cuts and infections may be more common on the legs.

The lower extremities are common sites for thermal trauma, accounting for the occurrence of erythema ab igne and toasted skin syndrome.

A variety of environmental exposures are related to skin conditions on the lower extremities. The toes are vulnerable to prolonged exposure to cold, causing frostbite. The warm-water-immersion foot is a well-established entity. The lower leg is a common site for insect bites and other infestations. Sweaty feet and contact dermatitis resulting from shoes and other footgear are commonly seen. Cosmetic practices such as leg shaving, pedicures, use of nail polish, and foot beauty aids (creams, lotions, powders) can also cause local reactions.

When we consider skin manifestations of systemic disease that appear on the lower extremities, the causal relationship is often puzzling. Studies of this distribution have not been accorded the emphasis they deserve. For example, are skin markers of systemic disease found on the lower extremities? The unequivocal answer is yes. The lower extremities reflect a wide spectrum of lesions that connote systemic disease. What is not clear is why and how they got there. This intriguing association has led us to propose several hypotheses that may account for such topographical predilection.[5] In this respect, we also have investigated skin tumors that show a selectivity for the lower extremities.[6]

Why do lesions connoting a systemic disease develop selectively on the lower extremities? What is responsible (the mechanism) for the localization? Is there a site-specific factor involved, or do these lesions develop

1

on the lower extremities by chance? It is our belief that repeated clinical observations of this relationship negate chance as a factor.

Various theories have been advanced to explain tissue reactivity in the lower extremity: anatomical-dependent position and circulatory, neural, hormonal/sex, and enzymatic factors. A single factor or several related factors can often explain the selective distribution. However, we believe that this conceptual framework must be amplified to account for the extent and varieties of lower extremity lesions. Certain questions come to mind: Is the skin on the lower extremities different from skin elsewhere? Is it possible that the skin is being told what to do? In the preface to our first edition we generalized that it is possible that tissue reactivity in the lower extremity is genetically coded to behave differently from how it does in other parts of the body.

We believe that the remarkably constant and limited localization of the lesions must be attributed to local phenomena peculiar to the skin of the lower extremities. Yet, why is one group of cells "sensitive" and another group not? According to Whimster, any group of cells under the influence of one neuron may, because of this, behave differently from adjacent similar cells which are influenced by other neurons.[10] Unfortunately, as Whimster continues, there is no adequate "wiring guide" in the skin to prove this.

We suggest another hypothesis. Can we presume that the lower extremity and its internal disease syndrome share certain distinctive characteristics that link them to form anatomical sets? Is this the result of development during embryonic life? Does localization result from a clone of cells with unique programming—cells that have become abnormal and keep producing abnormal cells—or is it the direct effect on cells from some endogenous agent? If "sensitive" cells are being triggered, what is the signal that initiates this cellular response, and what regulates the response once it is started? We know too little to explain this phenomenon.

On the other hand, recent studies have clarified mechanisms accounting for the selective distribution of some disorders to the lower extremities. Copeman suggests that the localization of cutaneous angiitis is based on a combination of factors which include the anatomical disposition of blood vessels, hemodynamic back pressure to which dependent skin is subjected, exposure and vulnerability to chilling on the peripheries, and constriction by clothing.[1] The pattern of livedo reticularis can be produced under various circumstances: in-flow obstruction (lupus erythematosus, hyperthyroidism); hyperviscosity of blood in capillaries and venules as occurring in polycythemia, thrombocythemia, and cold-precipitable proteinemias; and out-flow obstruction caused by immune and protein complex deposition or endotoxin damage.[2] Erythema nodosum appears to be an inflammatory response of the panniculus that reflects a delayed hypersensitivity reaction to an antigen.[11] We attribute this limited distribution to some local conditions peculiar to the legs. Were fat cells in this disorder coded to behave differently?

Anatemical organization of the lower extremity can also account for disorders of the panniculus. In acrocyanosis, pads of fat around the lower leg, particularly in women, often insulate this skin from heat in the core of the limb and predispose it to acrocyanosis.[4]

Cutaneous necrotizing vasculitides are frequently restricted to the lower extremities despite a range of pathogenetic mechanisms which include immune complexes, cellular hypersensitivity reactions, and involvement of C3 defects.[3,7–9,12] According to Ryan, "the legs are affected more often than any other part of the body in most forms of vasculitis, particularly in those at the purpuric and infarctive end of the spectrum. The most likely reason for this is the effect of the upright posture on the vasculature. The long-term effect of gravity on the vasculature of the lower legs is to dilate the deeper arteriovenous anastomoses through which blood is short-circuited; this leads to stasis in the capillaries even when supine."[4] Thus, the state of the vasculature of the lower extremity is important. It plays an active role in sickle cell ulcers wherein the abnormal red cell in sickle cell anemia may transit through a more sluggish circulation in the legs, give up more oxygen, and change its shape, to the extent that the altered cell will not move as readily through the vessels. The blood vessel progressively occludes, and the cutaneous tissues become devitalized and ulcerate. Macroglobulins may tend to aggregate under the same stagnated circumstances, likewise resulting in tissue necrosis and ulceration. Cold may cause excessive amounts of cryoglobulins or cryofibrinogens to precipitate and produce trophic changes in the skin.

Various tumors show a tendency to occur almost exclusively or regularly on the lower extremities. On the basis of our clinical experience, augmented by review of the literature, we noted at least 15 types of tumor predisposed to involve the integument and its appendages of the lower extremities.[6]

Is there an explanation for this topographical predilection? Is there a site-specific factor involved, or do these tumors develop on the lower extremities by chance? We know too little to explain this behavior related to tumors.

Speculating on possible predisposing factors that lead to topographical selectivity, we can consider internal and external factors, as well as heritable and acquired factors.

Viewed from this perspective, the hemodynamic uniqueness of the lower extremity is one example of an internal factor. Relative venous hypertension is conducive to the localization of infectious or noninfectious agents. Let us suppose that the Epstein-Barr virus were etiologic in Kaposi's sarcoma (if we consider this disease to be an infectious, granulomatous neoplasm). Under this supposition, it seems plausible that the relative venous hypertension in the lower extremities might lead to preferential early localization of the viral agent, producing the multicentric lesions seen on the legs.

An important external factor is the extreme variation in thickness of the stratum corneum as encountered on the soles. Plantar epidermis, as well as palmar, is a strong keratin-producer. We can deduce, for instance, that arsenical keratoses localize in these sites because arsenic has an affinity for keratinizing epithelium.

In another situation, we ask if a benign or malignant tumor can be localized because of external trauma. The plantar wart is an excellent example of a condition in which pressure plays a leading role. Trauma is considered essential in the localization of plantar fibromatosis and in the evolution of malignant melanoma arising *de novo* or in the junction nevus on the sole, especially in Blacks. Histiocytomas represent an inflammatory proliferation of histiocytes which may follow trauma; in many instances, arthropod bites have been incriminated as being antecedent.

Both heritable and acquired factors allude to the structural and anatomical conditions that account for subungual exostosis arising from the phalanx and presenting as a tumor of the nail bed. In that the integumentary covering of the nail bed has no substance to it, a tumorous growth of bone must arise, perforce, in a subungual location.

We can offer no hypotheses to explain why the eccrine poroma, the clear-cell acanthoma, and stucco keratoses seem to prefer the lower extremities.

It is apparent that explanations for the selective distribution of tumors or of lesions connoting systemic disease rest often on circumstantial evidence, and the causal agent in many cases cannot be precisely defined. The functional significance, if any, of these curious linkages remains to be determined. Nonetheless, these skin lesions of the lower extremities are diagnostic clues that may lead the "prepared mind" to elucidate further the pathogenesis of many local and systemic disorders.

CLASSIFICATION OF SKIN DISEASES

In order to differentiate cutaneous lesions that are strictly dermatologic entities from those that are the counterparts of lesions in internal organs, a simple classification may be used.

I. Heritable
  A. Inborn errors of metabolism (*e.g.,* hyperlipoproteinemias, "gouty" syndromes, acrodermatitis enteropathica)
  B. Biochemical defect still unknown (*e.g.,* epidermolysis bullosa, ichthyosis, mal de Meleda, keratoderma palmaris et plantaris).

II. Acquired
   A. External causes (*e.g.,* impetigo, contact dermatitis, dermatophytosis)
   B. Internal causes
      1. Skin lesions precede systemic disease (*e.g.,* necrobiosis lipoidica diabeticorum with diabetes, scleroderma preceding systemic sclerosis)
      2. Skin lesions secondary to systemic disease (*e.g.,* pyoderma gangrenosum with ulcerative colitis, leg ulcers due to hypertension, sickle cell anemia or diabetes, vesicles on the feet in hand, foot and mouth viral disease)
   C. Diseases limited to skin; strictly dermatologic entities of known and unknown origin (*e.g.,* psoriasis, lichen planus, x-ray dermatitis)

It is essential for one to have a reasonable knowledge of:

1. The anatomy of the skin,
2. The relationship between structure and function, and
3. The biochemical factors and physiologic alterations that play a role in causing the pathologic picture.

HUMAN SKIN

An understanding of human skin is incomplete without knowledge of skin functions in lower animals. The morphology and physiology of human skin is the outcome of a long period of phylogenetic development. None of the varied adaptive changes, such as the modification of the papillae of pads which is unique in different bird species, was necessary for humans and therefore is not present in the human foot. The comparison of footpads in nonhuman primates with soles in humans is pertinent. When man assumed the upright stance, a great burden was placed on the lower extremity. The soles of the feet helped meet this work load by presenting a thickened, tough stratum corneum.

Human skin totals about 10 pounds of weight for the average-sized man, about 7 pounds for the average woman. Estimates of the area of the human skin cover a wide range, up to 15,000 square inches, roughly the size of a 9' × 12' rug. It is a complex, flexible, fibrous structure that encases all the living tissues and organs of the body. It is the most accessible tissue of the body, it is by far the largest desquamating organ in the human body, and it may serve as an excellent model for multidisciplinary research.

The skin is divided into three layers: epidermis, dermis (corium), and hypodermis (fatty layer).

EPIDERMIS

The epidermis has a thickness approximately equal to a sheet of paper. Most of it does not exceed 0.2 mm, although it is much thicker in the palms and soles. This thickness is predetermined embryologically and not primarily by pressure and trauma, although these factors can increase thickness. When transplanted, palmar or plantar skin continues to be "palmar" or "plantar" skin morphologically, no matter where it is placed.

The epidermis is ectodermal in origin. It consists entirely of cells (anywhere from 10 layers of cells to several dozen). It contains no blood vessels or lymph channels and depends upon tissue fluid for its sustenance. It is the repository of the terminal ramifications of sensory nerve fibers and is anchored to the dermis by the papillae of the dermis, with which it is functionally interdependent.

The epidermis contains two distinct cell types:

1. Keratinocytes, which produce the fibrous protein keratin, possess A and B blood group antigens, and share in some immune reactions
2. Dendritic cells
   a. Melanocytes, the melanin-forming cells
   b. Langerhans' cells (LC), considered an antigen-processing cell. LC plays a macrophage-like role in contact allergic reactions and in other types of cell-mediated responses
   c. Indeterminate cells, which are similar to LC; their origin and function are unknown.

The keratinocytes are most numerous and comprise approximately 95% of the epidermis; the dencritic cells make up the other 5%.

On microscopic examination, the epidermis is separated into five layers—basal, prickle, granular, stratum lucidum (visible only on the palms and soles), and horny—representing distinct functional stages in the keratinization process.

The basal layer is innermost and consists of a single row of columnar cells. Scattered among the cylindrical cells, there is also an interconnecting network of dendritic cells (melanocytes) that branch among, and carry melanin pigment to, the adjoining epidermal cells. The ratio of active melanocytes to keratinocytes is about 1:36. Keratinocytes actively phagocytize the melanin-combining tips of melanocytic dendrites. Racial color differences are due to the number and size of mature melanosomes and the way they are dispersed in the keratinocytes. Frequently, melanin granules form a supranuclear cap in the basal cells.

The basal layer is the progenitor of all the other cells in the epidermis. The main source of regenerative activity is from the basal layer; mitotic activity is greatest at night and is accelerated as a response to removal of the stratum corneum, injury, and repair. The increase in cell population from normal mitotic activity produces a gradual outward displacement of all the cells toward the surface.

The prickle cell layer (stratum spinosum, malpighian layer) composes most of the epidermis and is made up of cells that are polygonal and form a mosaic. The cells are separated by spaces that are traversed by intercellular bridges or prickles. The spaces are perhaps functionally analogous to lymphatic vessels and play an important part in the nutrition and metabolic exchanges of the cells. Electron microscopy has demonstrated that the prickles are "attachment plaques" of the cell membranes of opposing cells; tonofibrils extend from the cytoplasm out to the plaques. The entire complex has been termed the **desmosome.**

The granular layer (stratum granulosum) consists of diamond-shaped cells filled with basophilic granules. The thickness of the stratum granulosum varies from one to three layers. It is most prominent where the degree of keratinization is most active. The cells are less hydrated, their nuclei are disorganized, and the intercellular bridges have all but disappeared.

The stratum lucidum is a narrow band of flattened cells that lack nuclei and is situated immediately beneath the horny layer. It is most prominent and visible on the palms and soles. It derives its name from the fact that it does not take usual histologic stains.

The horny layer (stratum corneum) is the outermost or surface layer of the epidermis. It is composed of compressed, parallel, homogenized, nonnucleated cells—dead epithelial cells that have become horny or keratinized. The lower part of the horny layer is compact and coherent (stratum compactum), but in its upper part the horny cells lose their coherence (stratum disjunctum). The horny layer varies in thickness from 10μ on the face, to 40 to 50μ on the trunk, to 400 to 700μ on the soles. The thickness is relatively constant when not affected by external forces. Based on a body surface area of 2 square meters, the amount of horny material produced is 0.5 to 1 g daily. In exfoliative dermatitis, the amount may reach 9 to 17 g daily.

Keratinization

The term "keratinization" denotes the morphologic and biochemical changes associated with the outward progress of cells from the basal layer to the horny layer. It has been estimated that it takes approximately 28 days for a cell to mature, that is, to progress from basal layer to final shedding.

Keratinization is the synthesis of fibrous proteins made up of amino acids embedded in an amorphous ground substance. The sequence of amino acids along the polypeptide chains is probably significant in determining the type of keratin. Keratinization is not synonymous with horny layer formation. The horny layer contains about 50% of other materials, by-products of keratinization, along with keratin and glandular secretions.

DERMIS

The dermis, or corium, the connective-tissue layer, along with its blood vessels and nerves, supports and is intimately associated with the overlying epidermis and separates it from the subcutaneous fat.

The dermis makes up the bulk of the skin. In humans, the whole mass of the dermis constitutes 15 to 20% of the total body weight. It is divided into two sections: (1) stratum papillare, the most superficial portion which projects as finger-like extensions (called papillae or papillary bodies) into the epidermis, and (2) stratum reticulare, the lower portion. The main constituents of the dermis are the collagenous, elastic, and reticular fibers. Collagen makes up about 95% of the dermis. Elastic fibers are found entwined among the collagen bundles. Reticular fibers, probably immature collagen, appear as a basketweave of fine elements. Occupying the spaces between fibers is the ground substance or matrix. Cellular elements consist of fibrocytes, histiocytes, mastocytes, melanocytes, and extravasated leukocytes.

Collagen is a tough, resistant fibrous protein consisting of three polypeptide chains wound into a triple helix. Its amino acid composition shows a high content of glycine and lesser amounts of proline and hydroxyproline. Elastic fibers are composed of elastin, a protein similar to collagen but having important differences. The ground substance is a viscous material whose main constituents are the mucopolysaccharides, hyaluronic acid, and chondroitin sulfate.

The dermis also contains a superficial (subpapillary) and a deep (reticular) vascular network, lymphatic capillaries, and vessels that accompany the veins, autonomic and peripheral nerves, the epidermal appendages, and the arrectores pilorum muscles.

HYPODERMIS

The subcutis (fatty layer) is the deepest skin layer and is characterized by closely packed lipocytes. This fatty layer varies in thickness and composition and shows a selective distribution throughout the body. Fat deposition is controlled by hormones, which include sex hormones and insulin. By simple syringe-biopsy technique, the composition of fat can be studied by gas-liquid chromatography for analysis of the adipose triglycerides.

SKIN APPENDAGES

Among the appendages, the sweat glands and nails are pertinent to the lower extremities. The ubiquitous eccrine sweat glands are coiled tubular glands situated at the dermal-subdermal junction, with ther ducts straightening out, piercing the dermis, and finally spiraling through the epidermis to the surface. Pertinent data relating to the eccrine glands are reviewed in the section on sweat disorders.

The nail organ is formed from an invagination of epidermis located on the dorsum of the distal phalanx of each digit. The invagination is first noted in the fetus at 9 weeks, and development of the nail plate is completed by the 20th week. The nail is formed by the matrix located at the floor of the posterior nail fold. It grows forward instead of upward because of pressure from the posterior nail fold. Nails grow continuously throughout life at an average rate of between 0.5 and 1.2 mm per week. Toenails grow at one-third to one-half the rate of fingernails. There is also some variation in the precise growth rate of the nails of the various individual digits; in general, the longer the digit, the more rapid the nail growth.

The formation of nail by the matrix is an active metabolic process and is therefore susceptible to local and systemic disorders. The nail plate is a dead structure, and defects of the plate represent the "scars" of previous damage to the matrix occurring when that particular portion of nail was being formed.

The nail normally appears pink because of the reflection of light from the underlying capillary bed throughout the translucent nail. Normally the epithelium of the nail bed does not keratinize. If as a result of a pathologic process, the nail bed produces keratin, the nail appears white rather than pink.

The nail changes seen in various diseases of the feet will be described as each clinical disorder is discussed.

HISTOPATHOLOGIC FACTORS

Epidermis

Pathologic processes primarily involving the epidermis may be

1. Congenital
   a. generalized, as ichthyosis vulgaris
   b. localized, as keratoderma palmaris et plantaris
2. Acquired
   a. limited, as a callus
   b. diffuse, as pityriasis rubra pilaris

Pathologic changes in the epidermis depend upon the involved cellular tissue: keratinocyte or melanocyte.

Keratinocyte

1. Alterations in function
   a. Hyperkeratosis. Increased keratinocyte activity as seen in the corn or callus in which the hyperkeratosis is due to stimulation of the epidermis by intermittent pressure
   b. Parakeratosis. Accelerated keratinocyte activity, usually seen in association with inflammatory diseases (*e.g.*, psoriasis) or neoplasia (*e.g.*, squamous cell cancer). The resulting cells are not completely mature and therefore retain their nuclei
   c. Dyskeratosis. Imperfect keratinocyte activity or abnormal cornification as the benign disorder Darier's disease, or as a malignant change in Paget's disease of the nipple, Bowen's disease, and squamous cell carcinoma
2. Alterations from injury. The malpighian layer is the principal site and is characterized by the blistering diseases
   a. Allergic contact dermatitis. Spongiosis (intercellular edema), widening of the intercellular spaces due to edema
   b. Autoimmune disease: Pemphigus. Acantholysis, loss of adhesion between epidermal cells resulting in clefts, vesicles, or bullae, which may be due to loss of intercellular cement or the intercellular bridges
   c. Viral infection, herpes simplex, herpes zoster, varicella. Ballooning degeneration (intracellular edema): marked swelling of the cells, which results in acantholysis, rupture of cell membranes, and the formation of multiloculated intraepidermal vesicles
   d. Friction, friction blisters, Weber-Cockayne disease. Vesicles occur in the prickle cell layer just beneath the granular layer
3. Alterations in growth
   a. Hyperplasia. Thickening of the epidermis due to increased number of cells
   b. Acanthosis. An increase in the thickness of the prickle cell layer
   c. Papillomatosis. Digitate projection of the epidermis above the skin surface (*e.g.*, verrucae, seborrheic keratoses)
   d. Anaplasia. Increased thickness of the epidermis due to malignancy; the cells have large, irregularly shaped and hyperchromatic nuclei and atypical mitotic figures (*e.g.*, basal and squamous cell cancer)

Melanocyte

1. Alterations in function
   a. Hyperfunction: postinflammatory hyperpigmentation, tanning, freckles, chloasma.
   b. Hypofunction: postinflammatory hypopigmentation (leukoderma)
   c. Absent function: albinism
2. Alterations in growth
   a. Benign
      1. Epidermal melanocytes: lentigo simplex, lentigo senilis, café au lait, and so forth
      2. Nevus cells: junction, compound, and intradermal nevi
      3. Dermal melanocytes: blue nevus, mongolian spot, and so forth
   b. Malignant
      1. Lentigo maligna, superficial spreading melanoma, malignant melanoma
3. Absence of melanocytes
   a. Genetic: piebaldism, Waardenburg syndrome
   b. Acquired: vitiligo

Langerhans' cell (LC)

Damage to LC (from substances released from sensitized lymphocytes and/or antigen-antibody complexes plus complement) leads to edema, spongiosis, vesiculation, bulla formation, and urtication, which characterize the early histologic changes in allergic contact dermatitis.

Corium

Pathologic changes in the corium are innumerable; in general, they may be described according to cellular connective tissue, and matrix.

Cellular Changes. Simple inflammations: acute or chronic; granulomas; neoplasias.

1. Acute inflammations: characterized by a perivascular infiltration usually around the pilosebaceous apparatus and sweat glands. The infiltrate is usually composed of polymorphonuclear leukocytes. Lymphocytes predominate in subacute and chronic inflammations; in deeper chronic inflammations, plasma cells are increased.
2. Granulomas: the cellular infiltrations characteristic of a limited number of slowly progressive, persistent diseases. Granulomas consist of plasma cells, epithelioid cells, and multinucleated giant cells.
   a. Nonspecific granulomas: from chronic mechanical or chemical irritation (*i.e.*, poor-fitting shoes, purulent exudates).
   b. Foreign body granulomas: due to substances inplanted in the skin such as metals, wooden splinters, oils, silicone, silica, or starch, or to substances formed endogenously such as keratin or urates.
   c. Allergic granulomas: due to delayed hypersensitivity to (1) Foreign substance or microorganism that is being phagocytized. Zirconium, beryllium, and dyes used in tattoos can produce allergic granulomas. Among the microorganisms inducing infectious allergic granulomas are *Mycobacterium tuberculosis, M. leprae, Treponema pallidum*, and deep mycoses. (2) Idiopathic: sarcoidosis and allergic granulomatosis.

The infectious granulomas have certain distinctive histologic features: for example, plasma cells in syphilis, lepra cells in leprosy, tubercles in tuberculosis, abscesses and sinuses in addition to plasma cells in mycotic granulomas.

3. Neoplasms (tumor cells): those primary in the corium are characterized by cellular infiltrations that conform to the cells of origin of their lineage. They may be benign or malignant: The fibroma is a benign alteration; the fibrosarcoma and reticulum cell sarcoma are malignant changes in the connective tissue cells. Carcinomas resemble those of either the basal cell or prickle cell layer of the epidermis, or they may be mixed. Around the invading edge of most malignant tumors, there is a tissue reaction consisting of plasma cells and leukocytes.

In melanomas, the tumor cells contain large, irregularly densely stained nuclei and nucleoli, the greatest activity being at the dermoepidermal junction.

Alterations in the Connective Tissue

1. Elastic fibers—may be degenerated, scarce, or absent (scars). In atrophic skin, the elastic fibers show marked changes, and fatty or calcareous deposits may occur.
2. Collagenous fibers—may be subject to a variety of chemical degenerative changes which give rise to altered staining reactions

Changes in the Matrix. These relate to chemical alterations in hyaluronic acid and chondroitin sulfate.

Hypodermis

Pathologic Changes in the Fatty Layer. These changes are divided into:

1. Noninflammatory disorders such as low-protein edema (cardiac, renal), high-protein edema (lymphedema, elephantiasis), and cold injury (immersion foot).
2. Inflammatory disorders such as traumatic (mechanical, physical, or chemical), infective (tuberculosis, syphilis, leprosy), pancreatic disease, and uncertain cause such as erythema nodosum, nodular vasculitis, or Weber-Christian disease.

STRUCTURE AND FUNCTION
OF THE SKIN

As man evolved, two critical cutaneous adaptations appeared: loss of most of his body hair and the development of eccrine sweat glands, which serve a thermoregulatory function. These evolutionary changes resulted in increased freedom of movement, but at the expense of protection. For man to survive in his environment, it was essential that he evolve adaptations of his cutaneous integument to provide an effective barrier against the continuous onslaught of radiation, chemicals, and microorganisms to which he is subjected and to prevent loss of water to the external environment. The human skin has successfully developed this bidirectional barrier function, thus preventing the egress of water and the ingress of noxious environmental agents.

Protection against mechanical trauma is provided by a two-phase integumentary system—tough yet resilient fibers imbedded in a pliable matrix—which is present throughout all layers of the skin. The stratum corneum provides a protective external barrier of great toughness over the entire body surface. The principal function of the epidermis is the replacement of the stratum corneum cells that are being continuously worn away or shed.

Water is an important constituent of the stratum corneum. At least 10% of water by weight is necessary for the skin to maintain its flexibility and strength. When the water content falls below 10%, the skin becomes chapped; it loses its mechanical pliability, cracks, and breaks down. Excessive hydration of the horny layer results in maceration of the skin. When the thick stratum corneum of the soles absorbs too much water, immersion foot results. Excessive hydration of the stratum corneum also alters its barrier function, allowing topically applied substances to become absorbed. (The clinical practice of occluding the skin with impermeable dressings utilizes this action.)

In protecting against chemical agents, the horny layer acts as a physical barrier. Through the darkening of pigment precur-sors, the subsequent increased production and migration of melanin, and the later thickening of the horny layer, the skin achieves some measure of protection against ultraviolet radiation.

The dermis is composed of collagen and elastin fibers within a ground-substance matrix. It functions as a support for the epidermis and binds the epidermis so that it conforms to the underlying tissues. The dermis contains up to a quarter of the body fluid, and the skin is the major organ for water storage.

The subcutaneous fat layer below the dermis provides a measure of insulation, protecting the body from excess external heat and decreasing heat loss when exposed to the cold.

CUTANEOUS CIRCULATION

The dermis and subcutaneous fat are supplied with blood through patternless masses of interlacing vessels. The number of blood vessels appears to be far in excess of the biological needs of the skin. The primary function of this extensive vascular network is temperature regulation.

Circulatory Patterns

Arterioles oriented perpendicularly to the skin surface branch in the upper reticular dermis into smaller arterioles. These ultimately divide into hairpin-shaped capillary loops in the dermal papillae. The pattern has the configuration of a candelabra.[4] Returning blood flows into a horizontally oriented plexus of venules in the subpapillary dermis, then into descending venules and collecting veins in the subcutaneous tissue.

The configuration of the papillary capillaries varies with disease, trauma, and aging. In acrocyanotic skin, the tips of the capillaries are dilated. The loops are elongated and coiled in acanthotic epidermal diseases. In psoriasis and on lower extremities' skin in association with gravitational stasis, similar changes are seen. In epidermal atrophy seen with scars, aging, chronic exposure to extremes of temperature and ultraviolet light, use of potent topical corticosteroids, scleroderma, and on the shins, there is a decrease in the number of the papillary capillaries. In many of these same conditions, an associated loss of supporting collagen and ground substance results in dilation of the horizontal venous plexus and remaining capillaries, producing telangiectasis. Where the skin is regenerating in wound healing, one sees a disorganized pattern of anastomosing capillaries.

Microscopic examination of the blood vessels on the skin of the lower extremities shows that they are generally thickened. Venules have increased amounts of smooth muscle, supporting adventitia, and even elastic tissue. These changes are even more pronounced in patients with hypertension and the pernioses. This arteriolization of venules endows them with a remarkable ability to contract and dilate.

The Capillary Network

As elucidated by Zweifach (Fig. 1-1) terminal arterioles eventually give rise to metarterioles or preferential channels with a single layer of smooth muscle surrounding them.[6] Capillaries consisting of an endothelial-lined tube arise from these preferential channels, anastomose, and terminate in collecting venules. Blood flow through the capillary is controlled by the precapillary sphincters and the muscular venules; contraction of the metarterioles diverts the blood through the arteriovenous anastomoses directly into the muscular venules. The capillary network is more dense in the upper dermis, around hair roots and sweat glands.

Arteriovenous Anastomoses

Cutaneous arteriovenous anastomoses are found predominantly in the upper part of the reticular dermis. They originate as branches of arterioles or arteries and connect directly to the accompanying venule or vein. In the tips of the phalanges and nail folds, these shunts or glomi have a characteristic appearance. The lumen is usually quite small, lined with endothelial cells which rest on thin reticulum fibers. The greatly thickened media consists of closely packed smooth-

muscle cells. Numerous autonomic nerves, probably both sympathetic and parasympathetic, innervate this contractile tissue. These channels are usually closed, permitting blood to flow from arterioles through the capillaries and veins, thereby serving the metabolic needs of the skin. Sudden increases in blood pressure and changes in temperature result in opening of the glomi. The shunts are also opened by progesterone, venous hypertension, and capillary obstruction.[5] In edema, the increased tissue pressure can prevent opening of A-V shunts. Increased blood flow through these shunts does not supply oxygen or nutrition to the skin. Although the skin may feel warm, it is undernourished.

Function

In general, the purpose of the circulatory system is to supply oxygen and nutrients to every cell of the organism and to remove the toxic waste products of cellular metabolism. Since different tissues have vastly different requirements under a wide range of conditions, the circulation must be subject to numerous controls. This local regulation of peripheral blood flow is achieved through the coordinated effects of several distinct systems, such as the sympathetic nervous system, local chemical substances in the tissues, and circulating factors acting on intrinsic properties of the vessels themselves.

Compared with other tissues of the body, the cells of the skin require a very low minimum blood flow to maintain their viability—roughly estimated as 0.8 cc/min/100 cc of skin tissue.[1] The blood flow of the digits can vary from a minimum of 0.5 to 1.0 cc/min/100 cc of tissue in full vasoconstriction to a maximum of 90 cc/min/100 cc of tissue in full vasodilatation. By heat acclimatization, this flow can be further increased to 122 cc/min/100 cc of tissue.[1] Thus, the blood flow through the skin can increase by a factor of 100 to 200. Short variations in blood flow can amount to as much as 20%, although they are much less during periods of extreme vasoconstriction or dilatation. Neither this tremendous range nor fluctuation of blood flow is necessary for the maintenance of cellular metabolic needs of the skin. The minimum

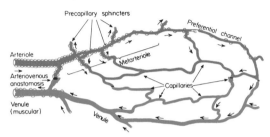

Fig. 1-1. Zweifach's concept of the basic structural pattern of the terminals of cutaneous vessels. The white humps on the walls of the vessels indicate muscle fibers. *(From Zweifach BW: Structural aspects and hemodynamics of microcirculation in the skin. In Rothman S (ed): The Human Integument, pp 67–76. Washington, DC, American Association for the Advancement of Science, Publication No. 54, 1959)*

flow would be sufficient for normal cellular needs; the maximal flow far exceeds the maximal requirements of the cells. The primary function of the cutaneous circulation is therefore to service the organism as a whole and not the skin itself. The numerous arteriovenous shunts in the skin of the acral areas play an important role in the ability of the cutaneous vasculature to dissipate or conserve heat as dictated by the needs of the organism.[3]

Temperature Regulation

Upon exposure to cold, the cutaneous blood flow is decreased by the vasoconstrictor effects resulting from stimulation of the sympathetic nerve endings, and heat is thereby retained. Conversely, an inhibition of sympathetic nerve discharges upon exposure to heat leads to cutaneous vasodilatation and increased heat loss. If this mechanism fails to produce a normal body temperature, the eccrine sweat glands increase their activity and body heat is dissipated through the evaporation of water from the skin surface.

Hunting Reaction

Although the major function of the cutaneous circulation is to serve the organism as a whole, mechanisms for fulfilling local metabolic requirements of the skin are provided as well. One of these mechanisms is the "hunting reaction" of Lewis, a cold-induced paradoxical cyclic vasodilation described in 1930.[2]

When a finger is immersed in water sufficiently cold to provide an adequate stimulus (0° C to 7° C), intense vasoconstriction occurs. The skin temperature drops to within 2 to 4 degrees of the water temperature. The digit appears pale and begins to ache, the pain increases in severity until the temperature stops falling. Within 2 to 10 minutes, the skin temperature begins to rise owing vasodilatation of the cutaneous vessels. As the temperature rises, the digit becomes more comfortable and warmer and then begins to burn and throb as the skin becomes red. With continued immersion, the temperature drops again in several minutes and may reach the original low point, although it usually does not. Over the next 4 to 6 minutes, the erythema fades and the pain subsides, only to recur again. This reaction is repeated over and over during continued immersion. The slow "hunting" of temperature is never quite rhythmic, and the rise is irregular in time and form.

Most believe that this vascular response to cold is a protective physiologic mechanism. It serves a useful purpose in protecting the peripheral parts of the body and integument against damage from exposure to cold at some presumed disadvantage to the organism. In acclimatized persons, experimental exposure to cold showed that the cycling time was shortened, faster cooling occurred initially, spontaneous rewarming occurred earlier and proceeded at a more rapid rate, higher and more labile final temperature levels were obtained, and pain decreased or disappeared on chronic exposure to cold. Blood flow was increased in chronically cold exposed digits. The ability of the blood vessels to constrict maximally was not destroyed but rather was reset at a different level of activity. In persons living in cold regions, the hunting reaction is very marked. These people suffer much less discomfort from the cold without any danger to the total heat economy of the body.

THE IMMUNE SYSTEM

The field of immunology is an important part of the continuing biologic discovery. For our purposes, it would be useful to understand immunology related to clinical practice.

The immune system is a vast network of communication in which the products of immune-response genes are used as surface-reactive molecules and as soluble transmitters for the triggering of receptors and the activation of cells.[7]

There are four major components of the immune system: B cells, T cells, the phagocyte system composed of mononuclear and polymorphonuclear leukocytes, and the complement system. Although each part is described here individually, *in vivo* the component parts act in concert.

Immunoreactive cells originate from a common stem cell in the bone marrow. Precursor lymphocytes influenced by the thymus become T cells. Those cells induced to mature through a bursal equivalent in man become B cells.

B and T cells differ notably in their surface antigenic structures: B cells possess surface immunoglobulin (Ig), which is the specific receptor for antigen recognition; T cells display little or no conventional Ig on their surfaces.[1]

The B cells are primarily concerned with humoral immunity. Five classes of immunoglobulins—IgM, IgG, IgA, IgE, and IgD—are produced by mature B cells or plasma cells. IgM and IgG play an important role in immunity against staphylococci, streptococci, and pneumococci. These two classes of immunoglobulins are also concerned with viral neutralization. They prevent viral infections, while still extracellular, from becoming established in the body. IgA, known as the secretory antibody, coats the mucosal surfaces of the nasopharyngeal and gastrointestinal systems. The presence of IgA prevents attachment of infectious agents in these areas of the body. IgE or reagin is found on the surfaces of mast cells and basophils; very small amounts are found in the serum. It is concerned with release of histamine and SRS-A from these cells to produce the clinical changes of hay fever, urticaria, asthma, and anaphylaxis. IgD is not found as a circulating immunoglobulin. Its role in humoral immunity is not known at present.

The T cells or the small circulating lymphocytes are concerned with cell-mediated immunity. There are two subpopulations of T cells: reactive T cells and memory T cells. T cells help to combat certain infections: those caused by the tubercle bacillus, fungi, especially *Candida albicans*, and intracellular viral infection such as varicella, vaccinia, and rubeola. These cells play an important role in the rejection of allografts and in tumor immune surveillance. They also mediate the inflammatory reaction characteristic of contact dermatitis and autoimmune disease. T cells also have both a helper and a suppressor function in Ig synthesis and immunologic response. A series of proteins known as lymphokines are secreted by T cells.[5] These substances are the mediators of T cell immunity. Migration inhibitory factor, chemotactic factor, cytotoxic factor, and blastogenic factor represent but a few of these substances.

Macrophages nonspecifically phagocytose and digest antigenic material. They debride wounds by disposing of damaged cells and cell debris. Macrophages are also important in the development of B and T cell immunity. They digest material into a form more suitable for linkage to the surface receptors of T and B cells, and present it to these immunoreactive cells. Macrophages are also the first line of defense against some intracellular organisms such as the mycobacteria.

Polymorphonuclear leukocytes, in addition to their phagocytic function, release lysozymes containing a number of proteases at the site of inflammation. These proteases degrade collagen, elastin, and basement membrane.

In addition to the specific elements of the immune system, immunoglobulins and lymphocytes, inflammatory processes bring into play a group of nonspecific plasma protein effector systems which may amplify immunologic inflammation.[1] These are the complement, coagulation, fibrinolytic, and kinin-forming systems.

The complement (and the properdin) system consists of approximately 20 plasma proteins that interact sequentially to mediate their inflammatory effects.[1] (They have been likened to cascades.) The reaction sequence in the classical pathway C1 through O9 is initiated by IgM, certain IgG subclasses, double- and single-stranded DNA, and other substances. The alternate pathway C3 through O9 does not require antigen-specific immunologic mediation. It may be activated by whole-antibody IgA, IgE, antibody fragments, some venoms, bacterial endotoxins, and cell membrane polysaccharides. In addition to cytolysis produced by C8 and C9, the other components of the complement system have important biological functions. C3a- and C5a-designated anaphylatoxins cause release of histamine from mast cells. Chemotaxis is provided for by C3a, C5a, C5b, V6, C7. C3b and C4 promote immune adherence. C3b facilitates phagocytosis, known as opsonization. C2 has kinin-like activity causing vasodilatation and increased vascular permeability.

Kinin-forming (bradykinin), clotting, and fibrinolytic activities are part of the Hageman factor system (HF). They exist as a second system of plasma proteins which possess considerable biologic activity.[1]

Some dermatologic disorders associated with complement defects are:

Hereditary angioedema—defective or absent C1 esterase inhibitor.
Lupus-like syndrome—deficiency of C2, C1r, and C4.
Leiner's syndrome—dysfunction of C5.
Gonnococcal syndrome—deficiency of C6.

Immunodeficiencies can be divided conveniently into primary immunodeficiency disorders and secondary immunodeficiency disorders. Primary immunodeficiencies are those in which the immunologic dysfunction appears to be the basic underlying disorder predisposing to the clinical condition; secondary immunodeficiency disorders are those in which the immunodeficiency appears to be a result rather than a cause of the disease process.[3]

Primary immunodeficiency disorders are rare, and those known have been classified and their dermatologic manifestations evaluated.[3,6] As for the secondary immunodeficiencies—and that which is germane to our theme—the skin provides a unique opportunity to observe a wide variety of immunologic responses. The ability of the skin to respond consistently to immunologic challenge is the basis for detection of many immunologically mediated illnesses which may primarily affect other organs or organ systems.[2] Although many facets of the responses remain to be elucidated, Table 1-1 shows the four classic types of immunologic responses, each with different hallmarks, that can be demonstrated in the skin.

Office evaluation of the immune status includes:[4]

B cell function
1. Quantitative estimation of immunoglobulins
2. Schick test after immunization.

T cell function
1. Total lymphocyte count
2. Skin tests with purified protein derivative (PPD), mumps, and deep fungi.

If these tests are abnormal, more specific tests should be performed.

It cannot be emphasized enough that knowledge of basic immunologic responses is essential for an understanding of many of the disorders discussed later in this book.

Table 1-1. TYPES OF IMMUNE RESPONSE

Type	Hypersensitivity	Antibody	Mediator	Disease
Type 1	Anaphylactic	IgE	Histamine SRA-A	Urticaria Angioedema
Type 2	Cytotoxic	IgM IgG	Complement	Pemphigus
Type 3	Immune Complex	IgM IgG	Complement	S.L.E. Serum Sickness Bullous Pemphigoid Leukocytoclastic Vasculitis
Type 4	Cell Mediated	T-lymphocytes	Lymphokines	Contact Dermatitis

HLA AND DISEASE

The main histocompatibility complex (MHC) is a remarkable system of genes that serve a variety of related functions, and that have been maintained together in a small chromosomal segment throughout a long period of evolution.[3] The importance of the MHC probably resides in its control of the immune response and its resistance to a variety of diseases. In man, MHC is called HLA (human leukocyte antigens), and HLA studies are providing new approaches to understanding various skin diseases (Table 1-2).

The clinical usefulness of histocompatibility antigen typing is evident from the ability to make earlier diagnoses of such disorders as ankylosing spondylitis and Reiter's syndrome. An association between HLA and certain diseases is recognized by the relative increase in frequency of particular antigens in diseased patients as compared with racially and ethnically matched control groups.

Four loci—HLA-A, B, C, and D—on the sixth chromosome contain 50 antigens that determine the histocompatibility of tissues.[1] A complement-mediated cytotoxic assay is used to type patients. Lymphocytes of the individual are incubated with antisera and complement and then examined for viability. Although HLA antigen inheritance is mendelian, diseases associated with specific HLA types do not follow this inheritance pattern. The presence of a specific HLA antigen probably represents at least a partial genetic factor in either exclusion from or being at risk for certain diseases.

REGIONAL VARIATIONS IN ANATOMY AND FUNCTION

It is clear to even the most casual observer that there are marked differences in the skin of the palms and soles as compared with glabrous skin elsewhere on the body.

The horny layer of the palms and soles is markedly thickened, measuring up to 1.0 mm, in contrast to the stratum corneum elsewhere, which is usually about 10 microns in thickness. In the palms and soles, the deeper portion of the stratum corneum, the stratum lucidum, is present as a distinct layer which

Table 1-2. SOME HLA ASSOCIATIONS OF IMPORTANCE IN DERMATOLOGY

Disease	HLA
Dermatitis herpetiformis	B8
Diabetes—insulin dependent	A8, BW 15
Keloids	B14, BW 16
Lichen planus	A3
Pemphigus	B13
Psoriasis (familial)	BW 17
Psoriasis (nonhereditary)	BW 17, B 13
Reiter's syndrome	B 27
Sarcoidosis	B 7
Systemic lupus erythematosus	B8, BW 15

is not noted in skin from other sites. This markedly thickened horny layer occasionally lends a yellowish appearance to lesions, leading to a possible mistaken clinical diagnosis of xanthomata. The thick stratum corneum also necessitates that biopsies of the palms or soles be much deeper than those taken from skin elsewhere.

Apocrine glands, sebaceous glands, and hair are absent from the palms and soles while eccrine glands are numerous. The ability of the skin of these areas to maintain a "grip" and avoid slippage is related to the absence of oil or hair and to the presence of moisture from the sweat glands.

The skin of the palms and soles, although distinctly diifferent from that of other portions of the body, is quite similar. However, as pointed out by Marples, our bipedal style of locomotion produces totally different environmental conditions in the two areas.[13] The hands are freely exposed and are in wide ranging motion, and the digits are relatively separated and mobile. By contrast, the feet are encased in rather impervious shoes, their movement is relatively restricted, large areas of the skin are compressed by the body weight, and the toes are fairly immobile. The skin temperature of the feet is lower than that of any other body area. The thick stratum corneum of the feet can absorb large quantities of water, and evaporation is decreased by the low skin temperature and the impervious coverings. These factors lead to maceration and an alkaline pH, which in turn favor the establishment of dermatophytes. Fungi are rarely isolated from the feet of people who habitually go barefoot, whereas they are recovered with such regularity from the feet of people who wear shoes that they might almost be considered a part of the normal flora of the toe webs.

The anatomical organization of the lower extremity can account for disorders of the panniculus such as in acrocyanosis. The state of the vasculature of the lower extremity plays an important role in the localization of lesions of vasculitis, sickle cell anemia, and cryoglobulinemia. These factors were discussed in an early part of this chapter. We also reviewed factors unique to the lower extremities that could explain the preferential localization of a variety of tumors such as arsenical keratoses, plantar warts, plantar fibromatosis, subungual exostosis, Kaposi's sarcoma, and melanoma.

There is a regional variation in immunoglobulin deposits, and the lower extremity is a favored site. Necrotizing vasculitis shows a predilection for the lower extremities, and in studies done by Sams et al, immunoglobulins and complement were demonstrated in the blood vessel walls of clinically normal skin 1 to 5 cm adjacent to lesions of active necrotizing vasculitis on the legs.[15] Can we hypothesize that cells in this region are coded for this selective distribution?

DERMATOGLYPHICS

Dermatoglyphics are furrows in the skin of the digital pads, palms, and soles and can be permanently recorded on specially treated paper with various techniques of imprinting. Fingerprinting has been known and utilized as a method of identification for years; however, more recently this procedure has become useful in clinical medicine and genetics. The differentiation of the skin ridges occurs in the developing fetus between the 13th and 19th weeks, with the hand developing somewhat earlier than the foot.

Dermatoglyphic patterns of the fingers and palms have been studied extensively in many disease states. The mechanism of their production is still not completely clear. Abnormalities have been described in such congenital disorders resulting from chromosomal defects as mongolism, trisomy

D, trisomy E, cri-du-chat, XXYY, XYY, and Klinefelter's syndrome and in such miscellaneous disorders as in-utero infection with rubella, psoriasis, von Recklinghausen's disease, pseudohypoparathyroidism, Wilson's disease, and schizophrenia.

In recent years, since the discovery of abnormal patterns of the ball area of the sole in cases of chromosomal anomalies, greater attention has been directed toward the dermatoglyphic patterns occurring on the sole. Abnormalities have been reported in such conditions as anonychia, nail-patella syndrome, zygodactyly, syndactyly, brachydactyly, polydactyly, Down's syndrome (mongolism), trisomy 13, 14 or 15, 17 or 18, Turner's syndrome, and Klinefelter's syndrome. Several characteristic sole patterns are shown in Fig 1-2. A clinical diagnosis, however, should not be made on dermatoglyphic features alone; the anatomic features serve to strengthen a diagnostic impression and may be useful as a screening device. (For detailed discussion of the normal and abnormal dermatoglyphic patterns of the sole, the reader is referred to Holt and Cummins and Midlo.[8,12])

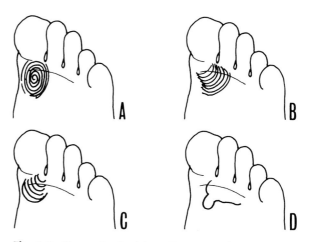

Fig. 1-2. Dermatoglyphic patterns on the soles. **(A)** Large whorl (Turner's syndrome); **(B)** Tibial arch (Down's syndrome, Trisomy E, Smith-Lemli-Opitz syndrome, deLange syndrome), **(C)** Fibular arch (Trisomy 15), **(D)** Arch Fibular S pattern (Trisomy D [Trisomy 13])

PLANTAR SKIN AS A RESEARCH TOOL

The skin of the foot, particularly the callus, can be utilized to study many aspects of cutaneous physiology, biochemistry, and microbiology including keratinization, blister formation, and percutaneous absorption.

KERATINIZATION

A major function of the epidermis is the production of keratin. Keratin is often classed as either soft, as in human skin, or hard, as in hair, horns, and so on. Keratins are fibrous proteins resistant to enzymatic digestion and to hydrolysis by acids and alkalis. They are crystalline structures, whose atoms are arranged in a regular repetitive pattern resulting in an x-ray diffraction pattern of an alpha type; when the normally folded keratin polypeptide chains are stretched, the x-ray pattern is of a beta configuration. Keratin has a high cystine content, and the level of cystine parallels the degree of hardness of the keratin. Since the production of keratin is the paramount function of the epidermis, and the maturation of the epidermal cells is paralleled by the appearance of keratin within the cells, further study of keratin will provide better understanding of the structure and function of the skin.

Topically applied agents can influence keratinization by either differentiation or desquamation of horny cells. Retinoids mainly affect differentiation, whereas the cohesiveness of horny cells is affected by salicylic acid and propylene glycol.[1,9,18] Lactic acid aids in normalization of the faulty epidermis in hereditary ichythyotic disorders.[21] Benzoyl peroxide has keratolytic activity, and sodium lauryl sulfate, a cutaneous irritant, produces nonspecific peeling.[21]

CALLUS

Numerous studies of cutaneous physiology and biochemistry have been carried out utilizing readily available callus. It has been legitimately questioned how appliable such results are to normal glabrous skin; nevertheless, studies using callus have yielded much worthwhile information. A very important basic finding was that dry callus remains hard and brittle in the presence of petrolatum or other oils but becomes soft and pliable if allowed to absorb some water. (For further information consult the classic studies of I.H. Blank.)[3,4]

FRICTION BLISTERS

Friction blisters are distinctive forms of reactions confined to the human species. These lesions occur with frequency and constitute one of the most common reactions to trauma, especially of the lower extremities. Studies have shown that extremes of dryness and wetness tend to decrease friction, whereas intermediate degrees of moisture at the rubbing surface tend to increase skin friction. Friction blisters do not usually occur clinically on thin skin because it lacks the thick and resistant stratum corneum for the blister roof. They also do not usually occur on loose skin because it lacks the tight adherence of the skin to underlying structures necessary for shearing effects to be produced in the epidermis.

Many factors have been implicated in the mechanism of friction blisters. Studies done by Sulzberger and his colleagues have yielded significant information and have pointed out new areas for further research.[7,20] Friction blisters can be produced by either a linear rubbing apparatus or by the twisting rubbing injury of a pencil eraser applied to the skin surface. Fluid accumulates within one hour after injury, and the blister is completely filled in two hours. Accumulation of fluid depends on arterial and hydrostatic pressure. Histologic examination of friction blisters shows a cleavage within the epidermis just beneath the stratum granulosum.

By reproducing in the laboratory under controlled conditions what is done to skin during marching, Comaish found that the effects of friction on skin can be mediated by a mechanical fatigue mechanism acting on epidermal cells in the mild and lower epidermis, perhaps in association with the damaging effects of increased tissue temperature.[5] The most important component of the friction stress is the shearing force horizontal to the skin surface; pressure, stretching, and ischemia seem to play no direct role in friction injury. Highley *et al* evaluated various parameters (hydration, oils, surfactants, and so forth) affecting skin friction using a rotational friction technique.[11] Their observations suggest that separate frictional events occur when materials are applied to the skin surface. The increase in friction observed upon wetting the skin involves two distinct phenomena; one is related to the surface tension of the aqueous phase, while the other, closely associated with hydration, is a consequence of physiochemical adhesion of the skin to the rotational friction probe.

Clinical disorders relating to friction blisters on the feet are discussed in Chapter 19.

PERCUTANEOUS ABSORPTION

A vital function of the skin is to act as a barrier—to prevent the absorption of noxious substances and to retard the outward passage of water. However, the effectiveness of this barrier function varies depending upon the material presented to the skin and upon other environmental factors present at the time. Thus, the presence of moisture increases absorption, as do surfactants; the absorption of acidic and basic drugs will be greatly influenced by the pH of the vehicle. Thickness of the skin and its temperature also affect the rate of absorption.

There is still much debate concerning the routes of absorption through the skin. Essentially, there are two routes, the transepidermal and the transappendageal (through the hair follicles, sweat glands, and sebaceous glands). Many observers now feel that early transient percutaneous absorption is through the hair follicles and ducts, and steady-state diffusion is primarily through the intact stratum corneum. Children are more susceptible to percutaneous absorption than adults because of their reduced body mass.

Numerous investigators, including Stoughton and Scheuplein, have contributed to our present knowledge of percutaneous absorption.[16,19] Despite these excellent studies, however, much remains to be elucidated about the barrier function of the skin. Such information has much practical importance, for intelligent formulation of dermatologic preparation depends upon a thorough understanding of percutaneous absorption, which includes the effect of skin disease on absorption, drug bioavailability, drug pharmacodynamics, the effect of drug vehicles, metabolism of drugs in the skin, and the effect of skin permeability. An excellent discussion of this multifaceted problem was reviewed recently and opens new avenues for research.[10]

PRINCIPLES OF DIAGNOSIS

The basic mechanisms of dermatologic disease will be better understood when we learn more about genetics, molecular biology, biochemistry, and physiology. Until this information is forthcoming, we shall have to concern ourselves with morphology and classification.

A practical approach to establishing an etiologic diagnosis utilizes the following:

1. Clinical findings
2. Histopathologic and histochemical studies
3. Laboratory studies
4. Special dermatologic procedures and skin tests.

CLINICAL FINDINGS
(History, Lesions, Topography)

History

A well-planned history is often essential for an etiologic diagnosis. One starts with the chief complaint, the date and site of onset, possible precipitating factors, the presence or absence of subjective symptoms, course, exacerbations, and recurrences. With experience, the history can be effectively directed. At times, these data may be sufficient to make a diagnosis. More often, an extensive thorough questioning will be necessary and may have to be reexplored at subsequent interviews. The following represent some aspects of the historical data.

Family History. The traditional history of the general health, or causes of death, of parents and siblings is of obvious importance. There is probably some genetic factor in almost all disease processes, but the extent of this component varies. The spectrum embraces rare disorders such as ichthyosis, mal de Meleda, epidermolysis bullosa, thalassemia, sickle cell anemia, porokeratosis of Mibelli, certain common skin diseases such as atopic dermatitis and psoriasis, and systemic diseases such as diabetes. Certain diseases such as scabies, furunculosis, and tuberculosis may show a high familial incidence without being hereditary.

Personal History. A history of systemic disease, recent and current illnesses, and past dermatologic illness probably provide helpful diagnostic clues. Certain skin diseases of the lower extremities are prone to affect particular age groups; for example, atopic dermatitis and papular urticaria in childhood and adolescence, pigmented purpuric eruptions, xerosis, and skin cancer in older people. Sex is an important determinant; for example, tinea pedis and Kaposi's sarcoma occur dominantly in males. Erythema induratum and lupus erythematosus mainly affect females.

Geographic Origin and Travel. Certain diseases are endemic in different areas of the world; for example, leprosy in the Philippines, China, India, Cuba, Africa, and South America; leishmaniasis in Israel, Iran, and other Near East countries; kwashiorkor in Africa and South America; miliaria in the tropics; chigger bites in southern United States; poison ivy dermatitis in the eastern half of the United States. Therefore, the present and past places of residence, as well as time spent in different areas on holidays and on long trips may be significant. "Tropical" diseases are appearing with increasing frequency among travelers who live in temperate zones.

Season of Year. Seasons may strikingly influence skin disease. Atopic dermatitis has spring and fall flares. Contact dermatitis due to plants largely occurs in spring and summer. Typical summer problems include insect bites, photosensitivity, and miliaria; ragweed dermatitis ococurs in the early autumn; winter brings chapping, xerosis, and pruritus.

Occupation and Avocation. In this list are the physical, biological, and chemical agents responsible for occupational dermatoses, the irritant and sensitizing chemical compounds contacted in our leisure activities, the reactions due to cosmetics and wearing apparel, and environmental exposures such as pesticides and cleansers. The most detailed interrogation may be necessary to establish a causal relationship.

Previous Medications. One must always be alert to the fact that the presenting skin lesions may be due to drugs. Almost any drug can cause an adverse reaction in certain persons. These drugs include self-medications, patent medicines, and those prescribed to be taken orally, by inhalation, and by injection. One can include in this category the host of flavorings and preservatives in various foods and the chemicals in soft drinks and foods. Adverse reactions to drugs such as antibiotics, analgesics, soporifics, tranquilizers, diuretics, and other common medicaments are common. Less frequently recognized are the many drugs capable of triggering photosensitivity reactions; for example, thiazides in diuretics, certain antibiotics (Declomycin, tetracycline), sulfonamides, tranquilizers (Thorazine), antiseptics (bithionol), antihistamines (Phenergan), oral hypoglycemic agents (Diabinese, Orinase), and griseofulvin. Of great importance is information relating to topical forms of treatment the patient had already used for his skin problem, including such measures as x-ray and ultraviolet light therapy, and medicaments used in the form of ointments, creams, lotions, or sprays. Common offenders are antibiotics, antihistaminics, fungicides, and local anesthetics. Reactions may be produced not only by the active chemical constituents in these medications but also by the vehicles and preservatives.

Psychologic Factors. Every skin disorder may have an associated emotional component. What is germane is to determine which feature is primary and to assess the exact role that the psychologic factors play in the presenting symptoms. Emotions probably have been overemphasized in the causation of disorders which still remain unexplained. Anxiety is usually a consequence, not a cause, of the skin disease.

Lesions

Careful inspection of the skin and characterization of the lesions provide the basis for developing the diagnosis. "Lesions are the alphabet without which nobody can read the language of the skin" (Darier). Meaningful concepts can be crystallized from these observations; at times, this alone is adequate for diagnosis. Proper examination of the skin always requires good lighting, preferably daylight. Adequate exposure of the entire skin and systematic examination is frequently necessary. The oral mucous membrane should be examined routinely.

There are three types of lesions: primary, secondary, and elementary. Primary lesions, which reflect the direct expression of the disease process, are the macule, petechia, papule, nodule, wheal, vesicle and bulla, pustule, and tumor. Secondary lesions are scales, crusts, excoriations, fissures, erosions, ulcers, scars, and atrophy. However, the differentiation is not always clear. The so-called elementary lesions—comedo, milium, burrow, lichenification, and telangiectasis—are instances of unique skin reactions.

The fact that one can diagnose a skin lesion is important; however, one must try to understand the mechanism responsible for its formation. *Why* did the lesion become manifest? Is there an external cause—a chemical, an insect, a fungus, a bacterium? Is the skin lesion part of a systemic disorder, as in dermatomyositis and lupus erythematosus? Is the skin reacting to an underlying abnormality; for example, bullae with porphyria, aphthae, and pyoderma gangrenosum with ulcerative colitis? Is the lesion a presenting symptom of a strictly dermatologic entity as in psoriasis and lichen planus?

What are the possible biochemical changes or physiologic alterations responsible for the structural change which manifests as the presenting lesion? *Why* in the alteration of function did such a structural change take place? Why was a macule the resultant lesion and not a vesicle or papule? Why was a crust formed and not a scale? *How* was such a lesion formed? Was something done on the exposed surface or was something wrong internally? Is this lesion congenital or was it acquired? Is it of a temporary nature or will it be permanent?

Some of these aspects can be elucidated almost at a glance, others require extensive additional studies. In essence, we see the effect, so we must seach for the cause.

Macule. A circumscribed alteration in the color of the skin, not visibly raised or depressed, or presenting any change in the consistency of the skin. Macules may be due to changes in blood vessels; for example, hyperemic or inflammatory macules, which are transient dilatations of blood vessels, and nevi such as nevus flammeus and nevus anemicus, which are the permanent enlargement or absence of blood vessels, respectively. Macules may also be due to changes in pigment (melanin), either to deficiency such as in vitiligo, or to an increase such as the café au lait mark, freckle, or fixed drug eruption. They may also be due to infection such as tinea versicolor, or to depositions in the skin produced internally by bile pigments, blood pigments, and iron; or externally from gunpowder or macule cerulae. Coloration produced by internal factors such as argyria and atabrine dermatitis and exogenous causes such as from silver nitrate are other factors.

Papule. A small elevation above the skin level. A papule has a solid center and can be felt, although on the palms and soles it is often flattened by pressure. It varies in size from a millimeter to a centimeter, and its shape depends upon the level of the underlying infiltrate. Papules may be produced by an increase in cells in the horny layer—warts; by edema in the epidermis—eczema; by edema, inflammatory changes, or cellular infiltrates in the dermis—lichen planus, tuberculids, and papular syphilids.

Nodule. A solid lesion larger than a papule and consisting of inflammatory cellular infiltrates (*e.g.*, erythema nodosum and erythema induratum), or neoplasms (*e.g.*, epitheliomata or tissue hypertrophies). Nodular lesions frequently show a destructive character and break down with suppuration (*e.g.*, gummas, erythema induratum, and Weber-Christian disease).

Wheal (Hive). An evanescent plateau-like elevation produced by edema in the upper corium and the extravasation of blood plasma through the vessel walls. Whealing or urtication may be produced either by external causes—reactions to insect bites or allergic responses to scratch and intracutaneous tests—or by internal factors—drug and food allergy. Wheals may be the same color as normal skin, redder if the superficial blood vessels are dilated and paler if the blood vessels are compressed by the extravasated fluid.

Vesicle. A circumscribed elevation of the skin containing fluid; a blister. On microscopic study, vesicles vary in pathogenesis and can be distinguished as being subcorneal, intraepidermal, and subepidermal. Impetigo presents as subcorneal separation; primary cell damage (intracellular) with ballooning cell forms is often due to virus invasion. Intercellular edema (spongiosis) is typical of contact dermatitis. Completely separated epidermal cells with loss of intercellular bridges is termed "acantholysis," of which the classical example is pemphigus. Subepidermal vesicles result from the separation between the epidermis and corium (*e.g.*, dermatitis herpetiformis, bullous pemphigoid, erythema multiforme, and epidermolysis bullosa). Vesicles are spherical and are characterized by their roofs, contents, and bases. They are usually tense and have a taut surface. If imbedded in thick skin, as in that of the palms and soles, they may be neither raised nor palpable.

Bulla. A large vesicle. Bullae are produced by extrinsic factors such as chemical (cantharides, adhesive), thermic (burns, frostbite), mechanical (friction), or internal factors as in erythema multiforme, pemphigus, pemphigoid, and porphyria.

Pustule. A circumscribed liquid accumulation containing free pus. Sometimes pustules start as vesicles, such as staphylococcic infection (vesiculo-pustules). Primary pustules are seen with such inflammations as folliculitis, periporitis, ecthyma, pustular psoriasis, pustular bacterids, acrodermatitis continua, and subcorneal pustulosis.

Tumor. A new growth of varying size composed of skin and subcutaneous tissue. Tumors may be benign (lipomas and fibromas) or malignant (basal and prickle cell epitheliomas, sarcomas, lymphomas).

Scales. The exfoliation of accumulated debris of dead stratum corneum resulting from imperfect cornification. Scales are characterized by their color (*e.g.*, the silvery or mica-like scales of psoriasis, loose or dry ones of exfoliative dermatitis and ichthyosis, greasy ones of seborrheic dermatitis and Darier's disease, branny ones of *T. rubrum* infections and pityriasis rubra pilaris, and adherent ones of discoid lupus erythematosus and actinic keratoses).

Crusts. Result from the drying of fluid, pus, serum, and blood in combination with scales, dirt, and bacteria on or in skin. Crusts may be thick, thin, bloody, or necrotic.

Excoriation. The loss of superficial substance of the skin as the result of scratching. Exposure of the corium and bleeding result from the mechanical removal of the epidermis.

Fissures. Lines or grooves due to the loss of continuity of the skin without any loss of substance. Normal fissures are preformed on the palms and soles; acquired fissures represent the loss of elasticity, usually sequential to an inflammatory infiltrate.

Erosions. Denuded areas due to the loss of all or part of the epidermis. Erosions are often the result of trauma to a primary lesion such as a vesicle or maceration secondary to ringworm of the toes. An erosion sequential to a bulla frequently presents a circular outline with a collarette of scales. Some postbullous erosions form vegetations instead of healing smoothly.

Ulcers. Produced by a destruction of skin with resultant scar formation. Ulcers are described by their size, depth, number, and by such features as induration and presence of underlying lesions. (See causes of ulcers on the lower extremities, in Chap. 14.)

Scars. Alterations of skin following destruction of the epidermis and cutis. Some scars become hypertrophic, of which keloids are a prominent example. They tend to occur in Blacks in certain areas of the body, especially the sternum. Hypertrophic scars are frequently provoked by burns. Irregular scars develop in syphilis and acne conglobata. New scars are pinkish in color; old ones white and shiny. Self-inflicted skin lesions, which can be produced in a variety of ways, end up as factitial scars, usually presenting as bizarre-shaped lesions and configurations.

Atrophy. Implies loss of tissue; either all or some of the tissues of the skin. Fragmentation and degeneration of the elastic tissue is a common pathologic finding. It is clinically manifested by a diminution of the actual thickness of the skin. Atrophic skin is more supple and thinner than normal skin, shows fine wrinkling, puckers like tissue paper, and has a parchment feel. Its color is pinkish to pearly white. Atrophy of the skin may be congenital (*e.g.*, congenital ectodermal defect and pseudoxanthoma elasticum). The acquired forms of atrophy may follow damage to the skin, as from x-ray dermatitis or from senile atrophy, in which the degenerative changes are caused by sunlight. Striae (linear atrophy) may follow cachexia and obesity or may be induced by the administration of ACTH, by application of topical corticosteroids, or in pituitary diseases. Post-traumatic or postulcerative types of atrophy appear as the final stages of interstitial pathologic processes. Many atrophic lesions are of unknown etiology (*e.g.*, the various macular atrophies, the diffuse picture of acrodermatitis chronica atrophicans, the poikilodermas, kraurosis vulvae, balanitis xerotica obliterans, and lichen sclerosus et atrophicus).

Lichenification. Infiltration of the skin horizontally rather than in depth, producing a thickened skin with accentuated skin mark-ings. The surface relief presents a coarsened appearance similar to that of shagreen. The color of lichenified skin may be red, more frequently pale and somewhat grayish. After a time, hyperpigmentation develops and may extend to the surrounding skin.

Telangiectasis. Visibly dilated, superficial blood vessels seen in connection with certain heritable diseases such as familial telangiectasis, associated with liver diseases and pregnancy, and as a sequel to x-ray treatment.

Skin lesions have certain attributes which are helpful in making a diagnosis.

Color Changes

The color of normal skin takes its origin from the pigments in various layers and from the state and amount of blood in the superficial vascular plexuses.

A. Pigments. *Natural pigments* include melanin, bile, carotene and lycopene from foods, and occasionally pigments in apocrine sweat. Localized increase of melanin occurs in freckles, chloasma, certain levi, café au lait spots, Peutz-Jeghers syndrome and in post-inflammatory reactions, *viz*, pyodermas, psoriasis, lichen planus, and syphilis. Decrease in melanin occurs in nevi depigmentosa, in vitiligo, and after inflammation. Jaundice reflects an increase in bile pigments. Carotenemia and lycopenemia due to the excess ingestion of carotenoid foods and tomatoes give a yellow to orange color, usually localized where the skin has a heavy horny layer (palms, soles).

Foreign pigments—tattoos are the best examples. The color tells the pigment—green due to chromates, red due to cinnabar and carmine, gray-black hues from gunpowder, or pictures peculiar to certain occupations such as that of miners and stonemasons.

Drugs taken internally can produce color changes; for example, the slate-gray color of argyria due to silver, the yellow color of gold (chrysoderma), the dusky gray-purple color of thorazine and Declomycin following sun exposure, the blue-gray line of the gums from bismuth.

Drugs applied externally may cause color changes; for example, tar, chrysarobin, anthralin.

Foreign Cells. Examples of characteristic color changes are the lemon yellow scutulum of favus, blackening of the horny layer due to dirt implanted in cracks and calluses on hands and feet.

Blood. Depositions of hemosiderin give rise to petechia, purpura, and ecchymosis.

Cells and cellular products. Keratin in the stratum corneum, depending on thickness, contributes yellowness; the stratum granulosum contributes whiteness. Cellular products in representative lesions of certain diseases show characteristic color tones: yellow-orange (xanthomatosis and necrobiosis lipoidica diabeticorum), ham (secondary syphilis), violaceus (lichen planus), silvery shades (psoriasis), red-brown or red-blue (lupus pernio color; sarcoid and tuberculoid lesions), black (black hairy tongue).

B. Blood Color. Color changes follow hyperemia or vasomotor changes; for example, erythema, cutis marmorata. Permanent increase or enlargement of blood vessels; for example, telangiectasis, angiomata, spider nevi, nevus flammeus, livedo reticularis.

Spatial Relationships of Lesions

Lesions present in different configurations. They may be solitary, discrete, grouped or herpetic, aggregate, or confluent. Lesions are described as localized or circumscribed, diffuse, generalized, and universal. A uniform eruption describes lesions of the same type. The term multiform, or polymorphous, is used for different types of lesions in the same eruption.

Descriptive Terms Relating to Lesions

Knowledgeable use of these terms provides a picture of what the lesion actually looks like.

Size

This should be expressed in millimeters and centimeters.

Shape and Configuration

They may appear round, oval, polygonal, square or irregular, linear, acuminate, filiform, spinulose, umbilicated, imbricated, rupial, condylomatous, vegetative, papillomatous, iris, serpiginous, circumscribed, discoid, circinate, annular, retiform, punctate, nummular, plaque.

Contents

The contents may be sweat, sebum, lymph, blood, horny material, foreign material.

Topography

In this text we have restricted ourselves to those diseases localized on the lower extremities. The known causes and speculative causes of this selective distribution have been considered in the first part of this chapter.

HISTOPATHOLOGIC AND HISTOCHEMICAL STUDIES

Histologic examination of the lesion is often necessary for diagnosis. Microscopic morphology may be diagnostically conclusive. The lesions are removed by a punch biopsy or scalpel excision, fixed, cut, and stained. Hematoxylin and eosin are almost universally used for routine work, but at times, special stains may be required.

Depending upon the history and clinical features, the clinician can request special studies which will utilize selective staining for histochemical alterations to identify special chemical substances (*e.g.,* glycogen, amyloid, and mucopolysaccharides).

Biopsies should be selective, that is, a representative lesion should be chosen. At times, multiple biopsies may be advisable. The ease with which skin biopsies can be performed enables the clinician to utilize them readily to assist in obtaining correct diagnosis. Unnecessary biopsies on the lower extremities should be avoided because of delayed healing in these areas, especially in patients older than the age of forty with peripheral vascular or degenerative diseases.

The techniques for biopsies are described under procedures.

LABORATORY STUDIES

Blood counts, urinalysis, and serologic tests for syphilis have been standard laboratory tests. Routine studies of the sedimentation rate, blood sugar, blood urea nitrogen, or serum uric acid may be indicated. Lesions in association with autoimmune diseases will require tests for rheumatoid factor, lupus erythematosus cells, electrophoretic patterns, and fluorescent antibody studies. In connection with myositis, serum enzyme activity and electromyographic studies may be necessary. A battery of lipid studies are essential for the lipoproteinemias. Special blood studies are required for anemias and lymphoblastomas; sophisticated biochemical studies for genetic disorders. In some instances, x-ray examination of joint, bone, lung, or gastrointestinal tract may be pertinent. In short, in any skin lesion which purports or reflects a systemic disease, use of the appropriate laboratory tests to give solid scientific support to the clinical judgment is imperative.

SPECIAL DERMATOLOGIC PROCEDURES AND SKIN TESTS

Diagnostic Clues

Auspitz sign. The appearance of pinpoint bleeding when the scale of a lesion of psoriasis is forcibly removed.
Nikolsky sign. The upper layers of the epidermis easily detached by slight pressure or trauma, pointing to an absence of cohesion in the skin. The sign is elicited in pemphigus.
Koebner or isomorphic phenomenon. The production of lesions, by means of physical trauma, of the same form that is characteristic of the eruption. Commonly observed in psoriasis and lichen planus.
Touching, feeling, and probing of lesions. To determine induration, thickening, atrophy, dryness, anesthesia, and caseation.
Movability of skin. Hyperstretchable in Ehlers-Danlos syndrome; distinct reduction in scleroderma.
Diascopy (glass pressure). To determine presence of intravascular blood and pigmentations and to detect the apple-jelly color in granulomatous lesions (e.g., lupus vulgaris). Lesions that consist of functioning blood vessels usually disappear in this procedure.

Cytodiagnosis

1. Tzanck test for bullous diseases and for

vesicular virus eruptions such as zoster, herpes simplex, varicella, and molluscum contagiosum. The identification of acantholytic cells in Tzanck smears made from pemphigus vulgaris, familial benign chronic pemphigus, and transient acantholytic dermatitis is easily made; cells that show the intranuclear "ground-glass" inclusions are typical for both varicella-zoster and herpes virus. A simple and accurate stain procedure for cytologic preparations has been described by Barr.[2]* The Tzanck test can be a rapid office tool to obtain a correct diagnosis.

2. Suspected basal cell epitheliomas. Touch preparations from neoplasms can be made from curettements or a shaving of the lesion, gently smearing or imprinting the tissue on a microscopic slide. Touch imprints by no means replace a biopsy, although tumor imprints provide fine cellular detail unobtainable with conventional formalin field, paraffin-embedded specimens[2]

Examination of skin scrapings with direct microscopy. Tineas (see Chapter 2).
Cultures. Mycologic, bacteriologic, virologic.
Use of ultraviolet light. To test for photosensitivity.
Wood's light. Erythrasma, tinea versicolor, detection of pseudomonas.
Exposure to cold and heat. To test for cold and heat hypersensitivity, Raynaud's phenomenon.

---

*Procedure for Tzanck test.
The scrapings are prepared by selecting an early intact vesicle or bulla. A blade is used to open the lesion, and the base is gently scraped to avoid hemorrhage. The material is placed on a clean, dry microscopic slide and gently spread. The slide is processed as follows: (1) It is fixed immediately in ordinary isopropyl alcohol, 70% for three minutes (immediate fixation is important to avoid drying artifact). (2) The slide is dipped five times in a mixture of 50% alcohol and 50% tap water (35% isopropyl alcohol). (3) It is dipped five times in 100% tap water. (4) Two to three drops of multiple stain solution (Polysciences, Inc., Warrington, Pa., 18976) are placed on the slide (enough to cover the smear) for five seconds. (5) The slide is then rinsed immediately in tap water. (6) Excess water is removed by blotting, taking care to avoid destroying the smear. (7) A drop of water is placed on the slide and then coverslipped for immediate interpretation.

Skin Testing

1. Patch tests. (Chapter 10.)
2. Immediate tests: Wheal test (scratch and intradermal) for atopic dermatitis.
3. Delayed intradermal tests (tuberculin, trichophytin, antigens of the deep mycoses such as histoplasmin, coccidioidin).
4. Long-delayed intradermal tests (Kveim, Mitsuda).

Skin Window Technique. A small area of skin is gently abraded, and a coverslip is applied but is removed at intervals and replaced by another. The coverslips are stained, and the cellular response can be evaluated.

Iontophoresis. A method of introducing into the skin substances that are ionized and carry an electric charge. Used as a research tool.

Immunofluorescent techniques have been a great aid in the diagnosis of certain cutaneous disorders. The direct immunofluorescent procedure is the most valuable one used in dermatology. Specific staining patterns are observed. In cases of pemphigus and pemphigoid, immunoglobulin deposits in skin sections serve to establish the diagnosis; IgA deposits at the dermoepidermal junction in patients with vesiculobullous eruptions are diagnostic of dermatitis herpetiformis; junctional deposits of immunoglobulins or complement, or both, in skin lesions and in apparently normal skin are highly characteristic of systemic lupus erythematosus; and more or less typical patterns of immunoglobulin and complement deposits in the lesion appear in discoid lupus erythematosus.[6]

Biopsy

Skin biopsies are specimens of tissue that are sectioned and variously processed by stains, and are examined with the microscope. The findings are extremely important for confirming or establishing a diagnosis. Unprocessed tissue specimens can also be used for bacterial and fungal cultures.

Biopsies are obtained by using a variety of techniques such as curettage, shave biopsy, punch biopsy, or surgical excision. The curet is a cutting instrument with a circular, loop-shaped cutting edge and a handle. It is available in varying sizes. Shave biopsies can be done with a razor blade.[17] Biopsy punches are circular instruments with a sharp cutting edge and a handle, and they are available in sizes ranging from 2 to 8 mm in diameter. The punch biopsy is the procedure used frequently by the dermatologist. Excision biopsies require suturing. On the lower extremities, excision (scalpel) biopsies are advisable for skin overlying joints and toes and on the shin area (*e.g.*, in erythema nodosum lesions), whereas the punch technique is used for a toenail biopsy. (Techniques for toenail biopsies are discussed in chapter 18.)

Basic steps for doing a biopsy:

1. Select a mature and well-developed lesion. For blisters, choose the earliest lesion available, preferably less than 24 hours old.
2. Clean the biopsy site with 70% isopropyl alcohol.
3. Anesthetize the area by injection of 1% lidocaine with or without 1:100,000 epinephrine around the lesion, and not in it. Epinephrine-containing solutions should not be used when anesthetizing the distal toes. A 1-ml syringe with a #25 or #27 needle should be used.
4. Determine type of biopsy by lesion depth.
   a. Epidermal lesion—curet or scalpel
   b. Dermal lesion—punch or scalpel
   c. Hypodermal lesion—scalpel.
5. Place flat specimens on filter paper or cardboard to prevent curling.
6. Place specimen in container with 10% buffered formalin. Attach pertinent clinical findings and patient's history, and submit for pathologic examination.
7. Use pressure, caustics, or electrodesiccation for hemostasis; for surgical excision biopsies, suturing is required (4–0 or 5–0 nylon or silk suture).
8. Biopsies on the legs and feet heal more slowly in patients older than 40, especially if the circulation is poor. Occasionally, an elastic bandage, to be worn for 1 to 2 weeks, might be required.

REFERENCES

LOCALIZATION OF LESIONS ON THE LOWER EXTREMITIES

1. **Copeman PWM:** Cutaneous angiitis. J R Coll Phys 9:103, 1975
2. **Copeman PWM:** Livedo reticularis. Brit J Dermatol 93:519, 1975
3. **Hendel DW, Roenig HH Jr, Shainoff J, et al:** Necrotizing vasculitis. Arch Dermatol 111:847, 1975
4. **Ryan TJ:** Microvascular injury. In Major Problems in Dermatology, p 44. Philadelphia, WB Saunders, 1976
5. **Samitz MH:** The "Tell-Tale Foot" or how observations on the lower extremities provide a unique opportunity to study systemic disease. J Am Pod Assoc 70:126, 1980
6. **Samitz MH, Lewis JE:** Skin tumors of the lower extremities. Int J Dermatol 17:558, 1978
7. **Sams WM Jr, Claman HN, Kohler PF, et al:** Human necrotizing vasculitis: Immunoglobulins and complement in vessel walls of cutaneous lesions and normal skin, J Invest Dermatol 64:441, 1975
8. **Sams WM Jr, Thorne EG, Small P, et al:** Leukocytoclastic vasculitis. Arch Dermatol 112:219, 1976
9. **Soter NA:** Clinical presentations and mechanisms of necrotizing angiitis of the skin. J Invest Dermatol 67:354, 1976
10. **Whimster IW:** Morbid anatomy and the skin. Trans St Johns Hosp Dermatol 54:11, 1968
11. **Winkelmann RK, Frostom L:** New observations in the histopathology of erythema nodosum. J Invest Dermatol 65:441, 1975
12. **Winkelmann RK, Schroeter AL, Kierland RR, et al:** Clinical studies of livedoid vasculitis. Mayo Clin Proc 49:746, 1974

STRUCTURE AND FUNCTION OF THE SKIN

1. **Burton AC:** Physiology of Cutaneous Circulation, Thermoregulatory Functions, In Rothman S (ed): The Human Integument, pp 77–88. Washington, DC, American Association for the Advancement of Science, Publication No 54, 1959
2. **Lewis T:** Observations upon the reactions of the vessels of the human skin to cold. Heart 15:177, 1929
3. **Rothman S, Lorinez AL:** Defense mechanisms of the skin. Am Rev Med 14:215, 1963
4. **Ryan TJ:** Pathophysiology of skin capillaries. Int J Dermatol 14:708, 1975

5. **Ryan TJ:** Microvascular injury. In Major Problems in Dermatology, p 288. Philadelphia, WB Saunders Co, 1976
6. **Zweifach BW:** Structural aspects and hemodynamics of microcirculation in the skin. In Rothman S (ed): The Human Integument, pp 67–76. Washington, DC, American Association for the Advancement of Science, Publication No. 54, 1959

THE IMMUNE SYSTEM

1. **Asthma and the Other Allergic Diseases.** Niaid Task Force Report, pp 41, 55, 57. US Dept Health, Education and Welfare, NIH Publication No. 79-387, 1979
2. **Beechler CR:** Skin immunology. Cutis 24:145, 1979
3. **Dahl MV:** Primary immunodeficiency diseases: Evaluation and cutaneous manifestations. Med Dig 17:31, 1978
4. **Hong R:** Immunologic assessment of the immunodeficient. J Allerg Clin Immunol 60:83, 1977
5. **Kreuger GG:** Lymphokines in health and disease. Int J Dermatol 16:539, 1977
6. Report of WHO Committee. Pediatrics 47:921, 1971. From Wansker BA: Clinical immunology. A simple primer for the practitioner. Cutis 20:247, 1977
7. **Talal N:** Systemic lupus erythematosus, autoimmunity, sex and inheritance. N Engl J Med 301:838, 1979

HLA AND DISEASE

1. **Carpenter CB:** The new HLA nomenclature. N Engl J Med 294:1005, 1976
2. **Danilevicius, Z:** HLA antigens—genetic markers of many diseases. JAMA 231:965, 1975
3. **Frelinger JA, Shreffler DC:** The major histocompatibility complexes. In Benacerraf B (ed): Immunogenetics and Immunodeficiency, pp 81–116. Baltimore, University Park Press, 1975
4. **Jajic I, et al:** HLA antigens in psoriatic arthritis and psoriasis. Arch Dermatol 113:1724, 1977
5. **Katz SI:** Histocompatability antigens in disease. Arch Dermatol 113:1715, 1977
6. **Lowe NJ, et al:** Antigens in lichen planus. Brit J Dermatol 95:169, 1976
7. **Ritzman SE:** HLA patterns and disease associations. JAMA 236:2305, 1976

REGIONAL VARIATIONS IN ANATOMY AND FUNCTION

1. **Baden HP:** The management of hyperkeratosis. In Frost P, Gomey EC, Zaias N (eds): Recent Advances in Dermatopharmacology, pp 219–242. New York, Spectrum Publications, 1977
2. **Barr RJ:** Cutaneous cytology. J Int Dermatol 17:552, 1978
3. **Blank IH:** Factors which influence the water content of the stratum corneum. J Inv Dermatol 18:433, 1952
4. **Blank IH:** Further observations on factors which influence the water content of the stratum corneum. J Inv Dermatol 21:259, 1953
5. **Comaish JS:** Epidermal fatigue as a cause of friction blisters. Lancet 1:81, 1973
6. Cooperative Study: Uses for immunofluorescence tests of skin and sera. Arch Dermatol 111:371, 1975
7. **Cortese TA, Sams WM, Sulzberger MB:** Studies on blisters produced by friction II. The blister fluid. J Inv Dermatol 50:47, 1968
8. **Cummins H, Midlo C:** Fingerprints, Palms and Soles. An Introduction to Dermatoglyphics. New York, Dover Publication, Inc, 1961
9. **Davies N, Marks R:** Studies on the effect of salicylic acid on normal skin. Brit J Dermatol 95:187–192, 1976
10. Dermatological needs in drugs and instrumentation. In Analysis of Research Needs and Priorities in Dermatology, Chap VII. J Inv Dermatol 73 (Part II): 473, 1979
11. **Highley DR, Coomey M, Den Beste M, Wolfram, LJ:** Frictional properties of skin. J Invest Dermatol 69:303, 1977
12. **Holt SB:** The Genetics of Dermal Ridges. Springfield, Ill, Charles C Thomas, 1968
13. **Marples MJ:** The Ecology of the Human Skin, p. 182. Springfield, Ill, Charles C Thomas, 1965
14. **Mills OH, Kligman AM:** Assay of comedolytic agents in the rabbit ear. In Maibach HI (ed): Animal Models in Dermatology; Relevance to Human Dermatopharmacology and Dermatotoxicology, pp 176–183. New York, Churchill-Livingstone, 1975
15. **Sams WM Jr, Claman HN, Kohler PE, et al:** Human necrotizing vasculitis: Immunoglobulins and complement in vessel walls of cutaneous lesions and normal skin. J Invest Dermatol 64:441, 1975
16. **Scheuplein RJ:** Mechanism of percutaneous absorption II. Transient diffusion and the relative importance of various routes of skin penetration. J Inv Dermatol 48:79, 1967
17. **Shelley WB:** The razor blade in dermatologic practice. Cutis 16:843, 1975
18. **Sporn MB, Dunlop NM, Newton DL, Smith JM:** Prevention of chemical carcinogenesis by vitamin A and its synthetic analogs (retinoids). Fed Proc 35:1332–1338, 1976
19. **Stoughton RB:** Some in vivo and in vitro methods for measuring percutaneous absorption. In Rook A, Champion RH (eds): Progress in the Biological Sciences in Relation to Dermatology-2, pp 263–274. London, Cambridge University Press, 1964
20. **Sulzberger MB, Cortese TA, Fishman L, Wiley HS:** Studies on blisters produced by friction. I. Results of linear rubbing and twisting technics. J Inv Dermatol 47:456, 1966
21. **Van Scott EJ, Yu RJ:** Control of keratinization with α-hydroxy acids and related compounds: I. Topical treatment of ichthyotic disorders. Arch Dermatol 110:586–590, 1974

2 MICROBIOLOGICAL DISEASES

Disease is not inevitable just because pathogenic microorganisms are present on the skin. Change in local resistance—alterations in immunity—is the dominant factor: Cutaneous infection depends on a balance between the attacking potentials of the organism concerned (its virulence) and the degree to which the host's defenses are compromised. The ecologic balance can be upset when trauma causes breaks in the skin, when antibiotic therapy leads to alterations in normal skin flora, or when systemic disorders, especially of the immunologic or metabolic variety (agammaglobulinemia, diabetes), or corticosteroid or immunosuppressive therapy predispose to infection. Ecologic factors in various regions of the skin can account for regional differences in susceptibility to transient as well as resident bacterial growth. Factors determining the type and distribution of microorganisms on the skin are water, skin lipids, exposure, and the microorganisms present on the skin.[9] The major defense against infection is the integrity of the epidermis. On the lower extremities, local factors such as moisture, mechanical trauma, friction and blistering, and the anatomy of the toe spaces can play important roles.

BASIC MICROBIOLOGY OF LOWER LEG SKIN

SKIN FLORA

Microbiologic studies of the lower leg are best understood from the ecologic standpoint. A variety of different microbial species

exist on the surface of the skin under environments ranging from the dry calf to the wet toe webs. These species include potential pathogens, even in the absence of lesions, which are prevented from multiplying to high densities by other members of the microbial community. Disturbance of the ecologic balance may occur spontaneously, or because of changes in the host, affecting the microbial environment, or as a result of therapy. The concept of a complex interacting flora changing as a result of outside influences, but retaining a strong homeostatic tendency, must replace the concept of one organism always causing one disease.[6]

Although the flora of the toe webs includes many species, many organisms in the general environment fail to colonize the skin. On the drier lower leg, the flora is quite restricted owing to the physical and chemical conditions on the surface and to the activities of the organisms already present. Different species differ in tolerance to dryness, pH changes, temperature, and specific and nonspecific chemical inhibitors, such as fatty acids from the skin and serum factors.[13] The relative importance of these factors in controlling the composition and density of the normal flora varies from site to site, but the overwhelming importance of moisture in favoring increased density over most of the skin has been well demonstrated.[7,14] Moisture has been found also to be of great importance in bacterial infections of the toes. Experimental studies showed that excessive hydration was required to produce a vesiculopustular rash of the toe webs by applications of *Pseudomonas aeruginosa*.[4] In a clinical study,

Pseudomonas cepacia, isolated in large numbers from the toe webs and sodden feet of troops after training in swamp conditions, was associated with macerated, hyperkeratotic lesions of the feet.[18]

The density and species variety of the toe webs appear to be greater than in the axilla, where more than 10^6 bacteria per sq cm can be recovered.[8] On the calf, the quantity of organisms is similar to the forearm, about 10^3 organisms per sq cm. The occurrence of *Corynebacterium minutissimum,* lipophilic and nonlipophilic diphtheroids, enterobacteria, *Pseudomonas, Mima-Herellea* and *Candida* species in the toe webs and axilla contrasts markedly with the dense coccal, *Corynebacterium acnes* flora of the head and the sparse coccal-lipophilic diphtheroid flora of the abdomen, leg, and arm.

A high density of a complex flora in intertriginous areas produces a higher pH than elsewhere. Urea and other nitrogenous compounds are metabolized with the release of ammonia, while the low availability of carbohydrates prevents much acid production. This contrasts with Marchionini's thesis of a protective "acid mantle" preventing colonization of the skin.

The low temperature of the lower extremity may also significantly alter the microbial flora. Some pathogens are unable to tolerate local temperatures of 37° C. Thus, *Mycobacterium marinum* and dermatophytes can flourish in an area which rarely becomes hotter than 35° C and is usually 4 or 5 degrees cooler, while many recognized pathogens cannot multiply.[6] The very large number of nonlipophilic diphtheroids in the toe webs that are only rarely recovered from the much warmer axilla may also be due to the low temperature.

TOPOGRAPHY AND NUTRIENTS

The relative importance of the substrate seems less in the lower extremities than elsewhere. The detailed anatomy of the skin surface is very similar to that of the arm. However, because of the custom of wearing shoes and the necessity for weight bearing, the local conditions of the skin are different, leading to retention of skin products, particularly water. The amount of fatty material from sebaceous glands arriving on the sole is less

than on the palm. From this a greater incidence of streptococci might be expected, but this is not seen. It has been suggested, though not proven, that low fatty acid levels on the foot may promote ringworm infection.[15] The lack of hairs in the toe webs and sole does not seem to diminish bacterial density, as would be expected if most bacteria inhabited the infundibular portion of hair follicles.[12] Using staphlococci under occlusion, Duncan *et al* found that it was easier to infect the lower leg or thigh than the arm and back, and speculated that circulatory factors in the lower extremities could account for this.[2]

INTERSPECIFIC INTERACTIONS

Because a very dense normal flora is carried on the moist skin of the toe webs, interactions between microorganisms have been clearly demonstrated in this region. Symptomatic interdigital "athlete's foot" is the result of interaction between resident diphtheroids and the ringworm fungus. Combined occupation by dermatophytes, *Staphylococcus aureus* and *Candida albicans* intensifies itching and aggravates the inflammatory response.[10] Protection against colonization by gram-negative forms, particularly *Pseudomonas,* has been demonstrated.[3] In the normal toe webs, *C. minutissimum* is very commonly found without lesions, yet erythrasma is a definite clinical entity. The reason a complex flora changes to permit a potentially pathogenic segment to cause lesions is usually unknown. Treatment enabling restoration of a normal flora often may be more effective than heroic antibacterial and antifungal treatment. Much more detailed study of microbial interactions is needed.[11,16,17]

ABNORMAL CONDITIONS

Tight interdigital spaces in which contact and friction between toes is unavoidable can initiate infections of the toe webs.[1]

Because the lower extremity is cool, moist, and usually dirtier than the upper extremity, dermatophyte and atypical mycobacterial infections are common. The increased incidence of minor trauma, often combined with poor vasculature, makes secondary infection of traumatic lesions common. Poor vasculature can lead directly to stasis ulceration or gangrene with secondary colonization, while neural involvement can produce similar lesions.

Excessive sweating of the feet can be responsible for the proliferation of organisms such as *Streptomyces* and *Coryne bacteria* found in patients with pitted keratolysis.[20]

Frequently in lesions of the lower extremity, secondary microbial infections prolong and intensity the lesion and cause difficulty in diagnosis. The presence of a dermatophyte does not indicate tinea pedis or *S. aureus* a pyoderma. Conversely, the ease with which significant colonization by these pathogens and *C. albicans*, *Pseudomonas*, and *C. minutissimum* from the toe webs can occur must be recognized.

PROTECTION

Critical investigation in this area has been rather limited. The mechanisms by which the skin protects against bacteria are still somewhat controversial, but desiccation appears to be the main defense against most bacteria occurring on the surface of normal skin, especially *E. coli* and *Pseudomonas*. In the case of streptococci, the antibacterial action of fatty acids, particularly oleic acid, seems most effective. An additional, and possibly very important, factor in protection of the skin against pathogenic microorganisms is the phenomenon of bacterial interference; for example, the presence of one strain of staphylococci at a cutaneous site prevents colonization of that location by another strain.

The prophylactic use of antimicrobial agents has been a controversial subject for many years. There is no evidence that combination of oral, topical, and parenteral antimicrobial agents reduces infection rates below those achieved by the use of any one route of prophylactic antimicrobial administration.[19]

Cleanliness is the best protection against bacterial infection of the skin.

EXPERIMENTAL APPROACHES

As with most bacteria, the mechanisms or factors responsible for virulence are, at best, only partially understood. With group A streptococci, resistance is type specific, depending usually on the surface antigens of the bacteria. Some distinctive features of the pyoderma streptococci have been delineated; however, why these strains have a propensity to infect skin and why some of these are nephritogenic is far from clear. Similarly, with staphylococci, the virulence of certain strains has not been fully explained. Recently, it has been shown that a toxin from phage group II staphylococci is responsible for bullous impetigo and staphylococcal scalded skin syndrome.[5]

It is clear that incidence data derived from group surveys are not the whole answer to the complex problem of microbially induced morbidity and its treatment. Quantitative techniques and detailed analysis of changes in the flora with treatment are in their infancy. However, the results of such studies are of practical value. Because examples of "athlete's foot" are readily available, detailed study of it can unravel both the pathogenesis of the various conditions lumped under this pseudodiagnosis and the activity of the various regimens prescribed.

BACTERIAL INFECTIONS

The cutaneous bacterial infections, pyodermas and erythrasma, occur frequently on the lower extremities. Bacterial infections are often conveniently divided into primary and secondary pyodermas.

A primary infection originates in normal skin. Primary cutaneous bacterial infections are due to either *Staphylococcus aureus* or Group A beta-hemolytic streptococci. Examples are impetigo, ecthyma, folliculitis, paronycia, and erysipelas.

Secondary cutaneous infections occur on skin sites that are involved by a preceding dermatitis. These infections are primarily caused by *S. aureus* and less frequently by streptococci or gram-negative organisms. Examples are infectious eczematoid dermatitis, infected intertrigo, and ulcers with secondary infection.

PRIMARY PYODERMAS

Impetigo

Impetigo is a contagious, superficial skin infection which may be caused by staphylococci or streptococci, or both. Certain strains of staph or strep cause impetigo but rarely cause other types of skin lesions (Fig. 2-1).

Impetigo Contagiosa—usually affects preschool-aged children; in developing countries, impetigo is a problem of major proportions.[5] It is quite contagious among infants, less so among older children and adults, but under adverse conditions, susceptibility is increased. Clinically, there are numerous thin-walled vesicles on an erythematous base which break readily and form yellowish crusts. Satellite lesions and peripheral extension may result in irregular serpiginous lesions. The crusts often become very thick and honey-colored with a "stuck-on" appearance, the hallmark of impetigo. After they dry, they separate, leaving residual erythema but no scarring. Such lesions usually occur on the face, especially around the nose and mouth, but they may occur anywhere on the skin except on the palms and soles.

Bullous Impetigo—a variant occurring in newborns and young children. Bullae that are less easily ruptured than the vesicles of impetigo contagiosa appear and tend to become larger. Eventually the bullae rupture and leave behind a "scaled skin" or "second degree burn" look to the skin. Peripheral extension occurs, and large portions of the body may be involved, becoming crusted and denuded. Low-grade fever is not uncommon. The most frequent causative organism is a Grade II phage type 71 strain of *S. aureus.* This strain and occasional other typable and nontypable strains elaborate a specific toxin known as exfoliatin that produces a superficial split in the epidermis just below the stratum corneum, which results in a superficial vesicle or bulla. The most severe expression of this toxin is toxic epidermal necrolysis (T.E.N.) or staphlococcal scalded skin syndrome.

Impetigo due to certain strains of streptococci may occasionally result in glomerulonephritis. In one series of patients with nephritis, 33.8% had had a history of recent impetigo, although the experience of most clinicians would suggest that this percentage is higher than usually encountered.[2] However, in the tropics or subtropics, skin infections due to nephritogenic strains of streptococci which cause glomerulonephritis are not uncommon.

A cornerstone of the therapy for impetigo is close attention to cleanliness with frequent washing of the lesions with an antibacterial soap. It is also essential that the crusts be removed by washing, compressing, or gentle debridement. A topical antibiotic cream or ointment should be applied several times a day. Systemic antibiotics are not usually necessary but may occasionally be required if the impetigo is extensive or associated with lymphadenitis or fever. Treatment for T.E.N. requires systemic antibiotics (erythromycin or penicillinase-resistant penicillins).

Ecthyma

Ecthyma (deep impetigo) is a streptococcal infection which occurs preferentially on the lower extremities (Fig. 2-2). In temperate climates ecthyma usually occurs in children. In the tropics it is much more common and may affect any age. All studies to date have concluded that environmental factors are important and that infections occur more frequently in hot, humid climates than in cool, dry areas. Crowded living and poor hygiene also predispose to infection. Streptococci do not survive well in intact human skin, and some injury such as a scratch or cut is essential for infection to occur. The initial lesion is a small vesicle or pustule which rapidly evolves into a punched-out ulceration (ecthyma) with an areola of erythema. A hard adherent crust forms which can be difficult to remove. Under the crust, a purulent irregular ulcer forms by extending into the dermis. Healing occurs in a few weeks with scarring and hypo- or hyperpigmentation.

Characteristically, lymphadenopathy develops early even with a single rather innocuous-appearing lesion. Certain strains (so-called nephritogenic strains) can result in postinfection glomerulonephritis, which is usually transient but can result in progressive, severe renal compromise. The pathogenesis of this complication involves circulating immune complexes which precipitate in the glomerulus and induce inflammation. Treatment is similar to that for impetigo;

however, systemic antibiotics are frequently indicated. Most effective is benzathine penicillin G; a single injection intramuscularly of 600,000 units will usually produce complete healing within a week. Since there is a tendency toward recurrences, protective measures to prevent trauma are advisable.

Folliculitis

Folliculitis is a pyoderma occurring within a hair follicle. The lesion may be either superficial or deep. The extremities are a frequent location for superficial folliculitis. If the lesions are neglected, they may extend more deeply into the hair follicle, and in the beard or scalp areas, the infection may become chronic.

Follicular pustules are invariably caused by *S. aureus*. Minor trauma, *e.g.*, leg shaving, is often an important contributing factor. Most patients will respond to either topical or systemic antibiotic therapy. In recalcitrant recurrent cases, one should consider colonization of the patients' anterior nares or the skin of the perineum as reservoirs for the offending organism. Occupational exposure to cutting oils and solvents may give rise to folliculitis, although the pustules are usually sterile.

Furuncles

Furuncles are erythematous tender nodules due to *S. aureus*. Presumably, these lesions start with follicular colonization by *S. aureus*, which then spreads into the dermis. Depending on the strain, a furuncle may be a fairly innocent, relatively asymptomatic lesion or a rapidly enlarging lesion which produces fever and other systemic signs. For the former, incision and drainage is often sufficient, while the latter requires systemic erythromycin or penicillinase-resistant penicillin. Recurrences are a sign to search for diabetes or a reservoir such as the anterior nares or the perineum.

Paronychia

Paronychia is a cellulitis of the nail folds. The disorder is usually caused by streptococci and results from invasion of skin dam-

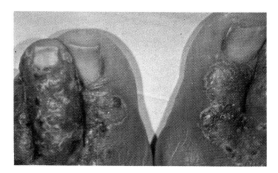

Fig. 2-1. Superficial pyoderma (impetigo).

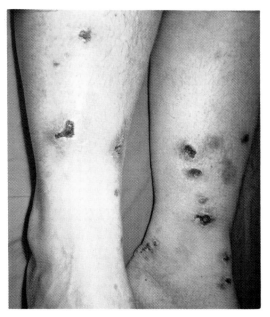

Fig. 2-2. Typical ecthyma. Group A streptococci recovered from lesions. A single injection of 600,000 units of benzathine penicillin G intramuscularly produced a rapid cure within a week.

aged by fungi, poorly fitting shoes, or other minor trauma. Swelling, erythema, pain, tenderness, and often a purulent discharge from beneath the nail fold occur (Fig. 2-3). Secondary dystrophic changes of the nail are often seen. Frequent exposure of the digit to moisture, sweating, friction, maceration, and systemic disorders, such as diabetes mellitus, will predispose to the development of paronychial infections and may cause acute infections to become chronic. In chronic paronychia, involvement with *Candida* may occur.

Therapy consists of encouraging dryness and avoiding trauma to the nail fold, control of any underlying predisposing systemic disease, systemic antibiotics as indicated by culture, and sensitivity tests. In addition, 2% or 4% thymol in chloroform applied by running a glass rod applicator along the edge of the nail fold several times daily will help maintain dryness and antibacterial activity under the separated nail fold. If a Candidal infection is present, specific topical antimonilial therapy (nystatin, amphotericin) should be instituted.

Cellulitis and Erysipelas

Streptococcal cellulitis appears as a sharply demarcated, erythematous, tender plaque with regional lymphadenopathy and fever. The most common area of involvement is the lower leg. A common reason for this predilection is a low-grade interdigital tinea pedis. The keratolytic activity of the fungus in the toe web damages the stratum corneum barrier sufficiently to allow a portal of entry for streptococci, which then find their way into lymphatics and initiate a host response. The management of streptococcal cellulitis of the lower leg should involve not only systemic penicillin or erythromycin but also treatment of any fungal infection of the toe web in order to minimize the chance for recurrences.

Erysipelas is a streptococcal infection causing a sharply demarcated, erythematous, tense edematous plaque which is brawny, hot, and tender. Vesicles may be present in the advancing margin. The infection is usually acquired by direct inoculation into the skin and tends to occur in newborns, the elderly, and others with lowered resistance. In adults, the leg is the site of involvement in 50% of cases (Fig. 2-4).

Without therapy, complications (*e.g.*, nephritis, subcutaneous abscesses, and septicemia) are common, and in infants the mortality rate may reach 40%. Therapy with penicillin is effective. Recurrent attacks may lead to progressively severe lymphedema and the ultimate development of elephantiasis nostra verrucosa (see Chap. 13). At times, low-dose prophylactic penicillin may be indicated to prevent recurrent attacks.

SECONDARY PYODERMAS

Skin affected with dermatitis routinely becomes colonized by S. aureus. For instance, several studies have shown that for atopic dermatitis, S. aureus is recovered from lesions in nearly 100% of cases. The strains involved appear to be less virulent than those responsible for primary pyodermas, and invasion of the skin to produce furunculosis, cellulitis, or bacteremia is decidedly uncommon in dermatitis. It has also been demonstrated that S. aureus colonization can aggravate dermatitis long before clinical signs of "infection" such as suppuration, fever, or lymphadenopathy appear. S. aureus in excess of 10^6 organisms per square centimeter is contributing to the signs and symptoms of the patient, and the use of an antibiotic, either topical or systemic, will produce clinical improvement. Since the primary problem is dermatitis, antibiotic therapy should be used as adjunctive therapy in the initial stages, while the main approach involves anti-inflammatory measures.

Infectious Eczematoid Dermatitis

Infectious eczematoid dermatitis is an eczematous inflammation resulting from the discharge of wet drainage seeping over the skin from an underlying cellulitis or pyogenic infection (Fig. 2-5). Autoinoculation often occurs. Therapy should be directed toward eradicating the primary site of infection. With control of the infection, the drainage ceases and the area of infectious eczematoid dermatitis clears.

Infected Intertrigo

Intertrigo is an inflammation of the skin resulting from the effects of friction, moisture, and sweat retention. These factors also predispose to bacterial invasion, and so it is not uncommon for some degree of bacterial infection to occur superimposed upon the intertrigo. Favorite sites of intertrigo are the axillae, crural regions, inframammary areas, and between the toes, where it is often misdiagnosed as tinea (Fig. 2-6).

Treatment consists of promoting dryness of the intertriginous areas by ventilation, cool drying compresses, and a bland, absorbent powder. The secondary infection is treated with the appropriate topical antibiotic in a lotion or compress form. Creams and ointments should be avoided.

Infected Ulcers

Ulcers of any cause may become secondarily infected. Studies of the role of "infection" in leg ulcers are difficult to conduct because of the problems of different etiologic factors, variance in severity from one patient to another, and patient compliance. Therapy consists of topical or systemic antibiotics and treatment of the underlying systemic or local cause of the ulcer itself.

Problems arise in trying to evaluate antimicrobial therapies. A currently widely used agent is benzoyl peroxide in concentrations ranging from 5% to 20%. This material, particularly at higher concentrations, stimulates granulation tissue and has a broad range of antimicrobial efficacy. Another useful agent is 1% acetic acid because of its drying or astringent effects as well as its antimicrobial effects particularly against gram-negative organisms. (See Chap. 14 for a detailed review of the subject.)

Miscellaneous Pyogenic Infections

Rarely many unusual organisms such as *Pseudomonas* and *Proteus* cause clinical pyodermic infections which are frequently resistant to the usual forms of antibacterial therapy. The causative organism and therapy should be determined by culture and sensitivities. Laboratory studies should be performed to determine the presence of any underlying systemic disorder such as diabetes, lymphoma, or immunoglobulin defect, which would predispose to the establishment of a cutaneous infection by these uncommon invaders.

Figure 2-7 shows a recalcitrant pyoderma of the foot due to *Pseudomonas* which was resistant to the usual topical and systemic antibiotics and responded to acetic acid soaks, erythromycin ointment, and Lassar's paste.

Erythrasma

For almost a century following its description, erythrasma was classified among the fungal disorders. However, in 1961, Sarkany and his coworkers described the causative organism to be a gram-positive bacillus and demonstrated that the clinical disease responded promptly to antibiotic therapy.[6,7]

Mild erythrasma is common in most populations, but a higher incidence has been observed in diabetics.[4,8] This complication is discussed in the section on diabetes.

The lesions themselves are irregularly shaped, dry, scaly, well-demarcated patches showing a predilection for the crural folds, the pubic area, the axillae, intergluteal cleft, inframammary areas, and the toe webs. The last-mentioned location is the most common site of erythrasma and accounts for many of the instances of maceration or scaling, or both, between the more lateral toes, which were not fungal in origin or due to intertrigo and were not "white psoriasis" (Fig. 2-8).

If the diagnosis is suspected it is confirmed rather readily, since the lesions show a characteristic coral-red fluorescence under the Wood's light.[3] The organism *Corynebacterium minutissimum* can also be seen in scrapings stained with PAS or Giemsa. The organism can be cultured on special media the crucial ingredient of which is 20% fetal bovine serum, and the colonies will also produce the reddish fluorescence due to a porphyrin.

The use of erythromycin either locally or systemically results in dramatic disappearance of the skin eruption, but recurrences may occur. Clotrimazole is also effective as a topical preparation.[1]

The proper recognition of this entity may result in prompt resolution of a previously intractable and incapacitating intertrigo of the feet.

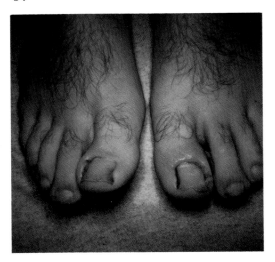

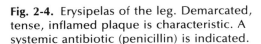

Fig. 2-3. Paronychia. Note erythema, swelling and purulent discharge beneath the nail fold.

Fig. 2-4. Erysipelas of the leg. Demarcated, tense, inflamed plaque is characteristic. A systemic antibiotic (penicillin) is indicated.

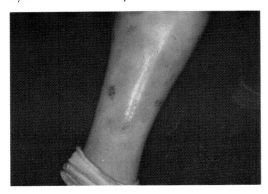

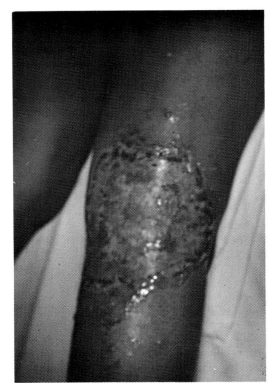

Fig. 2-5. Infectious eczematoid dermatitis secondary to underlying pyogenic infection. Therapy should be directed toward the pyogenic process; when the purulent drainage ceases, the dermatitis will clear.

Fig. 2-6. Intertrigo with superimposed streptococcal infection. Frequently misdiagnosed as tinea pedis.

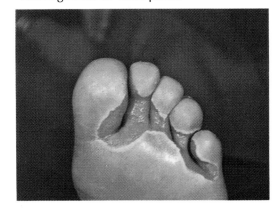

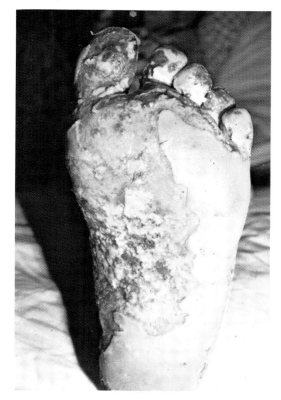

Fig. 2-7. Pseudomonas pyoderma. Systemic and local therapy were ineffective until acetic acid soaks were used. Laboratory studies did not reveal any underlying systemic disorder.

SYSTEMIC BACTERIAL INFECTIONS

A variety of bacterial infections may cause lesions of the skin and also have the potentiality for systemic involvement. Examples are diptheria, anthrax, erysipeloid, brucellosis, tularemia, tuberculosis, and leprosy.

The majority of these disorders show no predilection for the lower extremities and are therefore not reviewed. Erythema induratum is discussed under the nodose lesions (Chap. 4).

FUNGAL INFECTIONS— SUPERFICIAL AND DEEP MYCOSES; CANDIDIASIS

The fungi that affect man are relatively few, and their effect is often rather benign. They may, however, cause severe, even fatal, diseases.

The feet are particularly susceptible to the geophilic (soil-dwelling) fungi, especially in warmer climates where the feet are often bare. The legs and feet are also likely to come in contact with animals and their zoophilic fungi. In addition, the anthropophilic fungi are quite opportunistic and often find ideal conditions existing on the feet—warmth and moisture due to the occlusion of shoes, intertriginous maceration between the toes, moist hyperkeratosis of the soles, and the effects of aging, trauma, and vascular disease.

Since human beings are constantly exposed to fungal elements throughout most, if not all of their lives, clinical dermatomycotic infections would seem virtually unavoidable. Yet, in fact, such widespread infection does not occur because of wide variations in individual resistance and susceptibility. Why do some individuals quickly reject a fungal infection whereas others

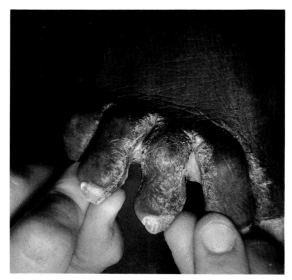

Fig. 2-8. Erythrasma. Note characteristic dry, scaly patches in toe webs.

maintain a chronic state of disease? Considerable work on epidemiology and environmental influences, and ongoing investigations into the immunology of dermatophytosis are now under review.

ACUTE INFECTIONS

Environmental Influences

The means by which fungal infections are acquired and transmitted are not entirely known. Ringworm fungi do not have a high degree of infectivity for normal healthy persons. Evidence for this is both clinical and experimental. Tinea pedis is not a highly contagious disease. There are few instances of acute tinea pedis among family members or of epidemics in institutions. Mere immersion of feet in a fungus-contaminated bath failed to produce clinical infections; only transient colonization of dermatophytes was established in 50% of the persons thus exposed.[4] Acute tinea pedis could be produced only by blistering the skin prior to immersion in the fungus-laden solution, by mechanical trauma, or by occluding the skin to increase moisture after massive exposure to dermatophytes.[1,3,14,16] These experimentally induced acute infections were transient and spontaneously regressed following removal of the predisposing cause. Occlusion appeared to play a significant role in rendering the skin susceptible to dermatophytic infection, and it has been postulated that the effect is related to concentrations of CO_2 on the skin surface.[18]

Frequent bathing decreases the chance of infection by removing a significant quantity of the infectious material and also by decreasing the amount of organic residues of perspiration upon which some fungi feed. Skin that is naturally thin, with little keratin, is more difficult to infect. Oily, moist skin is more readily infected than dry skin, which desquamates more readily. Wetness is basic to the symptomatic form of "athlete's foot"; it permits increased growth of resident diphtheroids and other normal bacterial flora, and on sites previously colonized by ringworm fungi, the clinical signs of acute tinea pedis appear. Conversely, when the bacterial population is suppressed through simple drying or topical antibacterial agents, the condition becomes asymptomatic.[12] (See Athlete's Foot Syndrome.)

The likely source of acute tinea pedis is a symptomatic infection of the soles and nails. These two sites are stable reservoirs of dermatophytes and serve as chief sources of acute attacks of interdigital tinea pedis. The anatomy of the toe webs, occlusive foot gear, and friction are *in vivo* counterparts necessary for induction of acute tinea pedis.

CHRONIC INFECTIONS

Immunologic Susceptibility

Many people are completely resistant to infection by some fungi. While local factors affect the likelihood of an individual's becoming infected, it is now apparent that the host's immunologic predisposition determines whether an infection heals spontaneously or spreads, becoming extensive and chronic.[11] In the study done by Jones *et al*, approximately 80% of chronically infected men failed to reject the infection for immunologic reasons. The responsible defect is a deficiency in cell-mediated immunity and may be either functional or actual, owing to cell-mediated tolerance. The remaining 20% of those with chronic dermatophytosis have apparently normal cell-mediated immunity but have persistent infections, possibly because of nonimmunologic factors peculiar to the skin.[11] The balance between the dermatophyte and its host is far from clear.

Intradermal testing with trichophytin has provided another procedure for evaluating immunologic responses in patients with dermatophyte infections: Patients infected with *Trichophyton rubrum* are more likely to show no reactivity or only immediate reactivity, while *T. mentagrophytes* patients are more likely to have delayed reactivity with or without immediate reactivity.[8] Thus, differences between the types of fungus and the cutaneous reaction to trichophytin antigen are evident. In addition to the relatively specific defect in delayed hypersensitivity to trichophytin in patients with chronic dermatophytosis, cell-mediated responses to other antigens may also be somewhat decreased.[15] The mechanisms of these responses are far from clear.

Several other factors may be important in the genesis of chronic dermatophytosis. A significant number of patients with chronic *T. rubrum* infections had elevated glucose tolerance curves.[10] Although serum fungistatic factors have been described, their exact role in clinical disease is not known.[7] On the clinical side, it appears that the continued presence of infecting dermatophytes may be responsible for a naturally occurring tolerant state.

UNUSUAL FUNGAL INFECTIONS

Extensive fungal infections, deep infections caused by dermatophytes, and infections due to nonpathogenic fungi have been described in patients receiving long-term systemic steroid therapy and in those with an immunologic defect resulting from disease or treatment.[6]

Tinea Pedis

Tinea pedis, the most common of the dermatomycoses, is usually due to *Trichophyton rubrum* or *T. mentagrophytes*, with *Epidermophyton floccosum* a less frequent causative organism.

The manifestations of tinea pedis vary widely but generally consist of two main clinical pictures: the acute inflammatory and chronic hyperkeratotic types.

Clinical Manifestations. *Acute Inflammatory Tinea Pedis.* In this form of fungal infection, the skin is involved with an oozing, macerated, vesicular eruption which leads to the loss of the epidermis, fissuring, pruritus, and occasionally secondary bacterial infection. Frequently, the initial area of involvement is in a toe web, usually the fourth interspace, where maceration and fissuring occur (Fig. 2-9). The process may then extend to other toe webs and may involve large areas of the sole (Fig. 2-10). *T. mentagrophytes* is the usual causative fungus in acute inflammatory tinea pedis, with *E. floccosum* being the etiologic agent less frequently.

Chronic Hyperkeratotic Tinea Pedis. In marked contrast to the acute vesicular inflammatory tinea pedia is the exceedingly chronic, scaling, often asymptomatic, hyperkeratotic type. In this disorder, the involvement is on the soles often extending onto the sides of the feet, the so-called moccasin distribution (Fig. 2-11). The toe webs are usually spared. This type of tinea pedis is almost always due to *T. rubrum*.

A peculiarity of chronic *T. rubrum* infections is their occasional tendency to persist as an asymmetric disorder. Only one foot may be involved for many years, and when the hands as well as the feet are involved, almost invariably only a single hand will be infected. The explanation for this behavior is unknown and is not related to the patient's being right- or left-handed.

Fungal Granuloma. Perifollicular granulomas (Majocchi's) caused by penetration of hairs infected with *T. rubrum* through breaks in the follicular wall are occasionally seen on the lower legs and ankles (Fig. 2-12). The condition occurs most frequently in women who have a diffuse tinea pedis and who shave their legs. The painless, inflammatory lesions may last for months and are commonly mistaken for a bacterial folliculitis. A rarely reported manifestation is a nodular granulomatous perifolliculitis, which also may be easily misdiagnosed.[9]

Onychomycosis. Fungal infections of the toenails (Fig. 2-13) may be the only manifestation of tinea pedis or may be present along with cutaneous involvement of the feet. The clinical appearances of onychomycosis caused by different species of dermatophytes are indistinguishable. There are three types of onychomycosis, based on the route of infection and clinical appearance: distal subungual, proximal subungual, and white superficial. The distal subungual is the most common variety. The primary site of involvement is the distal nail bed and hyponychium. The undersurface of the nail plate is involved secondarily. Opaque yellow discoloration, subungual keratosis, and onycholysis are early signs. The proximal subungual variety is less common. Infection begins under the proximal nail fold with minimal signs of inflammation. It may remain confined to the lunula or may grow distally as the nail grows. Yellowish discoloration and crumbling of the nail plate are early manifestations of infection. The white superficial infection called leukonychia trichophytica is commonly seen on the toenails. *T. mentagrophytes* is the organism most often isolated. The infection begins on the dorsal surface of the nail plate, showing well defined white islands. These may coalesce to involve the entire nail surface, which then becomes rough and crumbly. Late in the course of infection, the nail plate may be completely destroyed, at which time the three varieties are indistinguishable.

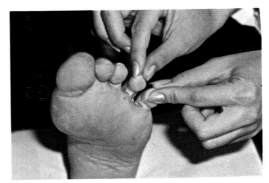

Fig. 2-9. Interdigital fungal infection characteristic of *T. mentagrophytes*.

Fig. 2-10. Tinea pedis: severe vesiculobullous reaction. *T. mentagrophytes* was cultured.

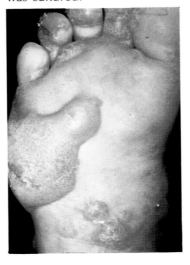

Allergic Manifestations. Dermatophytid or id reactions are secondary eruptions occurring on the fingers and hands of sensitized individuals as a result of the spread of fungi or their allergenic products from a primary site. The lesions usually present as tense discrete pruritic vesicles on the palms and inner sides of the fingers. Id eruptions can also occur on the trunk and lower extremities, where they may resemble other dermatoses. The reaction patterns seen on the lower extremities include an erysipelas-like picture, erythema nodosum, and a chronic variant of erythema multiforme. Id eruptions are usually seen in association with acute inflammatory fungal infections, often caused by *T. mentagrophytes* infections that have been irritated or overtreated. Fungi can be found in the primary lesion, but the secondary id lesion is sterile. The id lesions involute with the clearing of the primary focus; patients respond positively to skin tests with trichophytin.

While fungal infections are among the most frequent skin affections of the feet, many nonfungal disorders are misdiagnosed as tinea pedia (*e.g.*, intertrigo, erythrasma, contact dermatitis, dyshidrosis, neurodermatitis, and psoriasis appearing as marginated hyperkeratotic plaques, as "white" psoriasis of toe webs, or as pustular psoriasis). Tinea actually accounts for only about one-third of skin disease involving the feet. Onychomycosis must be differentiated from nail changes occurring in psoriasis, lichen planus, and alopecia areata, or as the result of recurrent paronychial infections and trauma. All clinical diagnoses of fungus infection of the feet should be confirmed by laboratory studies.

Diagnosis. The laboratory confirmation of tinea pedis and tinea unguium is relatively easy and should be carried out in all suspected cases. There are two basic techniques, the direct microscopic examination of samples of diseased skin for fungal elements, and fungal culture.

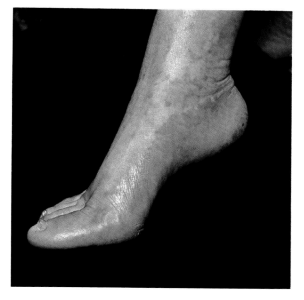

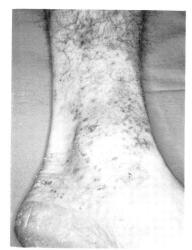

Fig. 2-11. *Trichophyton rubrum* infection of foot. Note characteristic mocassin distribution.

Fig. 2-12. Majococchi's granuloma *(T. rubrum)*. The follicular inflamed papules are distinctive in this form of tinea.

Fig. 2-13. Onychomycosis. KOH positive; *T. mentagrophytes* was cultured.

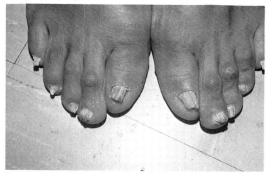

Examination of Skin Scrapings. Sponge the surface of the affected skin with 70% alcohol, let it dry, and then with a No. 15 bladed scalpel, scrape a small portion of involved tissue. It is advisable to take material from the more active portions of the lesions and to scrape deep enough to cause minimal bleeding. Place the flakes of keratin on a clean slide or implant onto culture media. If the skin is blistered, clip the top of a vesicle and place it, inverted, on a glass slide. In nail infection, scrape away the loose surface debris and take material from well under the nails (in the distal subungual type) or from the dorsal surface of the nail (in the proximal subungual and superficial white varieties). Add a drop or two of 10% potassium hydroxide, apply a coverslip, and gently heat the slide (over a Bunsen flame or alcohol lamp, or by placing on the lid of a heated sterilizer) for a few seconds to facilitate digestion of keratin. (More rapid digestion of the thick keratin of nails may be obtained by using a mixture of potassium hydroxide 17%, dimethyl sulfoxide 34%, and water 49%. Wet mounts prepared with this mixture should be examined when the keratin becomes soft, since further delay will result in digestion of the fungal elements.) Examine the slide under low power with subdued light. Fungal elements appear as branching, threadlike hyphae about 2 to 4 microns in diameter, somewhat double-walled and sometimes showing cross walls. If the first specimen results prove negative, repeat the examination with material from other areas of the lesion.

At times, it may be difficult to detect hyphae among epithelial cells and other debris, even with potassium hydroxide digestion, particularly since there are no color differences. Recently, a new rapid-contrast stain has been reported, greatly facilitating the reading of such microscopic preparations.[17] The contrast stain consists of two solutions: (1) one part 1% aerosol OTB, one part 10% potassium hydroxide, and 2 parts 1% ink blue P.P.; and (2) 0.5% rose bengal in buffered Shear's mounting fluid. Using this stain, on direct microscopic examination of scrapings, dermatophyte hyphae stain light blue against a background of rose-red keratinocytes. Candida hyphae and pseudohyphae stain blue; the cytoplasm of blastospores stains pink, the walls blue. The background is rose-red. Geotrichum, Trichosporon, and Aspergillus stain similarly.

Scrapings may also be placed on Sabouraud's agar and incubated at room temperature for 2 to 6 weeks. If growth occurs, this not only confirms the clinical diagnosis but also allows identification of the organism.

Taplin *et al* developed a fungal culture medium allowing identification of dermatophytes by simple observation of a color change in the medium.[18] The medium contains phenol red, which is yellow at the acid pH of the agar. The dermatophytes produce alkaline metabolites that raise the pH of the medium and change phenol red from yellow to red. This striking color change does not occur with saprophytes or with most candida strains. The agar contains additives that inhibit the growth of bacterial organisms. Experience in both the United States and Vietnam has shown this new medium to be at least 97% reliable. Nail scrapings containing large amounts of saprophytic fungi may give a false-positive color change; for this reason the new medium is not recommended for identification of dermatophytes from nails. An occasional strain of *Candida albicans* may produce the red color. The caps on the culture tubes should be kept loose, since false-negative reactions may occur if the caps are tightly closed. Cultures should be read within 14 days to decrease the chance of eventual growth of extraneous organisms, producing false reaction.

Since the dermatophytes show the characteristic color change in agar and are responsive to griseofulvin, the color change allows easy differentiation between those fungi that will respond to griseofulvin and those that will not. The medium is available commercially as the Pfizer Dermatophyte Test Medium (DTM).

Treatment. *Acute Inflammatory Exacerbations.* For acute inflammatory exacerbations with secondary eczematization, mild therapy should be used to control the dermatitis first, and the fungous disease should be treated later.

External Measures

Soaks or wet compresses should be applied for 20 minutes, 3 or 4 times daily.

Apply bland topical preparations such as Burow's paste (Burow's solution, 1 part, Aquaphor, 2 parts, Lassar's zinc paste, 3 parts) between soaks.

Topical antibiotics may be used if secondary infection is present.

Rest, partial or complete, is indicated; feet should be kept elevated if edema is present.

Open shoes or sandals are worn if patient is ambulatory.

Avoid fungicidal chemicals during this stage; they are often too irritating for eczematous areas and may cause id reactions.

Furthermore, there are no satisfactory data to show that antifungal agents are more effective than simple compresses in treating the inflammatory type of dermatophytosis.

Internal Measures When cellulitis or lymphangitis, or both, is present, broad-spectrum antibiotics should be used.

For severe forms of eczematization, oral corticosteroids may be indicated.

Subacute, Chronic, or Mild Infections. For subacute, chronic, or mild infections, the following should be done.

External Measures

Use powders, tinctures, or solutions during the day.

Antifungal creams or ointments are prescribed for night use.

Tolnaftate is primarily effective against dermatophytes; haloprogin, miconazole, and clotrimazole have a broader spectrum of activity.* These new antifungal drugs are available as powders, solutions, or creams.

Whitfield's ointment remains an old standby. The major difference between the new antifungal drugs and older measures such as Whitfield's ointment and Castellani's paint is the type of side effect produced; the older agents cause skin irritation, and the newer specific agents produce sensitization.

We give our patients a list of instructions to follow:

Directions for care of feet
1. Soak feet in solution prescribed, morning and evening and before retiring.
2. Dry your feet well.
3. Change socks twice daily, morning and evening. Socks should be cotton; avoid synthetic materials.
4. Change shoes twice daily, morning and evening.
5. Powder well your feet, socks, and shoes, twice daily.
6. Apply given medicine every night as directed.

Internal Measures Griseofulvin has revolutionized the therapy for fungal infections, but it is not without its drawbacks. The drug is fungistatic, not fungicidal. It operates by becoming incorporated into the keratin layer as it is formed and by inhibiting the fungus until the organisms are shed with the keratin. Treatment with griseofulvin must be continued 3 or 4 weeks in skin infections, 4 to 6 months for fingernail infections, and 18 to 24 months for toenail infections.

The dose of griseofulvin is 250 to 500 mg daily of the micronized type. The latest form of griseofulvin is ultra-microcrystalline, but there are no clinical efficacy data to indicate an advantage of one form over the others.

*Tinactin (tolnaftate), Schering Corp., Bloomfield, NJ 08003; Halotex (haloprogin), Westwood Pharmaceuticals, Inc., Buffalo, NY 14123; Micatin (miconazole), Johnson and Johnson, New Brunswick, NY 08903; Lotrimin (clotrimazole), Delbay Pharmaceuticals, Kenilworth, NJ 07003.

Some persons require 1000 mg, particularly those with chronic nail infections. The necessity for long-term treatment in onychomycosis should be stressed to the patient; "trials" of 3 to 4 months usually end up as disappointing treatment failures. It had been shown that intestinal absorption is enhanced by taking the griseofulvin after a fatty meal, but new evidence shows that this is an unnecessary requirement. Tinea pedis and onychomycosis may be persistent and recurrent in spite of therapy with griseofulvin or topical agents. Because of the problem of constant reinfection, success with griseofulvin (1 g/day) in onychomycosis is about 50% and about 80% following avulsion of the nails. Avulsion of nails is discussed in Chapter 18.

Side effects from griseofulvin include gastrointestinal distress, loose stools, headaches, and urticarial and morbilliform eruptions. Patients may be told to take griseofulvin at bedtime to reduce any disabling effects of the headache. In some patients, griseofulvin, particularly in large doses, may cause slowing of reaction time and interference with coordinated movements. The drug should therefore be administered with caution to airplane pilots and auto drivers. In rare instances, griseofulvin may cause hematologic alterations ranging from leukopenia to an LE syndrome, and by enzymatic interference may induce porphyria. Griseofulvin is a tumor-producing agent in animals, and although tumorgenicity is not documented in the human, the risk-benefit ratio must be considered. The drug should probably be prescribed with due caution for pregnant women, because toxic effects of the drug have been found in some fetal animal studies.

FUNGAL INFECTIONS IN SERVICEMEN IN TROPICAL ENVIRONMENTS

The importance of moisture in increasing the extent and persistence of dermatophyte infections has been graphically demonstrated among combat troops in Vietnam.[5] In the humid tropical environment, where many hours are spent in water with little or no opportunity to dry out, bathe, or put on clean dry clothes, skin problems have incapacitated as many as 25% to 40% of combat personnel, with fungous infections and tropical acne the major causes.

The most frequent dermatophytosis was *Trichophyton mentagrophytes* infection which, in the damp environment, frequently extended beyond the anticipated areas of involvement, such as the feet and crural areas, to cover widespread areas of the body surface. Frequently, dermatophyte involvement of the leg corresponding to the upper portion of the combat boots was as intense as the involvement of the feet. The widespread lesions often took the form of inflammatory folliculitis.

The organisms cultured and tested were sensitive to griseofulvin, and one would anticipate a tood response to this therapy. However, it was frequently impractical for men in the field to take an adequate dose for the necessary length of time.

A subsequent report clarified the source of infection: *T. mentagrophytes* infections acquired in Vietnam were possibly from rats; the risk of infection was directly related to the degree of exposure to wet clothing; and Americans were distinctly more susceptible to *T. mentagrophytes* infections than were adult Vietnamese.[3]

THE ATHLETE'S FOOT SYNDROME

Recent studies done by Leyden and Kligman have advanced a new interpretation for this common problem.[12,13] The concept that athlete's foot is strictly a ringworm infection of toe webs has been modified: Their experiments in volunteer subjects conclude that athlete's foot represents a continuum from a relatively asymptomatic, scaling eruption caused by fungi to a symptomatic, macerated, hyperkeratotic variety that is caused by an overgrowth of bacteria. Thus, symptomatic athlete's foot is a fungal-bacterial complex.

The clinical spectrum of interdigital athlete's foot ranges from mild scaling to a painful, exudative, erosive inflammatory process. The most familiar type is characterized by scaly, soggy, whitish hyperkeratotic toe webs associated with pruritus and foul odor.[13] These symptoms do not occur until there is an overgrowth of the normal bacterial flora,

especially Brevibacterium and the aerobic diphtheroids.

Wetness (hydration) enhances the growth of resident bacteria and is basic to the symptomatic form of athlete's foot. These factors provide a guide for therapy. Proper foot care, described under the treatment section, leads to a decrease in the amount of moisture and a corresponding clinical improvement. In their earlier study, the authors tested several aluminum compounds notable for their astringency and possibly for bacteriostatic or bactericidal action. Aluminum chloride in 30% solution proved to be most effective. Applied twice daily with a cotton-tipped applicator, the solution brought about relief of both itching and the foul odor within 2 or 3 days, and resolution of the toe-web lesions after 7 to 10 days.[12] Also, a pure antifungal drug such as tolfnaftate was less effective than agents such as miconazole or clotrimazole that have a broad spectrum of activity not only against fungi but also against the bacteria in controlling this collaborative infection.

CANDIDIASIS

Candidiasis, or moniliasis, is separated from the dermatophytes because it is caused by a quite different fungus. *Candida albicans* is a yeastlike fungus, occurring as a normal inhabitant of the gastrointestinal tract. Normal persons with normal skin are fairly resistant. It is an opportunistic pathogen and exerts its influence as a disease producer in altered physiologic states, such as prolonged or massive antibiotic therapy, diabetes, alcoholism, obesity, vascular stasis, excessive moisture, vitamin deficiencies, or endocrinopathies and cell-mediated immune deficiencies. While candidal infections are usually superficial, a chronic mucocutaneous or systemic form of candida infection will occasionally occur in the presence of a predisposing systemic disorder. Serious opportunistic infections caused by *C. albicans* in debilitated patients pose an increasing threat to their survival. The seriousness of the infection is roughly proportional to the degree to which the host's defenses are compromised. On the lower extremities, candidiasis may manifest itself as interdigital and intertriginous infections, paronychia and onycholysis, and candidal granuloma.

Intertrigo may occur wherever two skin surfaces are opposed to each other, thereby preventing adequate ventilation and evaporation of sweat. Intertrigo may occur between the toes of those persons who have thick, stubby, tightly opposed toes or in persons with normal-shaped toes who wear tight shoes and occlusive socks, preventing adequate evaporation of perspiration in warm weather. The candidal infection gives rise to white macerated tissue with fissuring and denuded areas, particularly in the fourth interdigital space, and is known as erosio interdigitalis blastomycetica. The eruption commonly extends to the dorsum of the foot.

Paronychia and onycholysis are commonly produced by candidal infections of the fingernails, but occasional involvement of the toenails occurs. The tissue adjacent to and including the nail fold becomes red, edematous, and tender. The posterior nail fold is raised from the underlying nail, and the nail becomes opaque and dystrophic. Harboring of moisture in this sulcus leads to further progression of the candidal infection. There may be further involvement distally separating the nail plate from the nail bed, possibly giving the nail the appearance of being depressed proximally and elevated distally. Only one nail may be involved, but more often several or all are affected.

A rare form of cutaneous candidiasis seen on the feet, as well as on the hands, face, or scalp, is the candidal granuloma.[2] In addition to the nail changes described previously, cutaneous horns may arise from the nail beds and face, and thick plaque-like hyperkeratotic lesions may appear on other skin areas.[3]

The cutaneous hallmark of systemic candidiasis is erythematous macronodular lesions which show mycelia in the dermis and blood vessels on histologic examination.[1]

The laboratory diagnosis of candidiasis is usually made rather readily. A potassium hydroxide preparation, as previously described, will show pseudohyphae and budding forms. Culture of the organism yields a soft, white, shiny colony which grows much more rapidly than the dermatophytes. Since candidal organisms are present on normal skin and only a few such yeast forms are necessary to yield a positive culture, however, the recovery of candida on Sabouraud's agar does not constitute proof of a significant fungus infection. Only when the potassium hydroxide (KOH) slide preparation shows the typical filaments and budding cells can the diagnosis of candidiasis be accepted.

Treatment of monilial intertrigo consists basically of bringing about and maintaining a dry environment through use of drying compresses, Castellani's paint, and proper aeration. Topical preparations of nystatin (Mycostatin), amphotericin B (Fungizone), miconazole, clotrimazole, or iodochlorhydroxyquin (Vioform) are of benefit; candida is unaffected by griseofulvin. Candidal paronychia or onycholysis responds well to the maintenance of a dry environment and topical application of a solution of 4% thymol in chloroform applied to the gap between the posterior nail fold and the nail plate twice daily. The free edge of the nail involved in onycholysis should be cut away to allow adequate drying and exposure of the nail bed to the same thymol in chloroform mediation. Candidal granuloma requires therapy with systemic amphotericin B.

In generalized or disseminated forms of candidiasis, as well as in localized infections—particularly those which are resistant or recurrent—it is obligatory to search for underlying metabolic or physiologic derangements that may predispose to this disorder.

DEEP FUNGAL INFECTIONS

In contrast to the dermatophytes producing primarily superficial infections, there are a group of pathogenic fungi that thrive in the deeper tissue and viscera, having the potential to produce systemic disease. They may become manifest on the lower extremities and are acquired by either inhalation, ingestion, or inoculation. Occasionally the disease, although acquired by way of the respiratory or gastrointestinal tract, may disseminate systemically and may manifest itself on the skin. If the infection is acquired by inoculation, it may involve more critical structures by direct extension, lymphatic spread, or dissemination by the blood stream.

Coccidioidomycosis

This is a deep fungal infection caused by the organism *Coccidioides immitis* and is usually contracted in the southwestern United States, and parts of Mexico and Central America, by inhalation of the spores of *Coccidioides immitis* in the dusty soil. The most common form of infection is asymptomatic, resulting in a positive coccidioidin skin test. About one third of exposed patients develop a transient grippe-like illness. Twenty percent of these patients develop erythema nodosum 2 to 3 weeks after onset of symptoms. Erythema multiforme is less frequently seen. In rare instances, it may become disseminated and produce clinical manifestations in the bones, central nervous system, or skin. On the lower extremities, the skin lesions may present as chronic abscesses or granulomas of a pustular, erosive, ulcerative, warty, or vegetating type which are frequently significantly infected secondarily. This disseminated form of coccidioidomycosis represents an inability of the individual to handle his disease immunologically, and carries a grave prognosis.

Another recently described, although very rare, form of coccidioidomycosis is the chancriform or primary inoculation type, often appearing in the lower extremities owing to contact with contaminated soil. The lesion is a painless indurated nodule or plaque with central ulceration, possibly accompanied by lymphadenopathy or nodules along the lymphatics. These lesions almost always heal within a few weeks with no treatment. If the lesion persists for months, it is unlikely that it arose by primary cutaneous inoculation.

The diagnosis of coccidioidomycosis may be made by demonstrating the organism in pus or biopsy material, but more definitively by culturing the organism. The coccidioidin skin test results usually become positive 3 or 4 weeks after infection, and remains positive for many years, perhaps for life. A false-negative reaction may be noted in overwhelming disease. The complement fixation test is also helpful in making the diagnosis and in following the results of treatment.

Coccidioides immitis is susceptible to the antifungal agent, amphotericin B. This is the treatment of choice in generalized infections.

On the lower extremities, abscesses may require excision or drainage in conjunction with systemic therapy.

Histoplasmosis

This is one of the most common systemic fungal infections. Usually the disease is pulmonary, although it may disseminate; cutaneous manifestations on the lower extremities are fairly rare. *Histoplasma capsulatum*, the causative organism, is found most frequently in North America, particularly in the North Central United States along the Mississippi and its tributaries, and is mainly acquired by inhalation of dust. There is apparently a relationship between infected soil and excreta from some birds and poultry.

The skin lesions of disseminate histoplasmosis are similar to the lesions of coccidioidomycosis, but occur much less frequently on the lower extremities. Mucous membrane lesions are not uncommon and may present as either ulcers or granulomatous masses. A rare primary cutaneous form of histoplasmosis acquired by direct inoculation presents as a chancriform lesion and follows a course similar to that described for coccidioidomycosis.

The diagnosis of histoplasmosis may be made by demonstrating the organism in the pus from cutaneous lesions, or by cultures on Sabouraud's agar at room temperature and blood agar at 37° C. The histoplasmin skin test is a reliable aid to diagnosis, and once positive, remains so for several years. In severe systemic histoplasmosis, the skin test result may be negative. The complement-fixation test has diagnostic and prognostic significance; a rising titer indicates a poor prognosis. A precipitin test is also available which correlates with the complement-fixation test. It tends to become positive earlier, within the first few weeks, and then to disappear.

Amphotericin B given intravenously is the treatment of choice for histoplasmosis.

Sporotrichosis

This is a deep fungal infection in which the lesions are manifested most frequently on the skin. The causative fungus *Sporotrichum* schenckii is found in soil and on many forms of vegetation. The disease is thus seen most frequently among farmers, gardeners, florists, outdoor laborers, and gold miners in South Africa. Approximately 60% of lesions occur on the hand or arm, 23% on the trunk, 11% on the legs. The organism must be inoculated into the subcutaneous tissue through a break in the skin, or through contamination of an open sore or wound.

The primary lesion begins days or weeks after contact and consists of a painless enlarging papule that forms an ulcerated, indurated lesion. After a week or more, the ulcer is followed by development of a series of erythematous, firm, painless nodules along the lymphatic chain draining the area, which may also break down to form ulcers. Although cord-like thickening of the lymphatics along which the nodules occur is common, lymph node involvement is rare. In general, the patient's health is not affected, but the localized lesions rarely heal spontaneously. In some cases, the lymphatic involvement may be minimal or absent. The primary lesion spreads in the skin itself, forming an erythematous flat plaque, either smooth or covered with silvery scales. When occurring on the knees, the lesion may take on a warty form sometimes with associated pustulation.

A disseminated form of sporotrichosis exists in which hematogenous spread gives rise to multiple subcutaneous nodular masses over the skin anywhere on the body. These soften and break down also to form chronic ulcerations.

The portal of entry may be an unrecognized cutaneous lesion, the lungs, or the gastrointestinal tract. An asymptomatic primary pulmonary form of the disease may occur in persons exposed to dust contaminated with S. schenckii.

The fungi from cutaneous lesions are easily grown on Sabouraud's agar at room temperature. On the other hand, organisms are rarely demonstrated in smears or biopsy specimens stained with P.A.S. after diastase digestion. Skin and serologic tests may help support the diagnosis but are rarely essential.

The disease responds remarkably to treatment with saturated solution of potassium iodide; 15 drops in milk or water 3 times a day is usually effective. Therapy must be carried out for at least 4 to 6 weeks after apparent clinical care.

Chromoblastomycosis (Chromomycosis)

This uncommon "deep" fungal infection, confined entirely to the skin, has been associated with five species of related fungi, *Phialophora verrucosa*, *Fonsecaea pedrosol*, *F. compactum*, *F. dermatitidis*, and *Cladosporium caprionii*. These are soil-dwelling organisms in all parts of the world. The distribution of the disease, however, is predominantly among barefooted farm laborers in the tropics. The majority of cases occur on the feet or legs below the knees, supporting the theory of inoculation from the soil. Occasionally, lesions occur on areas of the body that are normally clothed, and it has been postulated that these cases represent instances of cutaneous dissemination from a previously unrecognized primary focus in the lungs.

The initial lesion is a papule or pustule persisting unchanged for a prolonged period and then enlarging and ulcerating. Verrucous fungating lesions eventually develop which enlarge by peripheral extension with irregular central clearing and atrophic scar formation (Fig. 2-14). The lesions are often involved by secondary bacterial infection, which in turn may lead to lymphatic stasis and elephantiasis.

Systemic therapy for chromoblastomycosis is difficult and uncertain, since all the fungi involved are resistant to amphotericin B. Oral potassium iodide and calciferol or local perfusion with amphotericin B has occasionally resulted in apparent cures. Local treatment consists of excision of the involved area with primary closure or grafting. Individual lesions may respond to intralesional amphotericin B. Marked extension with debilitation of the individual has occasionally necessitated amputation.

Blastomycosis

This is a deep fungal infection due to *Blastomyces dermatitidis*, which at times may be confused with chromoblastomycosis. In most cases, the organism is probably inhaled as a dust, causing a primary pulmonary focus which is usually subclinical but occasionally may give rise to cutaneous lesions by dissemination.

Primary cutaneous blastomycosis, an extremely rare form of the disease, occurs apparently by inoculation directly into the foot or leg. Clinically, it resembles sporotrichosis including the lymphatic involvement.

The most common form is the chronic cutaneous type, probably caused by hematogenous dissemination from a fleeting or subclinical primary pulmonary blastomycosis. Other organs may be involved in the disseminated form, but it is the skin that is most often and primarily involved. The disease starts as an isolated erythematous papule or subcutaneous nodule that ruptures to form an ulcer, crusts over and spreads peripherally, eventually forming an elevated plaque. On close inspection, the margin of the lesion abruptly falls off to meet normal tissue, and the surface of the plaque may be studded with minute abscesses. Ulcers, subcutaneous abscesses, or sinus tracts may form. The central area of the plaque may clear spontaneously, giving rise to a circinate lesion with a highly active serpiginous border.

The organism may be found on microscopic examination of a 10% KOH preparation of pus or serous fluid as single budding yeast forms. Culture of the organism is readily obtained at either room or body temperatures. The blastomycin skin test and the complement-fixation test are of less diagnostic value than for histoplasmosis.

The treatment of choice is intravenous amphotericin B, to which the fungus is sensitive. Well-localized lesions on the lower extremities may be excised. However, because occult dissemination to other organs may be present, excision must be accompanied by systemic therapy with amphotericin B.

Mycetoma

This deep fungus infection is limited almost exclusively to the lower extremities. The feet are the most frequently affected sites, and this accounts for the name "Madura foot." It is a serious and disfiguring infection.

Mycetoma is a general term denoting a tumor that involves the skin, subcutaneous tissues, fascia, and bone in which the causative organism is eliminated through sinuses in the form of microcolonies called "grains." Two classes of organisms have been associated with the clinical syndrome: the bacteria-like Actinomycetes and the true fungi (Eumycetes). The organisms in the actinomycetes group include *Actinomyces israelii* Nocardia, and Streptomyces; *Allescheria boydii*, Cephalosporium, Madurella, and Phialophora are the true fungi. Thus, there are two types of mycetoma: Actinomycetoma and eumycetoma, and such a division is pertinent to the management of the patient.[1] Although the actinomycetoma and eumycetoma present with similar clinical manifestations, the term Madura foot (maduromycosis) should be reserved for designation of mycetoma caused by true fungi.

The disease is concentrated in scattered regions of the tropics and subtropics including Mexico, Guatemala, and South America. The mode of infection is inoculation of the involved organism through the plantar skin, aided by the fact that in the tropics, plantation workers, workers in rice paddies, or natives go barefoot throughout life, for pure comfort or lack of footwear. The disease is not contagious from man to man, or from animals to man. At the site of inoculation there arises a painless, indurated nodule which enlarges indolently and breaks down to form granulation tissue and sinuses which exude pus-containing tiny granules of varying colors. These granules are minute clumps of the fungus being extruded by the tissues. More nodules appear in adjacent areas, and connecting sinuses are formed. Through fusion of these lesions, the involved area may encompass a whole foot and part of the leg with tremendous swelling, hypertrophy, and multiple sinuses (Fig. 2-15). Some of the sinuses extend to the bone, and osteomyelitis may be extensive and quite destructive. These changes are readily detectable on x-ray examination, which shows evidence of periostitis and cavities within the bone. The foot may become so massive as to prohibit its use and its owner may fall victim to secondary infection, exhaustion, or malnutrition due to his immobility.

Diagnosis is made by demonstrating the grains extruded from the lesions and further identifying the causative organisms by culture. The color of the grains is at times of some diagnostic help. All black grains are due to true fungi and not to the actinomycetes, red grains are produced only by *A. pelletieri*, and light-colored grains may be results of either actinomycetes or true fungi.

More precise identification of the causative organism is afforded by culture and sensitivity studies. The aid of a trained mycologist should be utilized to obtain proper culture specimens and to interpret correctly any resulting growth. Fluorescent antibody techniques have been developed to diagnose *A. israelii* infections.

Treatment of mycetoma can be difficult because of fibrosis, abscess formation, and bony involvement. Conservative but vigorous medical therapy combined with surgical drainage and debridement should be carried out whenever possible, with amputation used only as a last resort.

In general, mycetoma due to the actinomycetes responds to therapy much more readily than that due to the true fungi.[3] Mycetoma due to *A. israelii* should be treated with at least 1,000,000 units of penicillin daily, with probenecid 1 g daily added to decrease renal tubular excretion of penicillin. *Nocardia asteroides* mycetoma should be treated with sulfadiazine in a dose sufficient to yield a blood level of 8 to 12 mg (100 ml of serum); dapsone has also been successful.[2] *N. brasiliensis* mycetoma responds best to the sulfonamides and diaminodiphenylsulfone (D.D.S.).

By and large, mycetomas due to the true fungi do not respond to any currently available therapeutic agents, although D.D.S. and the sulfonamides should be tried. Eventually, the treatment of choice for patients with fungal mycetoma is complete surgical excision of the affected tissues. Relapse is inevitable unless all traces of the infection are removed.

VIRAL INFECTIONS

VERRUCAE

Warts are a common nuisance that plague both physician and patient. They are caused by a specific virus (papova virus) that mul-

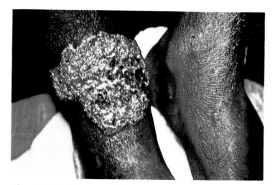

Fig. 2-14. Chromoblastomycosis. Typical verrucous, fungating lesion on foot.

Fig. 2-15. Mycetoma *(N. brasiliensis).* The granulomatous lesion contains multiple draining sinuses.

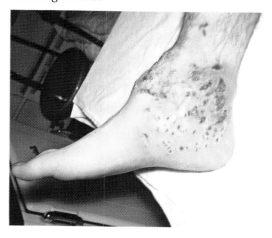

tiplies within the nucleus. Since the average incubation period after experimental inoculation ranges from 1 to 20 months, many generations of epidermal cells must undergo inapparent infection.

The virus almost certainly enters the skin directly. One clearly important factor influencing the localization of inoculation of the virus is trauma: nail-biting, occupational trauma, hyperhidrosis, or pressure points of the feet. Warts may be transmitted by close contact, but the long and variable incubation period and host resistance to infection frequently prevent clear-cut determination of epidemiologic pattern. In some patients, warts are readily autoinoculated. Group pools, gymnasium facilities, and locker rooms increase the likelihood of spread of plantar warts. Anogenital acuminate warts often, but not always, are spread by sexual contact.

Warts are rather uncommon in infancy and early childhood, reach their peak incidence between age 12 and 16, and then decline in frequency. Rook gives the incidence of the various clinical forms of warts as: common warts 70%, plantar warts 24%, plane warts 3.5%, filiform warts 2.0%, and acuminate warts 0.5%.[18] One of the remarkable features of warts is that they may suddenly disappear; the rate of spontaneous regression is probably in the region of 30% over a period of 3 to 6 months. The actual mechanism by which warts regress is still not known. Circulating antibodies to the virus in wart-bearing patients have been demonstrated. Their appearance probably represents a secondary phenomenon in wart rejection.[11] Of greater significance are specific immune responses against wart antigens. Some clinical evidence supporting this is the observation that the incidence of warts is increased during immunosuppressive treatment and in persons with cell-mediated immune defects.[12,16]

Common warts most frequently occur on the dorsal surfaces of the hands and on the fingers. They are also often seen on the legs, but they may occur on other areas of skin including the face and the dorsal surfaces of the feet and toes. A significant percentage (Rook quotes 65%) will disappear spontaneously in 2 years, but many persist indefinitely or require removal for cosmetic reasons or because of obvious autoinoculation.

Plane warts most commonly occur on the face, backs of hands, and the shins. The Koebner phenomenon is often noted. Plane verrucae may disappear within a few weeks or months, or may persist for years and are frequently resistant to therapy. Plane warts usually occur in young children and teenagers.

The types of warts seen on the feet are the common wart on the dorsum and toes, and the plantar wart with its variant the mosaic wart (Figs. 2-16, 2-17, 2-18). Common warts appear as grey or brown elevated firm papules with horny pitted surfaces. Thrombosed superficial capillaries may produce black or brown specks under the surface. Common warts are frequently multiple and may reach a size of 2 centimeters in diameter and one centimeter in height above the skin surface.

Plantar warts occur on the sole, and thereby certain distinctive features are imposed upon them. Besides exposure to the virus, pressure plays an important role, thus accounting for their frequent occurrence most often on weight-bearing areas. It has been noted that women have a higher incidence of plantar warts than do men; high heels could be a factor because the wearing of such heels produces increased pressure on the balls of the feet and big toe. Patients with structural foot deformities have a high incidence of plantar warts. Because they are subjected to frequent heavy pressure from the patient's standing and walking, plantar warts are pushed inward and sideways in the thickened epidermis of the sole and do not grow outward from the skin as is seen with common warts occurring elsewhere. Because of this inward growth and the pressure, plantar warts frequently are tender, occasionally markedly so.

Plantar warts can vary in size from a millimeter to several centimeters. The majority of patients who have plantar warts have a single lesion. Sometimes a cluster of small satellite warts having a vesicular appearance may develop around a larger wart, so-called mother-daughter warts. In other instances, warts may be clustered together to form a mosaic. When the plantar wart is gently pared, the horny margin is sharply outlined; if the paring is continued, capillary tips perpendicular to the surface are visible. Mosaic warts are often mistaken for calluses; however, paring reveals the angular outlines of tightly compressed individual warts that resemble a mosaic.

It is important to distinguish plantar warts from neurovascular corns and callosities. All three lesions occur at pressure points of the sole, but the prognosis varies with the diagnosis. Corns and callosities are cutaneous reactions to pressure; temporary relief from pain can be achieved by paring and application of 40% salicylic acid pads under occlusion. The use of corrective shoes, orthotics, or surgical reconstruction may be necessary to correct the structural foot deformity.

The myriad of therapies for warts attest to the lack of a truly satisfactory form of treatment. The choice will be influenced by the physician's previous experience and preferences, the number of verrucae, the location of the lesions, and the age of the patient. In prepubertal children, plantar warts may disappear in 6 months, but in older children and adults they often persist for years. Less aggressive techniques should always be used first, especially with children.

For some unknown reason, warts can be cured or "charmed" away by psychotherapy, suggestion, or hypnosis. There would appear to be no scientific basis for this effect, and it is impossible to assess the value of the influence of suggestion. Success probably depends on the tendency of warts to regress spontaneously. Nevertheless, if suggestion is applicable to the patient, especially children, it should be considered.

Curettage and light electrodesiccation is the most commonly used therapy for common warts and is generally satisfactory. The desiccation should be gentle to minimize risk of scarring.

Plantar Warts

Experimental evidence suggests that induction of inflammation with topical dermatologic treatment is the underlying mechanism by which lymphocytes become activated, causing involution of warts.[15] Topical treatment may therefore be considered as enhancing immunologic recognition on the part of the patient.

A large number of topical treatment modalities have been advocated for the plantar wart. Modifications of old measures and alternate methods are reported constantly in the literature: topical applications such as Fowler's solution, 0.5% idoxuridine, formaldehyde soaks, formalin with 50% salicylic acid plaster, 20% podophyllin and 20% linseed oil, vitamin A acid, escharotics such as Salisacom, intralesional bleomycin; treatment by blunt dissection and total

enucleation; and topical immunotherapy.[2,4,7,9,13,14,17,19-22] An assessment of methods of treating plantar warts by use of comparative treatment trials based on a standard design was reported recently by Bunney et al.[3] In this excellent study, these investigators reported that approximately 80% of simple plantar warts and 50% of mosaic plantar warts were cured within 12 weeks by applying a paint containing salicylic and lactic acids (SAL). This left a hard core of patients with resistant warts in which absent immunologic competence might be playing a role. On the other hand, there is increasing evidence that warts that resolve spontaneously or perhaps after some form of topical therapy may do so because of the development of circulating antibodies and, in some instances, because of cell-mediated immunity.[5]

In our clinics and offices, we carry out either a chemosurgical-occlusive or a surgical technique.

Examination of the patient's gait is made on the first visit. Patients with abnormalities should have podiatric or orthopedic evaluation, because abnormal pressure may be responsible for treatment failures.

Chemosurgical-occlusive technique. The surface of the lesion or lesions is shaved off with a scalpel to determine if the lesion is a wart, corn, callus, or scar. Following this, the therapeutic agent is applied. We prefer 40% salicylic acid plaster with adhesive tape (preferably 3M micropore surgical tape, No. 1530) or Duofilm* (16.7% salicylic acid, 16.7% lactic acid in flexible collodion). The softened tissue is then pared at regular intervals. This mode of therapy is usually painless; it does not restrict the patient's activity; and there is virtually no risk of scarring. Its only disadvantage is that several weeks to several months of therapy may be required. (Some of our colleagues use the same technique with alternative agents such as mono-, bi-, or trichloracetic acid, salicylic acid in petrolatum, phenol, and formalin.) Painful lesions should be padded with felt or moleskin. If the patient prefers home self-treatment, the following is recommended:

*Stiefel Laboratories, Inc., Oak Hill, NY 12460.

Soak the lesions in warm water for 20 minutes, then dry thoroughly. Apply the topical agent (formalin, salicylic acid plaster, or salicylic acid and lactic acid in flexible collodion) and cover with adhesive or moleskin, or both. The goal of therapy is the induction of chronic aseptic necrosis; the lesions turn black, or merely disappear.

Surgical Technique. Plantar warts that do not respond to the conservative approach or that have been present for one or more years (a stable wart population) can be treated with curettage. In this method, the lesion site is cleansed with 70% alcohol, and 1% Xylocaine (lidocaine) is injected around and in the wart. The wart is scooped out with a curet, and the overhanging skin edges are excised with scissors. Bleeding can be controlled with the application of Monsel's solution (ferric subsulfate) or with pressure exerted with a cotton-tipped applicator. Desiccation should not be used, because this procedure frequently delays healing and can enhance the pain response. A drop of an antibiotic ointment can then be placed in the cavity, which is covered with a dry dressing.

For mosaic warts, we prefer a simple regimen of painting the areas with Castellani's solution in the morning and "sanding" with sandpaper nightly. For mosaic warts associated with hyperhidrosis, the application of 20% aluminum chloride* or 10% glutaraldehyde to the soles twice weekly is helpful. (See Chapter 17.)

The surgical excision of warts is not recommended. The procedure is painful, and there may be a significant period of postoperative disability and occasionally a painful scar.

Treatment of Recalcitrant Warts by Immunologic Enhancement. Multiple plantar warts resistant to other modalities have been successfully treated by inducing an allergic contact dermatitis within the wart. Substances to which the patient is sensitive such as Rhus antigen or formalin can be used. Patients with no known contact allergies are deliberately sensitized to dinitrochloroben-

* Drysol. Person & Covey Inc., Glendale, CA 91201.

zene (DNCB).[8] Sensitization to DNCB should not be initiated without an explanation to the patient of the potential risks and benefits. The sensitizer is carefully applied to the wart after the overlying callus is removed with a scalpel and the surrounding skin is shielded with nail polish. The treated site is covered with elastoplast for 5 days. Local reaction ranges from pruritus and erythema to blister formation. Two to 12 applications at 2- to 4-week intervals are necessary for complete resolution of the warts.

Therapy for periungual warts can at times be very difficult. Curettage and electrodesiccation can be used, but there is a risk of nail deformity secondary to matrix damage resulting from the procedure. Cantharidin under occlusion, liquid nitrogen freezing, and 40% salicylic acid under occlusion can also be used. Liquid nitrogen is applied with a cotton-tipped applicator for 10 to 30 seconds with light or moderate pressure. This produces a blister in 1 to 3 days, and in about 7 days the wart, along with a piece of epidermis around it, may be lifted out. At times, the freezing will have to be repeated.

There is no rationale for the use of repeated smallpox vaccinations or any of the present-day agents administered systemically for the treatment of plantar warts. Wart vaccines have been found to be of no specific value. X-ray therapy carries a potential hazard and should not be used. Ultrasound has also been advocated.[10] However, experience is limited, and the effectiveness of this therapy relative to other forms of treatment cannot be judged.

MOLLUSCUM CONTAGIOSUM

Molluscum lesions are often confused with warts. Molluscum contagiosum is caused by a DNA pox virus. The disease is transmitted by direct contact through fomites and by autoinoculation. The incubation period ranges from 14 to 50 days.

The disease is characterized by firm, pearly white or pink, semitranslucent, smooth dome-shaped papules with a central dell. The average size of a lesion is 3 to 5 mm in diameter. They appear as solitary lesions but more often as scattered lesions or in clusters with a random distribution on the face,

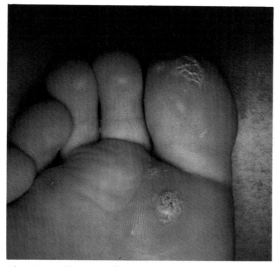

Fig. 2-16. Typical plantar verrucae.

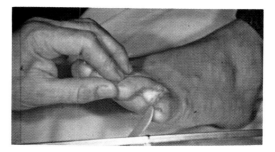

Fig. 2-17. Interdigital verruca. Warts in the web region are frequently misdiagnosed as tinea or maceration.

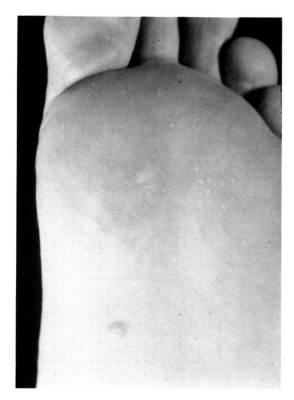

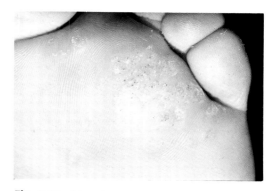

Fig. 2-18. Mosaic verrucae.

Fig. 2-19. Molluscum contagiosum on sole. The feet are rarely involved; therefore, a solitary lesion can lead to confusion in diagnosis. (Courtesy Dr. D. Baxter)

trunk, lower abdomen, pubis, and upper thighs. The feet are involved rarely, and a solitary lesion on the foot can lead to confusion in diagnosis (Fig. 2-19).[1] Molluscum infections are asymptomatic; occasionally, pruritus is a symptom. Untreated lesions persist from months to 3 or 4 years.

Diagnosis is readily made from the characteristic features of the lesion and is confirmed if a KOH wet mount of the crushed contents of a lesion show the typical molluscum bodies on microscopic examination.

Extirpation is a cure: curettage with or without ethyl chloride anesthesia, or dry ice; or the application of 0.9% cantharidin (Cantharone) alone or covered with plastic tape such as Blenderm (3M Co.) for 6 to 8 hours.

HERPES SIMPLEX

There are two distinct forms of herpes simplex infections: (1) primary herpes simplex infection, and (2) the common recurrent type. Herpes simplex is caused by a DNA virus. There are two distinct types of herpes virus: Type I, which is usually responsible for nongenital herpetic infections; and Type II, which is usually involved in genital infections. Type I is the agent involved in herpes simplex on the lower extremities.

Primary herpes simplex infection occurs in previously uninfected individuals without circulating antibodies. In a small minority of the population, the primary infection manifests itself in one of several forms, usually gingivostomatitis, vulvovaginitis, or keratoconjunctivitis. The infection is painful and disabling. After infection, specific antibodies appear and persist throughout the life of the individual, while a persistent carrier state of the virus in the skin is also believed to develop.

Recurrent episodes of herpes simplex occur in about 1% of the population who possess normal serum antibody levels. Such recurrent lesions usually occur on the face, especially around the mouth, but may develop anywhere on the cutaneous surface, including the feet.

In those persons who experience recurrent herpes simplex infections, one or more of several factors may trigger reactivation of the latent virus. These factors include fever, sunlight, trauma, foods, drugs, menstruation, and emotional stress. The association of herpes simplex with subsequent erythema multiforme has also been observed, and herpes simplex virus can be a cause of erythema multiforme. Many episodes occur without obvious cause.

The clinical appearance of the lesions of herpes simplex on the feet is the same as for other glabrous skin areas; that is, the sudden onset of small grouped clear vesicles on an erythematous base which subsequently dry and form crusts. Itching and burning accompany the appearance of the lesions. The Tzanck test is a rapid diagnostic test for herpes simplex—it is invaluable in confirming the diagnosis of an herpetic lesion in an unusual site such as the foot or leg. Healing occurs in 7 to 10 days with no resultant scarring. Lesions may occur on the dorsal aspect or sole of the foot. After the lesions appear, they are usually asymptomatic on most areas of the skin, but if on the distal portions of the extremities they may be associated with fever, pain, and lymphangitis.

Two particular forms of primary herpes simplex may occur on the foot: inoculation herpes simplex and eczema herpeticum. Direct inoculation of the virus into an abrasion or into normal skin may give rise, after an incubation period of 5 to 7 days, to deep-seated vesicles which are often extremely painful. Regional nodes are often enlarged, and the lesion is frequently mistaken for a pyogenic infection. Often, it is only after the lesions do not respond to antibacterial therapy that the diagnosis of a primary herpes simplex inoculation infection (herpetic whitlow) is considered. Herpetic whitlows usually occur on the fingers, especially of dentists, physicians, nurses, and dental assistants, but rarely on the toes. Eczema herpeticum, in which massive crops of vesicles and pustules occur accompanied by severe constitutional symptoms, results from herpes simplex infection in patients with preexisting skin disease. The virus enters the skin during the viremic phase, but it is felt that autoinoculation is not an important factor. Most cases occur in patients with atopic dermatitis; rarely it may be associated with Darier's disease, pemphigus foliaceus, ichthyosiform erythroderma, or other inflammatory dermatoses. Diseases that interfere with most responses, such as leukemia, also predispose to widespread and slowly healing herpes simplex infections.

Most lesions of herpes simplex involute without treatment in 8 to 10 days. For the relief of symptoms, simple measures such as the application of ice or an ice pack every 2 to 3 hours for 15 minutes at the onset of the eruption should suffice. Drying lotions are preferred during the early vesicular and oozing stage. After drying the blisters, a lubricating ointment can be used to soften the crusts, or an antibiotic ointment can be applied to reduce the possibility of secondary bacterial infection.

There are no preventive measures and no cure for recurrent herpes. A wide variety of treatments have been tried in the past decade—topical ether, topical 4% thymol in chloroform, topical interferon, photodynamic inactivation with antiviral dyes, 0.5% deoxyuridine cream (IDU), levamisole, oral L-lysine, Sabin's oral polio vaccine, and repeated smallpox vaccinations—but none is convincing.

HERPES ZOSTER

Zoster is caused by the same virus that gives rise to varicella. Varicella usually occurs in childhood and is regarded as the primary infection, while zoster occurs predominantly in adults and is felt to be the reactivation of a latent viral infection. Approximately two-thirds of patients with zoster are older than 45 years of age. Patients with lymphomas, particularly Hodgkin's disease, have an increased incidence of zoster, and the occurrence of gangrenous or disseminated zoster should raise suspicion of an underlying lymphoma.

The initial manifestation of zoster is often pain, which may be severe, localized to the area of one or more dorsal roots. After a few days, erythematous papules appear along one or two dermadromes, rapidly becoming vesicular and then pustular. The involvement is usually unilateral except in the rare cases of disseminated zoster. The regional lymph nodes are enlarged and tender. Recovery takes 2 to 4 weeks, but persistent postherpetic pain may be a troublesome or even disabling problem for months, especially among elderly patients. While zoster involves the thoracic, cervical, and trigeminal nerves in the great majority of cases, in unusual instances the lesions will involve one leg and extend down onto the dorsum or sole of the foot (Fig. 2-20). Paresis of the involved muscle groups is not uncommon.

Many initially enthusiastic reports about various therapeutic agents have appeared over the years only to fade soon into oblivion. At the present time, the major therapy is symptomatic for relief of pain. The skin lesions are treated much the same as an acute dermatitis: cool, astringent wet compresses applied for 20 minutes 3 or 4 times a day during the early stages of the eruption. After the lesions have dried, topical steroid creams or antibiotic ointments, when secondary bacterial infection is present, can be helpful.

Some observers feel that systemic steroids administered early in the illness may help to promote healing and reduce the incidence of postherpetic neuralgia; however, the fear of steroids causing dissemination of the viral disease has also been of concern. In a recent double-blind study done by Eaglstein and associates, patients with early severely painful zoster received either lactose placebos or triamcinolone.[6] The systemic steroids did not cause any worsening of the cutaneous eruption, did not result in quicker healing of the lesions, and did not lessen the pain during the first two weeks. However, such therapy did shorten the duration of postherpetic neuralgia in patients older than the age of 60. Post-zoster neuralgia often improved with intradermal injection of triamcinolone into painful areas.

HAND, FOOT AND MOUTH DISEASE

This disease is usually caused by Coxsackie A16 virus, but occasional outbreaks have been reported due to A5 and to other types. A painful stomatitis with irregularly distributed erosions is usually the most prominent feature of the disease. Skin lesions consist of thin-walled, light gray vesicles with narrow red areolae and may be present in as few as 25% of cases. When they do occur, they are usually located on the dorsal surfaces of the fingers and toes, especially around the nails. Lesions also occur on the palms and soles, in which cases they may be quite tender. Lesions tend to be limited in number and fade in 2 or 3 days, and the course of the entire disease is mild and lasts 4 to 7 days. There is no specific therapy (Figs. 2-21, 2-22).

FOOT AND MOUTH DISEASE

Foot and mouth disease due to one of the nonhuman picornaviruses is an epidemic disease of farm animals which rarely infects

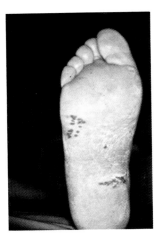

Fig. 2-20. Typical lesions of herpes zoster.

man. The disease is usually mild and consists of fever, headache, malaise, burning, and vesicles of the oral mucous membranes, tongue, and lips. Vesicles also appear on the palms, soles, and interdigital skin. The vesicles become ulcers, and there may be some pain and edema. There is no specific therapy.

SPIROCHETAL INFECTIONS*

Syphilis is caused by infection with the spirochete, *Treponema pallidum*, and is divided into 3 clinical stages—primary, secondary, and late. A complete classification is listed as follows:

Classification

Acquired
  Primary
  Secondary
  Early latent } Early infectious
  Late latent
  Late manifest
    Central nervous system
      Asymptomatic
      Symptomatic } Late noninfectious
    Cardiovascular
    Gumma
Congenital
  No primary
  Vesicular and bullous lesions } Early infectious
    may occur
  May have secondary-like lesions
  Stigmata } Late infectious
  Late manifestations

    The natural history of syphilis is outlined in the diagram on page 55.

*Charles L. Heaton, M.D., Department of Dermatology, University of Cincinnati contributed the classification of syphilis, the diagram of the natural history of syphilis, and the serology summary.

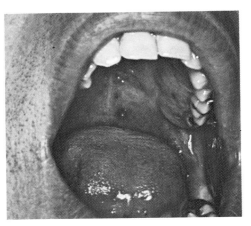

Fig. 2-21. Hand, foot and mouth disease: mouth lesions. Coxsackie A-16 virus was isolated.

Fig. 2-22. Hand, foot and mouth disease: foot lesions. Similar lesions were present on the hands. (Same patient as in Fig. 2-21.)

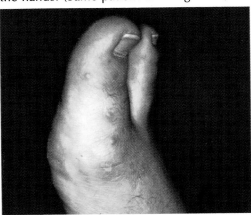

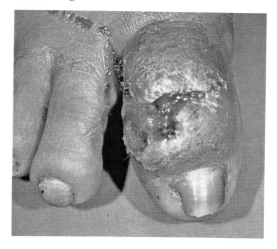

Fig. 2-23. Chancre on toe.

PRIMARY SYPHILIS

The chancre of primary syphilis occurs at the site of inoculation and penetration of the skin by the spirochete. Thus, the chancre is usually located on the genitalia; occasionally it may appear on the lips, where it may be mistaken for a malignant lesion. However, rarely the chancre may appear elsewhere, as on the toe in Figure 2-23. The chancre is an ulcerated or eroded firm papule which is painless. If the lesion is located where regional lymph nodes can be palpated, discrete, rubbery nontender enlarged nodes, the satellite bubo, may be found. The primary chancre will heal in 4 to 6 weeks without therapy, but treatment must be undertaken to prevent the disease from continuing its course.

Serologic tests do not become reactive until 1 to 3 weeks after the appearance of the

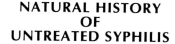

NATURAL HISTORY
OF
UNTREATED SYPHILIS

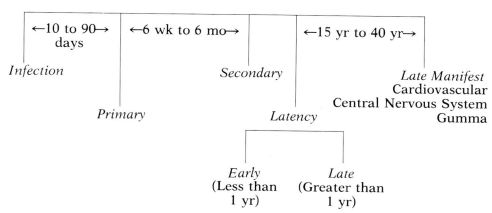

chancre. Thus, the tests may be nonreactive in the presence of a syphilitic lesion. Dark-field examination of a chancre will be positive if several attempts are made and if the patient has neither received systemic antibiotics nor applied topical antibiotic ointment to the chancre.

The therapy of choice is a long-acting intramuscular penicillin (Bicillin) given in a single individual dose of 2.4 million units— 1.2 million units into each buttock. In patients who are allergic to penicillin, tetracycline or erythromycin may be given in an oral dose schedule of 2 grams daily for 15 days, or 3 grams daily for 10 days.

SECONDARY SYPHILIS

Approximately 2 months after infection (range: 6 weeks to 6 months), or about 6 weeks after the appearance of the chancre, the lesions of secondary syphilis develop. The eruption is bilaterally symmetrical, rather widespread in distribution, and either maculopapular, papular, papulosquamous or, infrequently, pustular. In teen-agers or adults, the eruption is never vesicular or bullous. The palms and soles (Fig. 2-24) are commonly involved. Condyloma lata may occur in the anogenital region, around the mouth, or occasionally in the toe webs (Fig. 2-25). Lymphadenopathy, hepatosplenomegaly, and alopecia may be present. When present, they are often accompanied by constitutional symptoms such as fever, malaise, and sore throat. All moist lesions of secondary syphilis are highly contagious and darkfield positive. Serologic tests are virtually always reactive at this stage, often in high titer.

If untreated, the lesions of secondary syphilis will resolve without therapy. Treatment is indicated to prevent progression of the disease and is identical to that for primary syphilis.

LATENT SYPHILIS

In latent syphilis, no lesions either cutaneous or systemic, are present. The diagnosis depends upon the finding of a positive serologic test for syphilis, which is confirmed by one of the specific treponemal tests (TPI or FTA-ABS).

The treatment of latent syphilis of less than one year's duration is as described for the primary and secondary stages. The treatment of choice for latent syphilis of more than one year's duration is long-acting intramuscular penicillin G (Bicillin) given in a dose of 2.4 million units weekly for 3 weeks for a total dose of 7.2 million units. Penicillin-allergic patients may be treated with either tetracycline or erythromycin given in an oral dose schedule of 2 grams daily for 15 days.

LATE MANIFEST SYPHILIS

In contrast to the lesions of primary and secondary syphilis, the manifestations of late syphilis are not infectious but destructive. Imperfect immunity exists in the host, who may have cardiovascular or central nervous system involvement or gummatous lesions. Only in gummatous and central nervous system lesions, however, do lesions occur on the lower extremity. In neurosyphilis, there may be loss of proprioception, hypesthesia, or anesthesia of the distal extremities which, in turn, may lead to traumatic joint destruction (Charcot joints) and trophic ulcers of the feet. Gummata, which represent hypersensitivity reactions to the treponemes, may involve the viscera, skin, or bone. Biopsies of chronic granulomatous ulcers of the lower extremity may lead to the diagnosis of a previously unsuspected gumma (Figs. 2-26, 2-27). Gummas show dramatic improvement and healing after the initiation of specific therapy.

In late manifest syphilis the minimum indicated therapy is benzathine penicillin G, 2.4 million units intramuscularly weekly for 3 weeks, a total dose of 7.2 million units. Penicillin-allergic patients may be treated with either tetracycline or erythromycin given in an oral dose schedule of 2 grams daily for 15 days.

SYPHILIS SEROLOGY

It must be stressed that the titer of reactivity of serologic tests for syphilis determines neither the stage of syphilis nor the severity of the patient's infection. Syphilis serology can be summarized as follows:

Serology

Tests

Nontreponemal tests—Syn.: Cardiolipin tests

Flocculation—VDRL

Agglutination—RPRC (Rapid Plasma Reagin Card. Test)

Complement-Fixation—Wasserman, Kolmer

Treponemal tests

Whole body virulent viable—TPI

Whole body nonviable—FTA-ABS

Interpretation: Consider sensitivity, specificity, significance of titer changes, and sero-fast patients

Biologic False-Positive Tests

Acute

Chronic

The nontreponemal (cardiolipin) tests serve as screening tests, and are diagnostic of a treponemal infection only when there is a rapidly rising titer over a 7- to 10-day period. Once the diagnosis of syphilis has been established, these tests are most helpful in establishing the adequacy of therapy. Falling titers obtained sequentially at 2- or 3-month intervals indicate adequate therapy.

The specific treponemal tests (TPI and FTA-ABS) are used only to confirm the presence or absence of treponemal antibodies. They thereby confirm a diagnosis of syphilis and rule out a biological false-positive reagin test. They cannot be used to determine the activity of syphilis or the adequacy of the patient's therapy.

The reader, who may desire further discussion of serologic tests for syphilis, including sensitivity, specificity, and sero-fast states as well as acute and chronic biologic false-positive reactions, is referred to standard texts on syphilis.

MYCOBACTERIAL INFECTIONS

The atypical or anonymous acid-fast mycobacteria is a group of mycobacteria that differ from *Mycobacterium tuberculosis. Mycobacterium bovis* and *M. leprae* are capable of causing a variety of skin lesions in humans. Some of the characteristics that differentiate the atypical mycobacteria from *Mycobacte-*

rium tuberculosis are: *in vitro* resistance to standard anti-tuberculous chemotherapeutic agents, strong catalase activity, ability to grow at room temperature, and inability to produce progressive disease in guinea pigs after subcutaneous inoculation.[10] Mice are more susceptible than guinea pigs to some of the atypical mycobacteria.

Typical mycobacteria are animal pathogens and do not multiply outside their animal hosts. The atypical acid-fast mycobacteria have been found in nature in soil, water, and excreta. Runyon classified them into four groups.[10] Group I contains the organisms that produce pigment only after exposure to light (photochromogens): *M. kansasii, M. marinum* (balnei), *M. ulcerans.* Group II contains the organisms that produce pigment regardless of the presence or absence of light (scotochromogens): *M. scrofulaceum.* The pigment produced by Groups I and II is yellow or yellow-orange. Group III is characterized by the absence of pigment formation (nonphotochromogens): *M. intracellularis* (Battey bacillus). Group IV is characterized by the rapid growth of the organism (rapid growers, 3 to 5 days versus 2 to 3 weeks): *M. fortuitum, M. abscessus.*

M. avium, M. kansasii, M. intracellularis (Battey bacillus), and *M. fortuitum* primarily produce pulmonary disease in humans. Except with less common disseminated disease, draining sinuses, adenitis, and osteomyelitis, these rarely involve the skin of the lower extremity. *M. marinum* and *M. ulcerans* are well-known pathogens which infect the skin. The clinical, pathologic, and epidemiologic features of skin disease caused by *M. marinum* and *M. ulcerans* are often sufficiently distinctive to suggest an etiologic diagnosis.[6]

MYCOBACTERIUM MARINUM

In the United States, the most frequently recognized lesion is the swimming-pool granuloma caused by *M. marinum* (balnei). The lesions develop on traumatized skin and thus occur most frequently on the elbows, knees, and dorsal portions of the feet and hands (Fig. 2-28). After a 3- to 4-week incubation period, a small reddish papule(s) appears and slowly increases in size to become a hard purplish nodule(s). This nodule sometimes

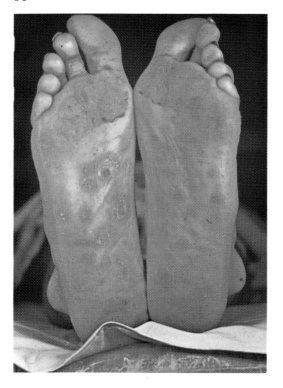

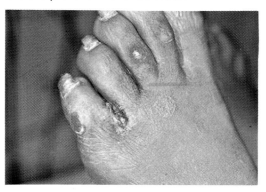

Fig. 2-24. Secondary syphilis. Note the characteristic "ham" color of the papular lesions.

Fig. 2-25. Secondary syphilis. Condyloma lata are present in the toe webs.

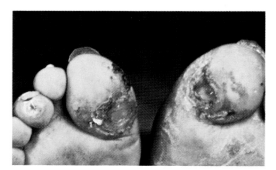

Fig. 2-26. Late syphilis: multiple gummas. Note the characteristically indolent, deeply infiltrated, punched-out ulcer that heals with an atrophic, noncontractile scar.

Fig. 2-27. Late syphilis: mal perforans.

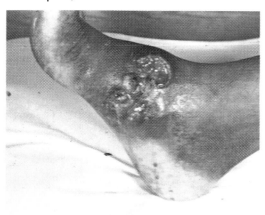

Fig. 2-28. Mycobacterial infection on the knee. *M. balnei* was cultured.

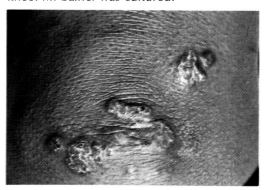

ulcerates and becomes covered with a crust or grayish exudate or becomes heavily crusted and verrucous in appearance. The lesions are usually asymptomatic and are not associated with lymphangitis or regional lymphadenopathy. Healing with scarring occurs after several months in most cases, although there are reports of lesions persisting for 4 to 45 years.[7,11]

In most cases, *M. marinum* has been isolated from crevices and grooves in the cement walls of the pools in which patients had been swimming. Local epidemics have occurred in Sweden, the United States, Canada, and Britain. Because of the association of this disease with fresh-water swimming, the designation "swimming-pool granuloma" has been used, although there are cases in which pools have not been the source of the organism.[4,12] The infection has also been related to swimming in salt water and exposure to tropical fish.[1,8,13]

Skin tests of a purified protein derivative (P.P.D.) of the organism usually show positive results; however, one of the most significant characteristics of the mycobacteria as a group is an antigenic relationship. Cross-reactivity with P.P.D. of other mycobacteria (especially tuberculosis) is quite common and may lead to confusion or a misdiagnosis.[5,7] Culture characteristics will distinguish between *M. marinum* and other mycobacterial infections of the skin.

As mentioned previously, most lesions heal without therapy. Antituberculosis therapy has been used, and in some cases "better" healing has been reported, even though the organism is resistant, as shown by sensitivity testing.[3] Except in persistent or severe lesions, antituberculosis therapy is not indicated. Minocycline hydrochloride has been effective in some cases of *M. marinum* infections. Excision of existing lesions may cause an exacerbation.[9] After establishing a diagnosis, masterful inactivity most often seems the wisest course of treatment.

MYCOBATERIUM ULCERANS

In the tropics, *Mycobacterium ulcerans* infections are highly prevalent in certain localities, especially near swamps and watercourses. Another epidemiologic charac-

teristic of the disease is its tendency to occur in outbreaks.[2] Most cases occur in children, with half the patients being between 5 and 14 years. Most lesions occur on the extremities, about one-half on the lower extremity, usually beginning on the anterior tibial area. Usually, the lesions are single and follow minor trauma. In the 3-week period following inoculation, induration develops and extends in diameter and depth. Hyperpigmentation of the overlying skin is usual. A rapidly enlarging area of ulceration ensues, followed by secondary infection, resulting in a granulation area covered with a foul exudate. The ulcer margins are irregular and undermining occurs, extending 10 to 15 cm with buried pockets of whitish necrotic material. Distinction between these ulcers and tropical ulcers is seldom difficult, since tropical ulcers are painful, do not have undermined edges, and are rarely seen above the knee.[2] Occasionally, small satellite lesions form with a narrow bridge of undermined skin separating the satellite ulcers from the mother lesion. Regional lymph nodes are rarely enlarged, and the patient's general health remains relatively unaffected in spite of the size of the lesion. The ulcer may last for years, healing eventually with a fibrotic scar which may cause deformity and lymphedema. Chemotherapy has been disappointing; surgical excision followed by skin grafting has been recommended. Trials undertaken to determine whether BCG vaccination confers protection against *M. ulcerans* infection appear promising.[2]

PARASITIC INFESTATIONS

The term "creeping eruption" refers to a parasitic larval infestation of the skin which is commonly seen in the southeastern United States, Central America, and many tropical areas of the world. The disorder is usually due to the migration through the skin of the larvae of the dog and cat hookworm *Ancylostoma braziliense* and *A. caninum* which produces a characteristic linear inflammatory reaction. The condition is also commonly referred to as "sand worm" or "larva migrans."

Cutaneous larva migrans resulting from exposure to nonhuman strains of *A. Brazil-*

iense has a widespread distribution through-out the sandy coastal areas of the United States from southern New Jersey to the Florida Keys of the Atlantic coast and along the entire coastline of the Gulf of Mexico. It extends inland in Texas as far as a line drawn north and south through Dallas and San Antonio. The largest number of cases, however, is found in the vicinity of Jacksonville, Florida. Many other tropical and subtropical coastal regions have reported cases, notably southern Brazil, Uruguay, and Argentina. Spain, southern France, South Africa, India, the Philippines, and Australia similarly have reported cases.

Exposure results from contact of the human skin with damp sandy soil where the larvae have developed after fecal contamination. Common sites of exposure are found both on bathing beaches and under houses, where workers may lie while repairing plumbing fixtures. It may also be picked up by children running barefoot in contaminated areas and may occur in children's unprotected sandboxes.

The initial sites of the lesions are usually on the uncovered parts of the body, hands, face, and feet (Fig. 2-29). Occasionally, lesions may be situated on the buttocks or genitals; rarely are the mucous membranes of the nose, mouth, and conjunctiva involved.

At each point where the filariform larva of *A. braziliense* invades the skin, it produces a red itching papule. In 2 or 3 days, the larvae produce a serpiginous tunnel at the dermal-epidermal junction. Manifestations arise from the progression of the larvae and appear as a serpentine linear inflammatory reaction. The larvae precede the inflammation by 1 to 2 cm and may migrate as much as several millimeters to several inches daily. The lesions are moderately to intensely pruritic, and secondary impetiginization may occur from scratching. Activity of the larvae may continue several weeks or months, resulting in severe skin involvement. The duration of the untreated disease seems to be related to the environmental temperature. Higher temperature apparently causes increased larval activity with a resultant shorter duration of the disease.

Treatment should begin with a discussion of the obvious: prevention. The wearing of protective clothing when in endemic areas is perhaps the most effective preventive measure. The predisposition of children to run barefoot during the spring and summer explains the high incidence of foot and leg involvement. Other protective measures would include proper covering of children's sandboxes, when not in use, so as to discourage visits by neighborhood animals.

Perhaps the most time-honored method of treatment is the application of freezing ethyl chloride spray or the application of dry ice to the "head" of the serpentine lesions. Clinically this is very effective; however, there is little evidence to suggest that this actually kills the larvae. It may be that the inflammatory reaction that follows the freezing aids in the destruction of the organisms.

Hetrazan orally, 2.0 mg 3 times daily, given after meals for 10 to 20 days has been recommended as a therapeutic measure. More recently, thiabendazole has been proven exceptionally effective in the treatment of creeping eruption. It is particularly useful where a patient has infestation which is difficult to manage topically. Side effects are not uncommon with this medication and nausea, vomiting, and dizziness frequently occur. In addition, anorexia and malodorous urine have been reported. The side effects, however, tend to be minimized on a thiabendazole dosage of 25 mg/kg of body weight for 3 or 4 days.

Pace subsequently reported success in injecting the advancing ends of the burrows with a thiabendazole suspension (100 mg/cc) using a jet injector.[5] No side effects were noted in his patients, and itching was relieved within a few hours after injection. The maximum number of burrows treated in any one patient was about 20. The small amount of drug given to each person (less than 10 mg per injection) probably accounts for the absence of side effects.

Eyster in 1967 reported success in the treatment of creeping eruption by occlusion of a thiabendazole suspension (Mintezol) and dexamethasone with a polyethylene film. The occlusive dressing was left in place 3 days.[3] Systemic side effects were absent; however, a few patients developed a symptomless perifollicular eruption which subsided soon after the occlusion was discontinued.

Davis and Israel reported a simple and effective way of using topical thiabendazole.[2] They applied Mintezol sparingly with the fingertips to all lesions 4 times daily. In all patients, pruritus was markedly decreased by the third day of treatment; on the seventh day all lesions were essentially healed. The local and systemic side effects noted in earlier methods of use were not seen, although two patients felt stinging when the medication was applied to denuded areas. It was not severe enough to stop treatment, however.

Thus, in the common form of creeping eruption, consisting of only a few burrows, simple freezing of the advancing end is a relatively effective method of treatment. In more severe infestations, the method of Davis and Israel for topical thiabendazole application appears to be a superior means of management.[2] Only in severe refractory cases should oral thiabendazole be used, since side effects occur rather commonly.

SCABIES

Scabies is an infestation with *Sarcoptes scabiei,* a barely visible mite. It has a universal distribution. In the United States, in urban and rural areas, the disease has increased noticeably in the past several years, and an expanding epidemic continues in most parts of the world.[4] Marked seasonal variations were noted, with a maximum number in winter and a minimum in summer.[1] No single factor has been identified that explains the cyclic occurrence of scabies in relation to time, the sex and age pattern, or the seasonal variation.

The pregnant female mite burrows into the stratum corneum forming tunnels and depositing eggs. The skin manifestations of scabies result from an allergy to the mite and its products. Scabies is characterized by nocturnal pruritus and a distinct distribution involving the sides of fingers, flexor aspect of the wrists, anterior aspect of axillae, genitals in men, and nipples in women. The finding of the burrow, a sinour gray ridge, is diagnostic.

The involvement of the lower extremities is limited. Few or many conical, often excoriated, papules may be found on the thighs.

The ankles are affected in extensive cases, but burrows are seldom found. The soles, not affected in adults, are often involved in infants; reddish macules, papules, and even bullae are commonly present. (See Chapter 8.)

Scabies is frequently seen in many guises that may be difficult to diagnose: scabies in the clean, scabies incognito, nodular scabies, animal-transmitted scabies, scabies in infants, scabies with syphilis, and Norwegian scabies.[4]

Diagnosis of scabies is made based on the history, morphology (the pathognomonic burrow), and identification of the mite in microscopic study of skin scrapings and in skin biopsies. Using mineral oil to scrape the burrows provides a technique for easier retrieval of the mite.

Treatment

Gamma benzene hexachloride, lindane (Kwell), in cream or lotion, is effective. It should be applied from the neck down and left on for 24 hours. Crotamiton (Eurax) in cream or lotion, also antipruritic, is preferred by some in the treatment of infants. The old-time remedy of precipitated sulfur (5% to 10%) with or without peruvian balsam (3%) in petrolatum is still a good alternative treatment. It is applied nightly for 3 nights. The linen should be changed, the clothing washed, and all affected members of the family treated simultaneously to prevent reinfection.

ARTHROPODS

The skin condition caused by arthropods often shows a predilection for the lower extremities. These disorders are reviewed in the section on skin conditions in the tropics.

LEISHMANIASIS

The increase in travel to endemic areas of South and Central America has led to an increase in the number of cases of cutaneous leishmaniasis diagnosed in the United States.[6,7] In our clinics, we have seen several cases of cutaneous leishmaniasis contracted in the Middle East (Israel, Iran, Pakistan).

Awareness of the patient's travels provided a clue in establishing the diagnosis (Fig. 2-30). For discussion and treatment of American leishmaniasis, the reader is referred to the section on skin conditions in the tropics.

SKIN CONDITIONS OF THE LOWER EXTREMITIES COMMON IN THE TROPICS*

In the tropics and subtropics, the lower extremities are often affected by skin diseases that are not encountered in temperate climates. Because of climatic and environmental conditions, some cosmopolitan skin diseases affecting the legs and feet present a distinctive clinical appearance.

For didactic purposes, some of the skin diseases of the lower extremities encountered in the tropics are divided as follows:

1. Skin conditions caused by arthropods.
2. Alterations in shape of the lower extremities.
3. The vegetating verrucous syndrome of the lower extremities.
4. Ulcerations common in the tropics.

SKIN CONDITIONS CAUSED BY ARTHROPODS

Arthropod bites and stings are exceedingly common in the tropics. They are more frequently seen in individuals from rural areas, especially those wearing sandals or going barefoot. The cutaneous response may result from: (1) an allergic reaction to antigens present in the saliva of the arthropod; (2) a toxic reaction caused by the venom injected; or (3) a mixed reaction to both previous mechanisms.

Insect bites may sensitize the individual, eliciting an immediate urticarial wheal type of reaction followed by an itchy papule—a delayed reaction of the cell-mediated type. Subsequent bites lead to a gradual desensitization with disappearance of the papular reaction and, eventually, even of the urticarial one. Thus, constantly exposed natives

*Contributed by Orlando Canizares, M.D., Professor of Clinical Dermatology, New York University College of Medicine.

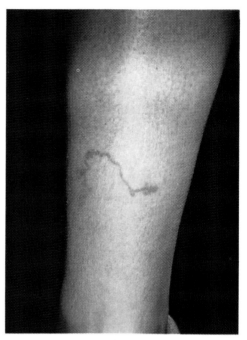

Fig. 2-29. Characteristic lesions of creeping eruption. Acquired by contact with contaminated sand; topical thiabendazole produced complete healing within 10 days.

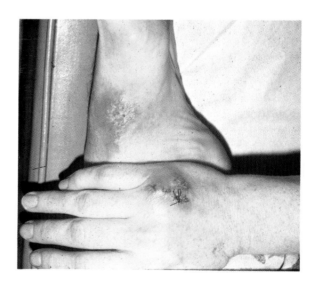

often become immune, while the casual visitor suffers from numerous and irritating bites on his ankles and lower legs. Children, especially those from lower socioeconomic classes, are frequent victims of arthropod bites. Affected adults are frequently farmers and ranchers exposed in fields and wooded areas.

Besides causing the local and systemic reactions, some arthropods are vectors of diseases. A few examples are malaria, dengue, and filariasis, which are transmitted by mosquitoes; leishmaniasis and bartonellosis, transmitted by sandfly bites, plague, by fleas; and so forth.

Clinical Examination. The response to arthropod bites varies depending on the agent, the age and degree of sensitivity of the victim, the number of bites, and the amount of antigenic saliva or poison injected. As a rule, in most insect bites, such as those of mosquitoes, chiggers, and fleas, there is an urticarial reaction with a central hemorrhagic punctum. The bites of scorpions, centipedes, flies, wasps, bees, and yellowjackets cause pronounced, painful swellings, which may persist a few days; mild systemic symptoms may develop. If the stinger remains in the skin, as often happens in tick bites, a persistent nodular granulomatous reaction may occur (tick-bite granuloma). Pruritus is a constant symptom is insect bites. It leads to scratching and excoriations; secondary bacterial infection is a common complication in the tropics. Highly sensitive individuals may develop a serious and even fatal anaphylactic reaction.

Treatment. Mild bites require simple antipruritic topical applications. Severe ones, like those of bees, centipedes, or scorpions,

need more care. If the stinger is still present, it should be scraped off with a blade. It should never be picked with a forceps because, if the sac is present, this will squeeze more poison into the wound. *Topically,* ice packs, cold compresses, corticosteroid lotions or sprays are helpful. If systemic reactions are pronounced, elevation of the limb and application of a tourniquet proximal to the affected area (released every 5 minutes) are indicated. A subcutaneous injection of 0.2 ml of epinephrine (1:1000 solution) repeated, if necessary, every 15 minutes is effective. Severe cases require immediate hospitalization, intravenous therapy, systemic corticosteroids, and oxygen administration.

Papular Urticaria

Papular urticaria, also called prurigo simplex, is an allergic response to insect bites. It may be caused by any biting insect, but fleas, mosquitoes, chiggers, sandflies, and bedbugs are the most common causes. Children are most frequently affected; adults may develop it when, by moving to a new locality, they become exposed to different insects.

Clinical Examination. The lesion begins as a wheal and soon becomes an itchy, firm, red papule, often with a vesicle at its apex (Fig. 2-31). This frequently becomes excoriated by

Fig. 2-31. Papular urticaria.

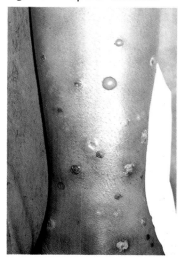

◄ **Fig. 2-30.** Painful red papules on the right hand and left foot that gradually enlarged and ulcerated. Patient had been on an archeological expedition in Pakistan and was subjected to many sandfly bites; a culture for leishmonads was positive. (*Courtesy of Dr. S. Gammer*)

scratching. Secondary bacterial infection is common. The distribution varies with the causative insect. The face, arms, and legs are affected by flying insects, while feet, ankles, and legs are mainly affected by fleas. The course is seasonal and chronic.

Treatment. Wide use of insecticides, treatment of flea-infested dogs or cats, and insect repellents are helpful. Topical corticosteroids and systemic antihistaminics relieve pruritus. Systemic antibiotics are indicated if there is secondary bacterial infection.

The cutaneous and systemic reaction to the bite or penetration into the skin of some arthropods requires special consideration.

Spiders

Spiders abound in tropical and subtropical regions. The two most harmful are:

Lactrodectus mactans, the black-widow spider, with a shiny black body and a distinctive red hourglass marking on its underside.

Loxoscela reclusa, the brown recluse spider, yellow-tan to dark brown in color. Spiders are found under stones and in wood piles, outhouses, and barns. They bite when disturbed or inadvertently trapped in shoes or clothing; children are often bitten on the toes.

Clinical Examination. The bite of black-widow spiders causes a pinprick sensation followed by pain which peaks in a few hours and persists 12 to 48 hours. There are two red puncture marks at the site of the bite but little local reaction. The neurotoxic poison causes muscular pain, spasm, a rigid painful board-like abdomen, and even convulsions. Death occurs in 4% to 5% of untreated cases. The bite of the brown recluse spider is relatively painless. Edema, redness, blister, and ischemia develop followed by a star-shaped, firm, deep-purple area with necrosis; the lesion heals with scarring in 2 to 3 weeks. Systemic symptoms are usually severe.

Treatment. Local treatment of spider bites is ineffective. In black-widow spider bites, administration of antivenom, 1 vial intramuscularly; calcium gluconate, 10% solution

10 ml intravenously; muscle relaxants; and analgesics are indicated. In brown recluse spider bites, immediate administration of intramuscular corticosteroids followed by oral therapy is the treatment of choice. Heparin and analgesics are helpful.

Tungiasis

Tunga penetrans, the chigoe, is a flea commonly found in tropical America, Africa, and parts of India. It lives in sand or dust around the houses and feeds on animals. The pregnant female burrows under the skin of the feet, usually between and at the tip of the toes, and the instep of the soles (Fig. 2-32). The lesion begins with itching and appears as a deep-seated inflammatory nodule with a central opening. Lesions may be grouped in a honeycomb appearance. Infection, necrosis, and ulceration may result. Other complications are abscesses, lymphangitis, lymphadenitis, septicemia, tetanus, and gas gangrene. Chronic lesions are verrucous and should be differentiated from plantar warts and calluses.

Treatment. The flea is killed with turpentine and is removed with a needle and gentle lateral pressure. Antibiotics are indicated if bacterial infection is present.

Scabies

Scabies is much more common in tropical regions, in some areas assuming epidemic proportions. When M. H. Samitz was in East Africa, he noted that scabies and pyoderma complicating scabies were the most common problems seen. For the discussion on scabies, the reader is referred to the section on parasitic infections earlier in this chapter.

ALTERATIONS OF SHAPE OF THE LOWER EXTREMITIES

Several tropical diseases cause changes in the shape of the skin and bone of the lower legs and feet. Some affect mainly the toes, others involve the feet and the lower leg. Mycetoma, usually involving a foot and causing pronounced deformity, is not included here, since it is discussed earlier in this chapter.

with a phenolized solution of leptomonas, which in 72 hours elicits an inflammatory papule. In early cases, the organism may be found in scrapings. Histologic examination shows a granulomatous reaction; organisms may be present.

Treatment. Two medications are effective: N-metil-glucamina (Glucantime) given in 10 to 20 intramuscular daily injections of a 1.5 g ampule; amphotericin B, more toxic, is given intravenously in resistant cases.

Vegetating Pyoderma (lymphostasis verrucosa, elephantiasis nostras)

This is a relatively common condition in the rural tropics (see Chap. 13.) It results from successive attacks of infection, usually due to beta-hemolytic streptococcus, causing lymphangitis, cellulitis, and erysipelas. Feet and legs are more often affected, but other parts of the body may be involved. Stasis dermatitis may be the portal of entry of infection. It develops slowly and progressively. The foot and leg become enlarged and hard; the skin is thickened, papillomatous, and verrucous; and fibromatous growths and ulcers may develop.

Treatment. Rest in bed, elevation of leg, and antiseptic wet dressings are indicated. Topical and systemic antibiotics should be administered. A maintenance dose of antibiotic therapy may help to prevent further attacks. Surgical excision of growths may be required.

ULCERATIONS COMMON IN THE TROPICS

All ulcers of the leg discussed in Chapter 14 may be encountered in the tropics. Their frequency varies with ecologic and climatic conditions and the races affected.

Sickle cell ulcers are common in Blacks, especially in Africa. When anemia is severe, swellings over the bones of hands and feet may develop. Hemolytic and abdominal crises often occur. Ulcerations of the legs in the tropics may be found in leprosy of the feet as plantar perforating ulcers, in yaws, as the portal of entry of Guinea worm infec-

tion, and secondary to other tropical dermatoses. Venous ulcers are less common in Asiatic and African individuals than in Caucasians.

Three ulcerations are peculiar to the tropical regions.

Tropical Phagedenic Ulcer

This is a painful, rapidly growing, sloughing ulcer, usually on the leg. It is found in the hot and humid tropics; malnutrition and debilitating diseases are predisposing factors. *Bacillus fusiformis* and *Treponema vincenti* are found in the early stage. The lower third of the leg and ankle are more frequently affected. It begins as a hemorrhagic vesicle that breaks down and rapidly enlarges, reaching several centimeters in diameter in a few weeks. The ulcer is painful and presents a crateriform appearance with bluish-red elevated borders. The surface shows a gray necrotic membrane which sloughs, showing a granulomatous base bathed in a foul-smelling serous and bloody discharge. In the chronic stage, the lesion is painless; the edge becomes fibrotic and the base appears cleaner. After several years, the ulcer heals with scarring. Carcinomatous degeneration may occur.

Treatment. The acute ulcer requires debridement, antiseptic wet dressings, and systemic penicillin or tetracycline therapy for 2 to 3 weeks. Occlusion with plaster or adhesive tape has been recommended for chronic ulcers. Surgical excision followed by skin grafting may be indicated. Recently, metronidazole (Flagyl) has been found effective.

Ulcer Caused by *Mycobacterium ulcerans*

(See discussion earlier in chapter.)

Cutaneous Diphtheria

Skin infection with *Corynebacterium diphtheriae* is common is some dry, hot, tropical areas. The ulcer often develops on a minor injury or an insect bite on legs and ankles. It is a few centimeters in diameter with rolled, purplish, undermined borders. The base is covered with a dark brown, heavy membrane. *C. diphtheriae* may be found in the lesion.

Treatment. Diphtheria antitoxic, 20,000 to 50,000 I.U., should be administered immediately intramuscularly. Systemic and topical antibiotics are recommended.

REFERENCES

MICROBIOLOGICAL DISEASES

1. **Ammonette, RA, Rosenburg EW:** Infection of the toewebs by gram-negative bacteria. Arch Dermatol 107:71, 1973
2. **Duncan, WC, McBride ME, Knox JM:** Experimental production of infections in humans. J Inv Dermatol 54:319, 1970
3. **Ehrenkrantz NJ, Taplin D, Butt P:** Antibiotic-resistant bacteria on the nose and skin: colonization and cross-infection. In Hobby G (ed): Antimicrobial Agents and Chemotherapy. Ann Arbor, Michigan, American Society for Microbiology, 1967
4. **Hojyo-Tomaka MT, Marples RR, Kligman AM:** Pseudomonas infection in hydrated skin. Arch Dermatol 107:723, 1973
5. Infections. In Analysis of Research Needs and Priorities in Dermatology. Chap V., J Invest Dermatol 73:452, 1979
6. **Marples MJ:** The Ecology of the Human Skin. Springfield, Ill, Charles C Thomas, 1965
7. **Marples RR:** The effect of hydration on the bacterial flora of the skin. In Maibach HI, Hildick-Smith G (eds): Skin Bacteria and Their Role in Infection, p. 33. New York, McGraw-Hill, 1965
8. **Marples RR:** Diphtheroids of normal human skin. Brit J Dermatol 81 [Suppl] 1:47, 1969
9. **Marples RR:** Bacterial infection. In Moschella, Pillsbury, Hurley (eds): Dermatology. Philadelphia, WB Saunders Co, 1975
10. **Marples MJ, Bailey MJ:** A search for the presence of pathogenic bacteria and fungi in the interdigital spaces of the foot. Brit J Dermatol 69:379, 1957
11. **Marples RR, Williamson P:** Effects of systemic demethylchlortetracycline on human cutaneous microflora. Appl Microbiol 18:228, 1969
12. **Montes LF, Wilborn WH:** Location of bacterial skin flora. Brit J Dermatol 81 [Suppl] 1:23, 1969
13. **Pillsbury DM, Rebell G:** The bacterial flora of the skin. J Inv Dermatol 18:173, 1952
14. **Rebell G, Pillsbury DM, de Saint Phalle M, Ginsburg D:** Factors affecting the rapid disappearance of bacteria placed on the normal skin. J Inv Dermatol 14:247, 1950
15. **Rothmann S:** Susceptibility factors in fungus infections in man. Trans NY Acad Sci Series II, 12:27, 1949–1950
16. **Savin JA, Noble WC:** Opportunism and skin infections. In Rook A (ed): Recent Advances in Dermatology, No. 4. New York, Churchill Livingstone, 1977
17. **Sprunt K, Redman W:** Evidence suggesting importance of role of enterobacterial inhibition in maintaining balance of normal flora. Ann Intern Med 68:579, 1968
18. **Taplin D, Bassett DCJ, Mertz PM:** Foot lesions associated with Pseudomonas cepacia. Lancet 2:568, 1971
19. **Van Scoy RE:** Prophylactic use of antimicrobial agents. Mayo Clin Proc 52:701, 1977
20. **Young CM:** Pitted keratolysis—a preliminary report. Trans St John's Hosp Derm Soc 60:77, 1974

BACTERIAL INFECTIONS

1. **Clayton YM, Conner BL:** Comparison of clotrimazole cream, Whitfield's ointment and nyastatin ointment for the topical treatment of ringworm infections, pityriasis versicolor, erythrasma and candidiasis. Brit J Dermatol 89:297, 1973
2. **McCullough GC, et al:** Acute glomerulonephritis: impetigo as an etiological factor. J Pediatr 38:346, 1951
3. **Michaelides P, Shatin H:** Erythrasma fluorescence under the Wood light. Arch Derm Syph 65:614, 1952
4. **Montes LF, Dobson H, Dodge BG, Knowles JR:** Erythrasma and diabetes mellitus. Arch Dermatol 99:674, 1969
5. **Samitz MH:** Dermatology in Tanzania—Problems and Solutions. J Int Dermatol 19:102, 1980
6. **Sarkany I, Taplin D, Blank H:** Erythrasma-common bacterial infection of the skin. JAMA, 177:130, 1961
7. **Sarkany I, Taplin D, Blank H:** The etiology and treatment of erythrasma. J Invest Dermatol 37:283, 1961
8. **Somerville DA, Lancaster-Smith M:** The aerobic cutaneous microflora of diabetic subjects. Brit J Dermatol 89:395, 1973

FUNGAL INFECTIONS

1. **Abdallah NA:** The role played by mechanical trauma in dermatophyte infection. Mykosen 14:595, 1971
2. **Allen AM, King RD:** Occlusion, carbon dioxide, and fungal skin infections. Lancet 1:360, 1978
3. **Allen AH, Toplin D:** Epidemic trichophyton mentagrophytes infections in servicemen. JAMA 226:864, 1973
4. **Baer RL, Rosenthal SA, Litt JZ, Rogachefsky H:** Experimental investigations on mechanisms producing acute dermatophytosis of the feet. JAMA 160:184, 1956
5. **Blank H, Taplin D, Zalas N:** Cutaneous trichophyton mentagrophytes infections in Vietnam. Arch Dermatol 99:135, 1969
6. **Burgoon CF, Blank F, Johnson WC, Grappe SF:** Mycetoma formation in trichophyton rubrum infection. Brit J Dermatol 90:155, 1974
7. **Carlisle DH, Inouve JC, King RD, Jones HE:** Significance of serum fungal inhibitory factor in dermatophytosis. J Invest Dermatol 63:239, 1974
8. **Hanifin JM, Ray LF, Lobitz WC:** Immunological reactivity in dermatophytosis. Brit. J, Dermatol 90:1, 1974
9. **Hazelrigg DE, Williams TE, Rudolph AH:** Nodular granulomatous perifolliculitis. JAMA 233:270, 1975
10. **Jolly HW, Carpenter CL:** Oral glucose tolerance studies in recurrent trichophyton rubrum infections. Arch Dermatol 100:26, 1969
11. **Jones NE, Reinhardt JH, Rimaldi MG:** Immunologic susceptibility to chronic dermatophytosis. Arch Dermatol 110:213, 1974
12. **Leyden JJ, Kligman AM:** Interdigital athlete's foot. Arch Dermatol 111:1004, 1975
13. **Leyden JJ, Kligman AM:** Interdigital athlete's foot. The interaction of dermatophytes and resident bacteria. Arch Dermatol 114:1466, 1978
14. **Rosenthal SA, Baer RL:** Experiments on the biology of fungous infections of the feet. J Inv Dermatol 47:568, 1966
15. **Sorenson GW, Jones HE:** Immediate and delayed hypersensitivity in chronic dermatophytosis. Arch Dermatol 112:40, 1976
16. **Straus JS, Kligman AM:** An experimental study of tinea pedis and onychomycosis of the feet. Arch Dermatol 76:70, 1957
17. **Swartz JH, Medrek TF:** Rapid contrast stain as a diagnostic aid for fungous infections. Arch Dermatol 99:494, 1969
18. **Taplin D, Zaias N, Rebell G, Blank H:** Isolation and recognition of dermatophytes on a new medium (DTM). Arch Dermatol 99:203, 1969

CANDIDIASIS

1. **Bodey GP, Luna M:** Skin lesions associated with disseminated candidosis. JAMA 229:1466, 1974
2. **Hauser FV, Rothman S:** Monilial granuloma. Arch Dermatol Syph 61:297, 1950
3. **Kirkpatrick CH, Smith TK:** Chronic mucocutaneous candidiasis: Immunologic and antibiotic therapy. Ann Intern Med 80:310, 1974
4. **Wilson JW, Plunkett OA:** The Fungous Diseases of Man, p 168. University of California Press, 1965

DEEP FUNGAL MYCETOMA

1. **Barnetson R, Milne LVR:** Mycetoma. Brit J. Dermatol 99:227, 1978
2. **Rogers RS, Muller SA:** Treatment of actinomycetoma with dapsone. Arch Dermatol 109:529, 1974
3. **Zaias N, Taplin D, Rebell G:** Mycetoma. Arch Dermatol 99:215, 1969

VIRAL INFECTIONS

1. **Baxter DL, Carson WE:** Molluscum contagiosum of the sole. Arch Dermatol 89:471, 1965
2. **Bremmer RM:** Warts: treatment with intralesional bleomycin. Cutis 18:264, 1976
3. **Bunney MH, Nolan MW, Williams DA:** An assessment of methods of treating viral warts by comparative treatment trials based on a standard design. Brit J Dermatol 94:667, 1976
4. **Carslaw RW, Neill TJA:** Linseed oil in the treatment of plantar warts. Brit J Dermatol 75:280, 1963
5. **Coskey RJ:** What's new about warts. Cutis 18:527, 1976
6. **Eaglstein WH, Katz R, Brown JA:** The effects of early corticosteroid therapy on the skin eruption and pain of herpes zoster. JAMA, 211:1681, 1970
7. **Ecker HA:** Salisacom treatment as preoperative preparation in plantar warts. Plastic Reconstr Surg 37:461, 1966
8. **Golhman-Yahr M, Fernandez J, Bootswein A, Convit J:** Unilateral dinitrochlorobenzene immunopathy of recalcitrant warts. Lancet 1:447, 1978
9. **Iacobellis F:** Plantar warts: treatment with topical vitamin A acid. Cutis 12:248, 1973

10. **Kent H:** Warts and ultrasound. Arch Dermatol 100:79, 1969
11. **Keogh G Von:** Warts: Immunologic factors of prognostic significance. Int J Dermatol 18:195, 1979
12. **Koranda FC, Dehmel EM, Kahn G, Penn I:** Cutaneous complications in immunosuppressed renal homocraft recipients. JAMA 229:419, 1974
13. **Lewis HM:** Topical immunotherapy of refractory warts. Cutis 12:863, 1973
14. **Manilla GT, Hood TK, Eakin NR:** Treatment of plantar warts. Rocky Mountain Med J 62:42, 1965
15. **Morison WL:** Cell-mediated immune responses in patients with warts. Brit J Dermatol 93:533, 1975
16. **Morison WL:** Viral warts, herpes simplex and herpes zoster in patients with secondary immune deficiencies and neoplasms. Brit J Dermatol 92:625, 1975
17. **Pringle WM, Helms DC:** Treatment of plantar warts by blunt dissection. Arch Dermatol 108:79, 1973
18. **Rook A, Wilkinson DS, Ebling FJG:** Textbook of Dermatology, p. 753. Oxford, Blackwell Scientific Publications, 1968
19. **Sutton RL Jr:** Plantar warts. Shoch letter, 26:10, 1976
20. **Tromovitch TA, Kay DM:** Plantar warts: treatment with formalin and salicylic acid tape occlusion. Cutis 12:87, 1973
21. **Ulbrich AP, Koprince D, Arends NW:** Warts: Treatment by total enucleation. Cutis 14:582, 1974
22. **Vickers CFH:** Treatment of plantar warts in children. Brit Med J 2:743, 1961

MYCOBACTERIAL INFECTIONS

1. **Adams RM, Remington JS, Steinberg J, et al:** Tropical fish aquariums; a source of *Mycobacterium marinum* infections resembling sporotrichosis. JAMA 211:457–461, 1970.
2. **Barker DJP:** Micobacterial skin ulcers. Brit J Dermatol 91:473, 1974
3. **Cott RE, Carter DM, Sall T:** Cutaneous disease caused by atypical myocabacterium: report of two chromagen infections and review of the subject. Arch Dermatol 95:259, 1967
4. **Dickey RF:** Sporotrichoid mycobacteriosis caused by *M. marinum* (balnei). Arch Dermatol 98:385, 1968
5. **Edwards LB, Krohn EF:** Skin sensitivity to antigens made from various acid-fast bacteria. Am J Hyg 66:253, 1957
6. **Feldman RA, Hershfield E:** Mycobacterial skin infection by an unidentified species. Ann Intern Med 80:445, 1974
7. **Gould WM, McMeekin DR, Bright RD:** Mycobacterium marinum (balnei) infection.

Arch Dermatol 97:159, 1968
8. **Jolly HW, Seabury JH:** Infections with *Mycobacterium marinum*. Arch Dermatol 106:32–36, 1972
9. **Mollohan CS, Romer MS:** Public health significance of swimming pool granuloma. Am J Public Health 51:883, 1961
10. **Runyon EH:** Anonymous mycobacteria in pulmonary disease. Med Clin N Am, 43:273, 1959
11. **Sommer AF, Williams RM, Mandel AD:** Mycobacterium balnei infection. Arch Dermatol 86:316, 1962
12. **Walker HH, et al:** Some characteristics of "swimming pool" disease in Hawaii. Hawaii Med J 21:403, 1962
13. **Zeligman T:** Mycobacterium marinum granuloma: A disease acquired in the tributaries of Chesapeake Bay. Arch Dermatol 106:26, 1972

PARASITIC INFESTATIONS

1. **Christophersen J:** Epidemiology of scabies in Denmark, 1900 to 1975. Arch Dermatol 114:747, 1978
2. **Davis CM, Israel RM:** Treatment of creeping eruption with topical thiabendazole. Arch Dermatol 97:325, Mar 1968
3. **Eyster WH:** Local thiabendazole in the treatment of creeping eruption. Arch Dermatol 95:620, 1967
4. **Orkin M:** Today's scabies. JAMA, 233:882, 1975
5. **Pace BF:** Creeping eruption treated by jet injection (Letter to the editor). JAMA 196:599, May, 1966
6. **Price SM, Silvers DN:** New World leishmaniasis. Arch Dermatol 113:1415, 1977
7. **Rav RC, Dubin HV, Taylor WB:** Leishmania tropica infections in travelers. Arch Dermatol 112:197, 1976

SKIN CONDITIONS OF THE LOWER EXTREMITIES COMMON IN THE TROPICS

1. **Biery TI:** Venomous Arthropods Handbook. Washington, DC, US Printing Office, No. 008-070-00397-0, 1977
2. **Canizares O (ed):** Clinical Tropical Dermatology. Oxford, England, Blackwell Scientific Publications, 1975
3. **Frazier CA:** Insect Allergy and Toxic Reactions to Insects and Other Arthropods. St. Louis, WH Green, 1969
4. **Maegraith B:** Exotic Diseases in Practice. London, W Heinemann Medical Books, 1965
5. **Prado Sampaio, Sebastiao de A.:** Dermatologia Basica. São Paulo, Brasil, Estudo e Pesquisa Editora, 1970

3 VASCULAR DISORDERS

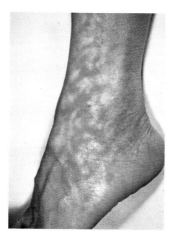

Fig. 3-1. Erythema ab igne.

Fig. 3-2. Toasted skin syndrome. There is a history of chronic heat exposure. Pigmentary changes (hyper- and hypopigmentation) occur predominantly in elderly black patients. *(Courtesy of Dr. J. Witkowski)*

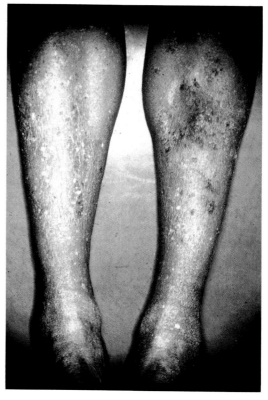

ERYTHEMA AB IGNE: "TOASTED SKIN" SYNDROME

This condition occurs most commonly in women past middle age. It is a common disorder of the legs of elderly black people in the United States. The topographical distribution and skin features are characteristic. The condition is found predominantly on the inner and outer aspects of the shins. In light-skinned patients, a persistent reticulate erythema-checkered pigmentation and dilated superficial vasculature are seen (Fig. 3-1).[2] Burning and itching often accompany the early skin changes. Because erythema is not prominent on dark skin, the term "toasted skin" syndrome is descriptive: Mottled hyper- and hypopigmentation with scaling occurs in black patients. This may be followed after many years by pigmented hyperkeratotic papules, plaques, verrucous nodules, and ulcers (Fig. 3-2). The potential to develop malignant lesions must not be overlooked.

Erythema ab igne is caused by repeatedly heating the skin just short of burning by means of heating pads, hot water bottles, or exposure to the long-wave infrared light from open fires or coal or wood stoves.

The histologic changes in the skin are similar to those resulting from chronic exposure to the sun. They range from elastosis, dyskeratotic epidermal changes, and carcinoma *in situ* to frank squamous cell cancer.[1,3]

Late sequellae can be prevented by protection and the uses of emollient preparations. Topical use of 5-Flurouracil is useful in the treatment of thermal keratoses and Bowen's disease. Squamous cell cancer requires electrosurgical or surgical removal.

THE STASIS LEG: STASIS DERMATITIS

The stasis leg is one of the most representative disorders of the lower extremities, and its cutaneous component—stasis dermatitis—is readily recognizable. The condition is caused by a disturbance of the normal blood flow resulting in an impairment of local tissue physiology and nutrition. The stasis leg occurs in multiple variations: It is manifested by eczematization (stasis dermatitis), pigmentation (hemosiderosis), edema, and varicosities (Fig. 3-3). Later, induration (fibrosis) and inflammation occur with or without subsequent ulceration and scarring. The clinical picture of stasis dermatitis can vary from an acute or subacute reddish and oozing type with marked inflammation to the chronic discolored and lichenified type. A prerequisite for stasis dermatitis is either perforator vein incompetence or large superficial varicose veins, or both.

The site of predilection is the lower leg just above the internal malleolus of the ankle, the left more often than the right. It occurs in those middle-aged or older, in women more than men. About one-third of the patients give a definite or suggestive history of deep phlebitis of the limb related to pregnancies, surgery, trauma, or a prolonged illness. In others, varicosities of the primary type or those resulting from increased intra-abdominal pressure (pregnancy, neoplasms, and so forth) are present. After a prolonged period of increased pressure in the saphenous system, incompetent perforating veins develop at or near the ankle.

Pigmentation is almost invariably present early. It results from the deposit of melanin and of hemosiderin following rupture of small venules and presents as a small area of light-brown macules which slowly enlarges as a single patch or by coalescence with other similar areas. Later in the disease, the color is a homogenous darker brown and may cover a very large part of the leg, with the lighter brown macules still visible at the periphery. A cyanotic erythema appears, associated with more or less edema which is generally accompanied by pruritus. Scratching may lead to secondary changes, the area becoming thickened and scaly, vesicular or exudative. It is at this time that the injudicious use of topical preparations to combat the pruritus and "infection" presents a major hazard. Sensitization or primary irritant reactions, or both, are commonly encountered in this situation and are often severe, sometimes with the appearance of distant eczematous patches on the trunk and upper extremities. Once such reaction has occurred, there appears to be a "broadening of the base" so that the patient develops multiple sensitivities.

Edema may not be apparent early, but sooner or later it becomes a prominent feature. It is a basic manifestation of venous insufficiency and leads to a progressive deterioration by mechanically interfering with an already impaired circulation to the local area. Edema from other causes, especially in those with obese legs, is an aggravating factor in many patients. Persons whose occupations require standing for long periods of time, and those who live in a hot and humid environment, are more prone to manifest clinical disease than they would under more favorable circumstances.

Prolonged edema eventually results in fibrosis manifested clinically as an induration or hardening of the tissues. Recurrent episodes of superficial phlebitis add an inflammatory component which, together with the induration, has been referred to as "chronic indurated cellulitis."[3] With each subsequent attack of "cellulitis," fibrosis increases, further impairing local tissue nutrition, and slightly retracted whitish sclerotic areas may appear within the hyperpigmented areas. The clinical picture presents as a dermatosclerosis (Fig. 3-4).

Ulceration may result from an episode of "cellulitis," appearing as a superficial, well-demarcated, avascular area. This may heal with scar formation or progress to form a deeper ulcer with soft irregular margins, surrounded by deeply pigmented sclerotic skin. The base is often necrotic, and a malodorous discharge is present. Rapid extension with undermining of the edges should arouse suspicion of an infectious process, perhaps of the symbiotic type. In this situation, anaerobic and aerobic cultures, using an adequate inoculum, are almost mandatory. In general, however, infection plays a minor role in stasis ulcer.

A history of slight trauma preceding the appearance of an ulcer is obtained in many patients. The lesion does not heal, and there is a slow or rapid extension so that large areas of the lower half of the leg may become involved. Recalcitrant post-traumatic ulcers are more commonly encountered when the disease process has been present for some time and advanced fibrosis and edema are present. It is not unusual to find the new ulcer adjacent to scars of healed lesions.

MANAGEMENT OF STASIS DERMATITIS

The management of stasis dermatitis must be directed at the correction of the basic abnormal physiology of the local tissues and any superimposed complicating factors such as infection or contact dermatitis. The prognosis depends on (1) how early (or late) in the course of the disease the patient is seen; (2) the patient's ability and desire to cooperate; and (3) the skill and knowledge of the therapist.

The prevention of iliofemoral thrombophlebitis would appreciably reduce the incidence of stasis dermatitis. This effort rightly falls into the domain of the surgeon, obstetrician, and internist, who are making encouraging progress toward this end. Early ambulation especially has contributed to a lower incidence, and prompt attention to other predisposing factors when edema first appears, often only detectable in the evening, is of the utmost importance. This may require the development of new habits or even a change in occupation, if necessary, to eliminate long periods of standing without relief. Periods of lying down or sitting with the feet elevated to the level of the heart are recommended and can be readily accomplished with the aid, for instance, of the newer reclining chairs. The patient must understand that the normal sitting position, with the feet on the floor or low ottoman, provides no advantage over standing.

When the patient presents with well-established stasis dermatitis, whether recent or of long duration, with or without ulceration, the reduction of edema and its subsequent prevention is the first order of importance. When swelling is severe, it may be necessary to put the patient on bed rest, with the foot of the bed elevated 6 to 8 inches, until all swelling has subsided. This period should be as short as possible, preferably no longer than 2 or 3 days, since prolonged inactivity may favor thrombophlebitic processes. The period of bed rest provides an excellent opportunity to correct local infection or any eczematous dermatitis, or both.

Local treatment will depend upon the stage of eczematization. For the acute weeping stage:

Moist cool compresses applied every 3 to 4 hours for 20 minutes. The following solutions are suitable in most cases: (1) isotonic saline solution (0.9 percent); (2) Burow's solution (1:32 or 1:16). Impervious dressings should not be applied because they prevent evaporation, and maceration of the skin may result. Avoid overtreatment. If indicated, Burow's paste may be applied between compresses. Antibiotic therapy, local or systemic, is only rarely indicated, and its use must be decided on for the individual patient. Avoid aggressive treatment.

For the subacute or chronic stages:

Corticosteroid creams may be alternated with wet dressings and later, with improvement, used alone. Following involution of the stasis dermatitis, the integrity of skin texture can be maintained by a hydration regimen (see under asteatotic eczema).

If secondary sensitization or irritant reactions develop, it is advisable to discontinue all topical applications except simple compresses. Because patients with stasis dermatitis are readily sensitized by topical agents, the clinician should avoid using such agents as lanolin, benzocain, tars, iodochlorhydroxyaquin, mercurials, and neomycin. Systemic corticosteroid therapy may be indicated in selected cases.

After the edema has subsided, adequate compressive support of the leg is applied just before the patient gets out of bed. There are many methods of supportive therapy, each with its own advocate and, indeed, used successfully by those well versed in their proper application. In the presence of an exudative and inflammatory dermatitis, for which continuation of local therapy is desirable on an ambulatory basis, the use of the elastic bandage is preferred. This can be adjusted with each application whether a paste or other dressing is used under it. The new ACE bandage with Spandex appears to be an improvement over the previous types. In hot weather the use of the all-cotton type may be better tolerated. The bandage must be applied smoothly without any wrinkles, beginning at the base of the toes and extending to the

Fig. 3-3. Stasis dermatitis, showing cyanosis, edema and eczematization.

Fig. 3-4. Stasis dermatitis: chronic stage. Characterized by fibrosis and dermatosclerosis.

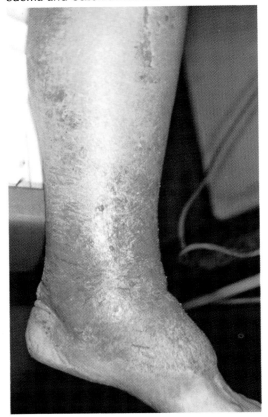

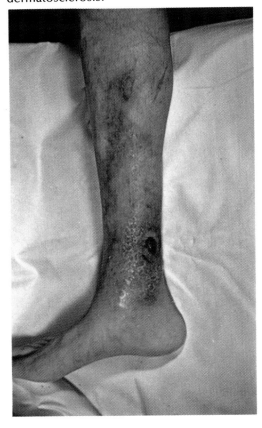

knees, overlapping half of a width each turn. Inclusion of the lower part of the thigh has been recommended by some, but from a practical point of view, this is difficult to do well and is rarely accomplished. Proper application is the keystone to the success of this treatment, but most patients readily accomplish this feat. These bandages must be washed frequently, so that several are required. It is important to replace bandages when they begin to lose their elasticity.

Under certain circumstances, the use of an elastic bandage may be inadvisable (e.g., when the patient lacks the ability to master its application or will not cooperate fully). In such situations, the use of an Unna Paste Gelatin Boot is an excellent substitute. Its proper application by the physician ensures a safe adequate support and provides for periodic follow-up inspection, preferably weekly, although the initial boot or two may have to be replaced sooner. Active infection must be cleared before starting the therapy. Prepared gelatin bandages (Dome-Paste, Gelocast, and so forth) are available and greatly simplify the application of a boot. They should be applied directly to the skin without underlying dressings, even though there still may be active exudation present. Enough layers of the bandage must be used to insure sufficient thickness for adequate support and to prevent creases. To those trained in their proper application, a plaster of paris cast is also effective. This approach has recently been advocated by Menendez, who allows them to remain in place for one month, and as long as two months if necessary.[2]

After healing of the dermatitis (and ulcer) has been accomplished, a properly fitted elastic stocking can be prescribed. To be effective, this requires a customized fitting, which is possible in most cities. Pressure-gradient support (Jobst) is more satisfactory and effective when prolonged use is necessary. The use of stock elastic stockings is rarely satisfactory and cannot be recommended.

One should dissuade patients from wearing high-heeled shoes because the muscle pump does not function properly even in normal persons under such conditions.[1] Another part of the regimen is exercise, with the leg properly bandaged. Walking in comfortable low-heeled shoes is the best exercise.

In selected patients, surgical intervention by a knowledgeable surgeon can be of immeasurable help, but the results will depend on the aforementioned factors.

PIGMENTED PURPURIC DERMATOSES

The differential diagnosis of purpura occurring in the legs embraces a wide spectrum of disease states. The pigmented purpuric eruptions, though somewhat uncommon, are by no means rare; frequently, however, they are not recognized by the general physician. If a pigmented purpuric dermatosis is suspected clinically, then a comparatively few screening tests (CBC, platelet estimation, ESR, serum electrophoresis, immunoelectrophoresis) are indicated to rule out other forms of purpura and to establish the diagnosis. A simple classification is presented in Table 3-1.

Originally each of the pigmented purpuric dermatoses was described as a separate entity because the authors considered the clinical morphology of the eruption to be distinctive. Additional observations, however,

Table 3-1. PIGMENTED PURPURIC DERMATOSES OF THE LOWER EXTREMITIES

I. **Common**
  A. Schamberg's progressive pigmentary dermatosis
    1. Eczematid-like purpura of Doucas and Kapetanakis
    2. Itching purpura of Loewenthal
    3. Transitory pigmented purpuric eruption of the lower extermities (Osment et al)
  B. Majocchi's purpura annularis telangiectodes
II. **Infrequent**
  A. Pigmented purpuric lichenoid dermatitis of Gougerot-Blum
  B. Angioma serpiginosum of Hutchinson
III. **Morphologically similar but etiologically unrelated***
  A. Hyperglobulinemic purpura of Waldenstrom
  B. Stasis dermatitis

*Not usually included in etiologic classifications of pigmented purpuric eruptions.

Table 3-2. FOUR CLASSICAL PIGMENTED PURPURIC DERMATOSES OF THE LOWER EXTREMITIES

Features in Common
1. Etiology: unknown
2. Hematologic studies: normal
3. Course: chronic
4. Prognosis: benign
5. Histology: capillaritis (angioma serpiginosum controversial)

Differences
1. Morphology: variable

Table 3-3. HYPERGLOBULINEMIC PURPURA

Features in Common With Pigmented Dermatoses
1. Course: chronic
2. Prognosis: benign
3. Morphology

Differences
1. Etiology: presumably different, related to hyperglobulinemia
2. Hematologic abnormalities
   (a) elevated gamma globulin
   (b) elevated sedimentation rate
   (c) anemia

raised questions about the uniqueness of each of these dermatoses (Figs. 3-5, 3-6, 3-7). Although theoretically each of the pigmented purpuric eruptions is quite distinctive, clinically there are often not enough characteristic features to distinguish one from another.[9] Common features in the pigmented purpuric dermatoses are shown in Tables 3-2, 3-3, and 3-4. The eczematid-like purpura of Doucas and Kapetanakis, itching purpura of Loewenthal, and transitory pigmented purpuric eruption of the lower extremities have been included under Schamberg's disease in Tables 3-1 and 3-4 because many dermatologists regard them as merely atypical cases of Schamberg's disease.[2,7]

The microscopic changes consist essentially of a chronic capillaritis with swelling, degeneration, and proliferation of the endothelial cells, extravasation of erythrocytes, and a pericapillary lymphocytic infiltrate in the upper dermis. Hemosiderin may also be found. The net result is capillary fragility resulting in purpura and pigmentation.

Table 3-4. DIFFERENTIAL DIAGNOSIS OF PURPURIC ERUPTIONS

	Schamberg's disease	Majocchi's dermatosis	Dermatitis of Gougerot and Blum	Angioma serpiginosum	Hyperglobulinemic purpura
Primary lesion	"Cayenne pepper" punctum	Punctum due to capillary ectasia	Reddish papule	Angiomatous papular punctum	Pinhead petechia
Age at onset	Adults	Adults	Adults	80% before age 20	Adults
Sex	Males 5:1[a]	More frequent in females	More frequent in males	Females 9:1	Females 3:1
Distribution	Legs unilateral	Legs bilateral symmetrical	Legs bilateral symmetrical	Legs unilateral(?)	Legs bilateral symmetrical
Purpura	+	+	±/+	0	+ +
Pigmentation	+ + +	+	+ (?)	0	+
Telangiectasia	0	+ +	0/+	+	0
Pruritus	0[b]	0	+ +	+	0
Lab. studies[c]	Normal	Normal	Normal	Normal	Normal[d]

[a]Exceptions: Itching purpura, equal sex incidence; transitory pigmented purpuric eruption, equal sex incidence.
[b]Exceptions: Itching purpura, significant pruritus; transitory pigmented purpuric eruption, mild pruritus.
[c]Normal studies include: Hgb., Hct., W.B.C., differential, platelet count, bleeding time, clotting time. Tourniquet test positive in 50–75% of cases of each dermatosis.
[d]Abnormal blood findings: Elevated gamma globulin and erythrocyte sedimentation rate; anemia.

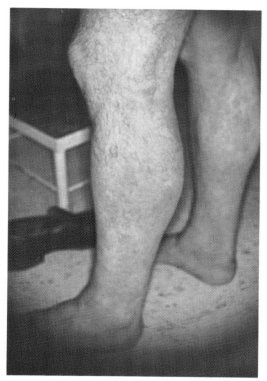

Fig. 3-5. Pigmented purpuric dermatosis (Schamberg's).

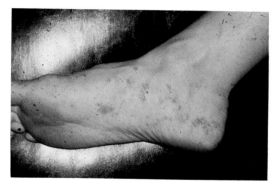

Fig. 3-6. Pigmented purpuric dermatosis (Majocchi's purpura annularis telangiectodes).

Fig. 3-7. Pigmented purpuric dermatosis (Gougerot-Blum).

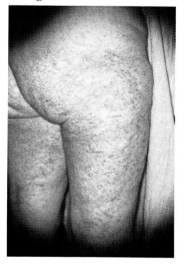

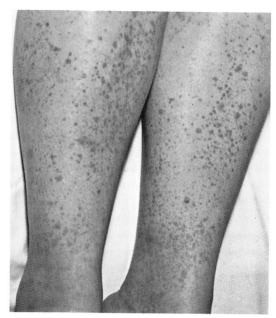

Fig. 3-8. Hyperglobulinemic purpura of Waldenstrom.

The general consensus at present is that the separation of these four eruptions into distinct diagnostic entities is unwarranted. However, Barker and Sachs pointed out that the pigment, purpura, inflammatory changes, and histologic findings of a vasculitis seen in varying degrees in Majocchi's,

Schamberg's, and Gougerot and Blum's dermatoses are not present in angioma serpiginosum. The authors consider angioma serpiginosum to be a "minute vascular neoplasm of angiomatous or telangiectatic nature" and would classify it as a "nevoid condition or form of vascular nevus."[1]

Therapy for all the dermatoses is empiric and symptomatic. Since the eruptions are benign, if any form of therapy is attempted, it should be very conservative. Variable results have been reported with ascorbic acid, bland antipruritic emollients, and fluocinolone acetonide cream with Saran wrap occlusion.[3] Clearing of the cutaneous lesions has been reported following the systemic administration of corticosteroids but there would not seem to be any valid reason for the institution of such therapy in these banal disorders.[13]

IDIOPATHIC HYPERGLOBULINEMIC PURPURA

Waldenstrom in 1943 introduced an entity characterized by chronic purpura of the legs appearing in recurrent attacks over many years, an elevated serum gamma globulin level with a normal albumin content, and an elevated erythrocyte sedimentation rate.[13] The majority of patients are female. The patients often have a low-grade fever and occasional arthralgia in the knees and ankles. A mild-to-moderate normochromic normocytic anemia, which is refractory to therapy, is usually present. Bleeding studies are normal. Pruritus is usually absent.[5] Clinically the disease has some similarities to multiple myeloma, from which it must be distinguished, since hyperglobulinemic purpura is usually a benign disorder. Rarely do patients with hyperglobulinemic purpura develop multiple myeloma.[10,11] Other systemic disease states associated with an elevated gamma globulin level and purpura (e.g., lupus erythematosus, sarcoid and Sjogren's syndrome) must be excluded.[12]

Hyperglobulinemic purpura is characterized by transient urticarial papules associated with tenderness and burning of the skin. The lesions become petechial within 30 minutes; they appear after prolonged standing, exertion, and wearing of constrictive clothing. After repeated showers of purpuric lesions over a period of years, the skin of the legs may show residual mottled brownish pigmentation, which probably represents hemosiderin deposits (Fig. 3-8). The purpuric eruption of hyperglobulinemic purpura may thus mimic the pigmented purpuric dermatoses; the possibility exists, as pointed out by Goltz and Good, that some persons may have been incorrectly classified as having one of the pigmented dermatoses when analysis of their serum proteins might reveal that they have hyperglobulinemic purpura.[4]

Two common disorders with features clinically similar to pigmented purpuric eruptions are stasis dermatitis and contact dermatitis caused by the rubber antioxidant isopropyl phenyl phenylenediamine (IPPPD) found in elasticized clothing, bandages, and rubber boots.

The morphologic picture of stasis hemosiderosis is often identical to the clinical expression of the pigmented purpuric eruptions. The presence of venous incompetence and diagnostic measures such as infrared photography, Doppler ultrasound, plethysmography, and phlebography would help to separate stasis from these syndromes. Stasis dermatitis is discussed more completely earlier in this chapter.

In the rubber antioxidant reactions, the clinical picture is a petechial dermatitis at the site of contact with disseminated purpura. Patch tests with 1% IPPPD show a petechial and eczematous response after 48 hours in sensitized patients.

THE HUNTING REACTION

The clinical expression of this unique vascular reaction was described in 1969.[1] (The physiologic mechanisms of the hunting phenomenon are discussed in Chapter 1.) The syndrome presented with erythematous, swollen, tender toes, associated with a sensation of burning, stinging, or pain, without preliminary blanching or subsequent cyanosis (Fig. 3-9). The clinical features were either absent or markedly reduced on arising, progressed during the day, and reached maximum intensity in the late afternoon and evening. A marked increase in symptoms was experienced upon exposure of the feet to a cold environment, particularly when going outdoors in winter. Occasionally, partial relief was noted by wearing slippers. The symptoms markedly regressed or completely disappeared during the spring and summer with the onset of warm weather and the wearing of sandals or loose shoes.

The patients were middle-aged, and in our series of cases, all were women. They showed no evidence of peripheral vascular disease, venous stasis, connective tissue diseases, dysproteinemias, or neurologic disorders. Pernio and acrocyanosis are not consistent with the clinical picture presented by these patients, since these syndromes are manifested by definite cyanosis and often exhibit associated hyperhidrosis. In addition, infiltrated macules and papules which may be later accompanied by vesicles and bullae and ulceration are observed in pernio. Some clinicians state that acrocyanosis is not painful or associated with burning or stinging sensations, although others do describe pain as a part of the syndrome.

Thus, occasionally a normal protective physiologic mechanism might become excessively active or hypersensitive to the point where the person would experience, in exaggerated form, the sensations that accompany the hunting reaction. Thereby he would develop unpleasant symptoms of pain and throbbing along with color changes of the digits upon slight exposure to cold or pressure from shoes. Control of these factors, protection against cold, and proper foot gear help in preventing and allaying the symptoms.

LIVEDO RETICULARIS

Livedo reticularis is not a disease—it is a clinical sign, a reaction pattern of the skin with a predilection for the lower estremities and which may indicate significant systemic disease or may be purely local. The point to emphasize is that the cutaneous pattern should alert the physician to investigate the patient to determine whether systemic disease exists.

Clinical diagnosis is not difficult: The disorder presents as a purplish, mottled vascular pattern, often described as marbling or fishnet-like, usually occurring on the lower extremities (Fig. 3-10), but also occasionally appearing on the buttocks, arms, or trunk. The discoloration persists even after the skin has been warmed, in contrast to cutis marmorata. The clinical signs derive from stasis of blood in the superficial venous drainage systems of the skin.[6]

Renaut in 1883 and Unna in 1896 postulated that the arterial supply to the skin was arranged in cones 1 to 3 cm in diameter. An area of anastomosis with neighboring cones was assumed to occur at the periphery of each cone. In these areas a relatively diminished blood supply was believed to exist. Skin temperature studies tend to support its presence. The basic mechanism of production of livedo is dilation of the minute vessels of the subpapillary venous plexus with subsequent marked slowing of blood flow. At times the blood flow may actually cease or even reverse direction, and thrombosis may occur. The resultant ischemia outlines the anastomotic areas between the cones as a violaceous reticulated network. Clinical observation confirms that the darker areas are relatively ischemic; in those patients with livedo reticularis who develop ulceration, the ulcers always originate in the dark areas. As a consequence of stasis, immune complexes and bacterial toxins are deposited in the dark areas. Vasculitis caused by these agents often presents with a livedoid pattern.

Many factors can delay the flow of deoxygenated blood away from the skin, notably hyperviscosity of the blood itself and obstruction due to disease affecting dermal arteries, capillaries, or venules. Copeman tabulated the mechanisms responsible for systemic disease relationships on an anatomic and rheologic basis.[5,6]

Livedo reticularis (systemic disease)*
In-flow obstruction
Arteriosclerosis; multiple small emboli; polyarteritis nodosa; temporal (giant cell) arteritis; systemic lupus erythematosus; "arteritis" of rheumatoid disease; hyperparathyroidism and hypercalcaemia.

*Courtesy PWM Copeman MD

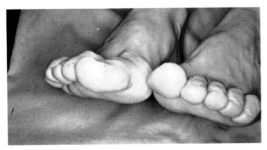

Fig. 3-9. Hunting phenomenon. Patient's feet show slight edema and congestion in the distal portions of the toes.

Fig. 3-10. Livedo reticularis. Typical marbling or fishnetlike appearance.

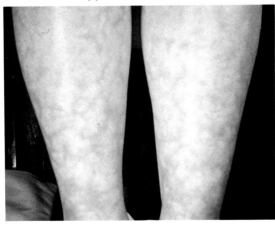

Hyperviscosity of blood and blood stasis in capillary-venules

Cells: polycythaemia, thrombocythaemia.

Plasma: cold precipitable proteinaemias of all types (cold agglutinins, cryofibrinogens, cryoglobulins, and so forth); macroglobulinaemias.

Ill defined hypercoagulable states (decreased fibrinolysis or increased fibrin deposition).

Locally in blood vessels.

Generally in blood.

Neurological disease or injury.

Drugs acting on blood vessels directly (physiological, toxic, immunological)

or via the autonomic nervous system. Liberation of natural vasoactive pharmacological agents (carcinoid syndrome).

Primary pathology in vessels, e.g., cutis marmorata telangiectasia congenita.

Out-flow obstruction

Immune and protein complex deposition ("drug rashes," "connective tissue" disorders, and so forth). Cryoglobulinaemic venulitis. Cutaneous venulitis (angiitis), 'livedoid' vasculitis, erythema elevatum diutinum.

Endotoxin damage (generalized or local Shwartzman reactions). Enzyme damage, e.g. acute pancreatitis.

Infections (syphilis; tuberculosis; meningococcaemia, streptococcaemia; rickettsia; viruses)—immune mechanisms often operating also.

Deposition of crystals: hypercalcaemia, hyperoxaluria.

Out-flow obstruction will be accentuated by haemodynamic back pressure as in heart failure and dependency. The several causes of 'venous gangrene'. Many of the conditions are self-perpetuating. Infections: microorganisms may act directly upon the vascular endothelium or indirectly through allergic mechanisms or occasionally in both manners.

Heat exchange defects

Thermal damage (chilblains, and radiant heat injury).

We have adapted a classification of livedo reticularis based on clinical pictures as follows:[3,7]

Classification of Livedo Reticularis

Physiologic

Cutis marmorata

Pathologic

Generalized (symmetric)

Congenital livedo

Idiopathic (acquired livedo reticularis)

Focal (asymmetrical)

Vascular

Perniosis

Arteriosclerosis

Intra-arteriolar occlusion—Embolization: thrombocythemia, caisson's disease, cholesterol and cholesterol esters.

Increased blood viscosity: cryoglobulinemia, cryofibrinogenemia, polycythemia

Infections: tuberculosis, rheumatic fever, syphilis, Rocky Mt. spotted fever

Connective tissue diseases: dermatomyositis, systemic lupus erythematosus, rheumatoid arteritis, polyarteritis nodosa

Neoplasms: Mycosis fungoides, acute lymphocytic leukemia

Drugs: amantadine, phenylbutazone

Miscellaneous: pancreatitis, hyperparathyroidism and hypercalcemia

PHYSIOLOGIC FORMS OF LIVEDO RETICULARIS

Cutis Marmorata

This is a physiologic response to cold seen in the majority of normal children and is of no significance. (See Chapter 8.) It may be seen in some adults, particularly in women, and is more prominent in the presence of debilitating illness. This condition has been reported in cases of perniosis in association with acrocyanosis and erythrocyanosis and has resulted in ulcerations, particularly during the winter months.

PATHOLOGIC CAUSES OF LIVEDO RETICULARIS

Congenital Livedo

This term is reserved for a relatively rare group of cases in which an irregular mottling is present at birth. It may be confined to one limb or may be generalized. It is quite prominent in appearance, and the skin may be atrophic. Although some fading may occur in time, the eruption is likely to persist indefinitely. Systemic involvement has not been reported. It is likely that this represents a developmental anomaly.

Idiopathic Livedo Reticularis

A large group of patients may be seen in which no associated cause may be found. They are frequently women in the 25- to 45-year age group. Unlike the patchy asymmetric livedo in patients with arteritis, this type is more likely to be diffuse. The condition is often progressive, and increasing ischemia of the skin may lead to disabling ulceration. Usually this is worse in winter, but in a number of cases the ulcers appear during the summer and are preceded by edema.

A small minority of the idiopathic cases do demonstrate widespread arterial disease and may be accompanied by cerebral thromboses, intermittent claudication, angina pectoris, and even renal involvement.

Perniosis

This is often associated with mottling of the skin; the mechanism of this response of the blood vessels to cold is unknown.

Arteriosclerosis

This may, in unusual instances, be associated with livedo reticularis.

Intra-arteriolar Occlusion

Champion and Rook reported three cases of thrombocythemia presenting with circumscribed areas of livedo and gangrene of single toes.[4] The livedo of thrombocythemia may be reversible and may clear with prompt treatment. Early recognition of this condition may preclude later development of hemorrhage and thrombosis, which is sure to occur if treatment is delayed. An interesting example reported recently is a focal form of livedo reticularis and digital ischemia (blue toe syndrome) caused by cholesterol or cholesterol ester emboli from ulcerating atheromatosis plaques in the aorta, its major branches, or abdominal aortic aneurysms.[8]

Increased Blood Viscosity

Localized areas of livedo may result from the intravascular precipitation of serum proteins, as in cryoglobulinemia and cryofibrinogenemia. (discussed later in this chapter). We have followed several patients with cryoglobulinemia that had livedo reticularis as the initial presenting symptom.[2]

Infections

In rare instances, infections such as tuberculosis, rheumatic fever, syphilis, and Rocky Mountain spotted fever show livedo reticularis.

Connective Tissue Diseases

Livedo reticularis in association with dermatomyositis, systemic lupus erythematosus, rheumatoid arthritis, and polyarteritis nodosa is discussed in Chapters 7 and 4.

Neoplasms

Livedo reticularis has been reported occasionally with mycosis fungoides and acute lymphocytic leukemia.

Drugs

An allergic response to drugs such as amantadine and phenylbutazone can damage venules, and as a secondary nonspecific effect, it causes blood stasis, clotting, and other flow disturbances of the microcirculation of the superficial dermal plexus, producing skin lesions often distributed in a reticular manner.[6] Photosensitive livedo reticularis, triggered by quinidine, has also been reported.[10]

Miscellaneous

Sigmund and Shelley reported a case of pancreatitis associated with a patch of livedo reticularis of the abdominal wall apparently due to vascular damage from pancreatic enzymes.[11] Progressive reticulated ecchymoses of the legs with infarction due to deposition of calcium in the media of the muscular vessels in the deep dermis of subcutaneous fat have been reported.[9,12] The basic diseases were hyperparathyroidism and chronic renal disease.

Bard and Winkelmann have described a segmental hyalinizing vasculitis which presents as ulcerative disease of the legs, the ulcerations developing in a reticular pattern.[1] The typical mottling of livedo reticularis is absent; however, the pattern of ulceration so resembles that seen in livedo reticularis at times that the condition has been described as "livedo reticularis with ulcerations without livedo reticularis." This disorder is now considered a separate entity and has been named "livedo vasculitis."

Livedo reticularis may at times be confused with *erythema ab igne*. For a differential diagnosis, the reader is referred to the beginning of this chapter.

The histologic picture of the cases, with or without systemic disease, is similar. The pathologic changes are confined to the intima, which is greatly thickened so that it may obliterate the lumen of the vessel. Some thickening of the media may be present, but there are no inflammatory changes.

TREATMENT

Idiopathic livedo reticularis and ulceration is treated with long-term anticoagulant therapy, low-molecular-weight dextran given intravenously, and sympathectomy.

For secondary livedo reticularis one should treat underlying disease.

CRYOBULINEMIA; CRYOFIBRINOGENEMIA; CRYSTALGLOBULINEMIA

These disorders present with distinctive lesions on the lower extremities; in some cases, livedo reticularis is a prominent feature.

Cryoglobulinemia

Cryoglobulins are cold precipitable proteins that migrate with the gamma globulins on electrophoresis. They are immune complexes in which the antibody is an immunoglobulin and the antigen is either another immunoglobulin or DNA. Most cryoglobulins as IgG, IgM, or IgA. In 30% of the cases, cryoglobulins are combinations of IgG—IgM or IgG—IgA and are associated with connective tissue disease.

There are two types of cryoglobulinemia—idiopathic and secondary. The latter are diseases associated with hyperglobulinemia, as follows.

Malignancy—multiple myeloma, carcinoma (breast and colon), lymphoma (leukemia, Hodgkin's, lymphosarcoma).
Connective tissue disease—lupus erythematosus, polyarteritis nodosa, rheumatoid

arthritis, Sjögren's syndrome, rheumatic fever, hemolytic anemia.

Infections—bronchiectasis, rheumatic fever, kala-azar, subacute bacterial endocarditis, malaria, leprosy, syphilis, infectious mononucleosis.

Plasma cell dyscrasia—macroglobulinemia. Clinical features precipitated by exposure to cold include:

. Livedo reticularis, acrocyanosis, purpura
. Raynaud's phenomenon with or without ulcerations of digits and gangrene
. Hemorrhagic bullae which become ulcers (necrotizing vasculitis)
. Urticaria which becomes purpuric macules on rewarming of the skin
. Bleeding from the gums, nose, GI tract, retinal blood vessels
. Thrombosis of retinal veins
. Deafness
. Glomerulonephritis

Laboratory findings are elevated ESR, inreased rouleaux formation, and low values or serum complement and cryoglobulins. Skin biopsies show a lymphocytic vasculitis, brin, and immunoglobulins in blood vessels n direct immunofluorescence.

Cryofibrinogenemia

This disorder is caused by a cold precipitable protein fibrinogen fraction. A gelatinous flocuulent material precipitates when heparinized plasma is chilled to 4°C.

The clinical features are similar to cryoglobulinemia.

Crystalglobulinemia

This condition is caused by a homogenous gG cryoglobulin (IgG3) that spontaneously orms crystals. The disorder can occur with nultiple myeloma and periarteritis nodosa. Purpura, acrocyanosis, and ulcers on the ower extremities are the skin features.

VASCULITIDES (NECROTIZING)

The concept of vasculitis is summarized succinctly by Fauci *et al:* "Vasculitis is a clinicopathologic process characterized by inlammation and necrosis of blood vessels.

Certain disorders have vasculitis as the predominant and most obvious manifestation, whereas others have various degrees of vasculitis in association with other primary disorders. Within the entire spectrum of vasculitis virtually any size or type of blood vessel in any organ system can be involved. Most of the vasculitides can be associated directly or indirctly with immunopathogenic mechanisms. In this regard, immune complex mediation is being increasingly recognized as the underlying mechanism in several of the vasculitides. With clinical, pathologic, and immunologic criteria, certain vasculitic disorders can be clearly recognized and categorized as distinct entities, whereas in others there is an overlap of different diseases within a broader category."[7] Adding to the complexity of the disorders included under the term "vasculitis" is the confusion engendered by the proliferation of synonyms, eponyms, and pseudoentities ascribed to clinical variations.

In 1952, Zeek reviewed the problem of periarteritis nodosa and stated that much confusion had been created by including under that term a conglomerate of syndromes, many of which were probably separate entities. She suggested the term "necrotizing angiitis" and advocated its use because (1) no particular etiologic factor was implied and (2) the term was applicable to any type or size blood vessel anywhere in the body.[23] Under this generic term, she included five diseases: periarteritis nodosa, hypersensitivity angiitis, rheumatic arteritis, allergic granulomatous arteritis, and temporal arteritis.

Another group of diseases was characterized by granulomatous vasculitis, including Wegener's granulomatosis, lethal midline granuloma, and allergic granulomatosis; the relation of these states to one other and to the necrotizing angiitides was, and still is, not clear.

Other forms of necrotizing vaculitis have been reported under the names arteriolitis allergica of Ruiter, dermatitis nodularis necrotica, nodular dermal allergid, anaphylactoid purpura, acute parapsoriasis, allergic angiitis, erythema elevatum diutinum, extracellular cholesterosis, and pyoderma gangrenosum.

These numerous syndromes were believed

to be related to one other by the histologic common denominator of necrotizing angiitis. Microscopic examination reveals a marked inflammatory infiltrate in and around the vessel walls, consisting predominantly of polymorphonuclear leukocytes, including numerous eosinophils. The leukocytes become fragmented, and nuclear debris is seen (leukocytoclasis). Extravasation of erythrocytes is an important feature. Necrosis takes place in the wall of the blood vessels, and hyalinization in and around the vessels is seen. Often a wide band of homogenization of connective tissue appears around involved blood vessels.

In the past decade, there has been an increased interest in the problem of cutaneous vasculitis. Old information has been recycled, and now the dermatologist seeks to explain the disorders with terms such as hyalinizing vasculitis, livedoid vasculitis, necrotizing vasculitis/angiitis, and leukocytoclastic vasculitis/angiitis. Old syndromes are being reclassified; for example, atrophie blanche is identical to the end stage or healing stage of livedoid vasculitis, erythema elevatum diutinum is a form of leukocytoclastic vasculitis, and an immunoglobulin-mediated vasculitis is considered in the pathogenesis of granuloma annulare.[5,8,22] Over the years various classifications of vasculitis have been proposed.

CLASSIFICATIONS

Vasculitis is based primarily on histopathologic criteria: The size of the blood vessels involved (small-vessel vasculitis or large-vessel vasculitis), the types of inflammatory cells (polymorphonuclear leukocytes, lymphocytes, or granulomatous cells), and the evidence of or lack of necrosis of blood vessel walls.[14]

Clinically, the vasculitis syndromes can be divided into three primary categories: leukocytoclastic vasculitis, Schönlein-Henoch purpura, and the more recently described hypocomplementemic vasculitis. These three categories also suggest an increasing potential severity. Leukocytoclastic vasculitis is usually a cutaneous manifestation with very little systemic disease. Schönlein-Henoch purpura has increasing invovlement, es-

timated between 20% and 30%. Some of the cases of hypocomplementemic vasculitis have involved extensive systemic disease and this represents a much more severe disorder.[12]

Copeman and Ryan presented an interesting classification and discussion of cutaneous vasculitis based on the factors that initiate and then enhance fibrin and platelet deposition and the subsequent pathologic changes resulting from such deposition.[4] Yet they point out that the varied manifestations of the syndromes grouped as cutaneous vasculitis or angiitis are not discrete disease entities and are not confined to the skin, but rather are often manifestations of one of several systemic disorders, such as malignancies or collagen diseases. Further attempts to classify these syndromes clinically or histologically have been unsatisfactory, since no individual clinical or histologic feature is a unique or even a consistent part of any single syndrome.

Thus, the diverse manifestations of vasculitis must depend on a number of variables including the type and intensity of the reaction in the vascular wall, the location of the vessel, the duration of the disease, the location and distribution of lesions, the persistence of etiologic agents in the body, and the degree to which the reaction may have been modified by therapy with corticosteroids. Through various combinations of these variables, differing clinical syndromes may result, although the basic pathogenic mechanism may be similar in all cases.

Numerous causes of necrotizing angiitis have been postulated. A significant number of patients have an unmistakable drug reaction (e.g., to penicillin, sulfonamides, other antibiotics, phenylbutazone, propylthiouracil) at the time of onset of vasculitis. Recently, necrotizing angiitis has been reported to be associated with drug abuse.[2] The exact cause in these cases is not clear; however, methamphetamine appears to be a common denominator. Other patients have an antecedent streptococcal infection whose onset is closely related to the appearance of the vasculitis. Winkelmann has reported cases of vasculitis resulting from exposure to chlordane, lidane, and 2,4-D, after injection of bacterial desensitization products for

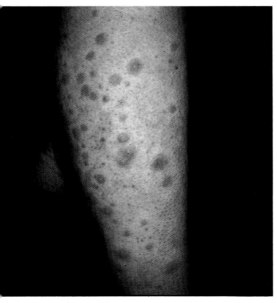

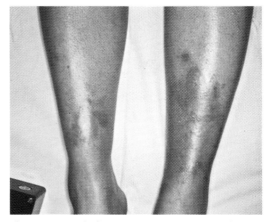

Fig. 3-12. Early lesions presenting as a broad mat of erythema. The lesions broke down subsequently into extensive ulcerations.

Fig. 3-11. Polymorphous eruption in asculitis. Palpable purpura is a distinctive feature.

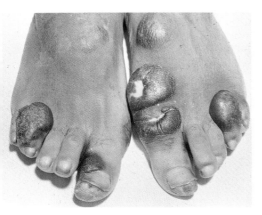

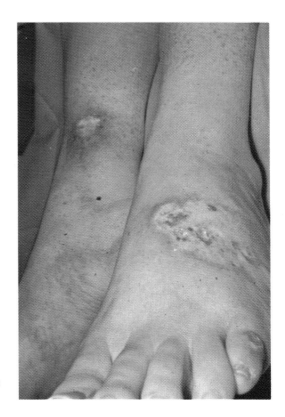

Fig. 3-13. Erythema elevatum diutinum. This are disorder is now considered a form of eukocytoclastic vasculitis.

Fig. 3-14. Atrophie blanche. Note characteristic white scar.

chronic sinusitis and after injection of trypsin.[21] A large number of other chemicals have
also been implicated.

Significant advances have taken place in
the last few years in our knowledge of the
pathologic mechanisms causing these syndromes and of their role in systemic disease.
New and pertinent information is accumu-
lating owing to the development of immunofluorescent techniques and an understanding of antigen-antibody complexes. The
demonstration of immunoglobulins, complement components, and fibrinolytic activity
in the cutaneous blood vessels has suggested
pathophysiologic mechanisms in vasculitis.
As in so many multisystem diseases in which
immunologic mechanisms are involved,
there are far more theories than facts. There
is an extensive literature on the subject;
Copeman succinctly described the mechanisms responsible for the clinical signs of
individual lesions of the vasculitis rash.[3]
Sams *et al*, Handel *et al*, Dodman *et al*, Soter,
Austen, and Gigli, Soter *et al*, Braverman and
Yen, to name a few, have provided new data
and concepts, but precise explanations still
elude us in many situations.[1,6,9,16,18–20]

Leukocytoclastic angiitis is the most frequently encountered form of necrotizing vasculitis. The disorder is considered to be an
immune complex disease. According to
Sams, several factors distinguish leukocytoclastic vasculitis from all other forms of
necrotizing vasculitis and justify it as a distinct entity.[15,17] Foremost is that the clinical
syndrome has a much wider spectrum of
manifestations and is less uniform than the
others. Also, small rather than large vessels
are involved; thus, vessels within organs
rather than those supplying an organ are
affected. Exudation and hemorrhage are the
prominent clinical features; palpable purpura is almost always present in the cutaneous array of lesions. In the cutaneous-sys-
temic form, arthritis and arthralgias are
frequent associations; respiratory and gastrointestinal tracts may be involved. Renal
disease is generally a poor prognostic sign.
Proteinuria and hematuria should be evaluated. Leukocytoclastic vasculitis also sometimes develops during the course of rheumatoid arthritis, systemic lupus erythe
matosus, or lymphoma.

The diagnosis of necrotizing vasculitis i
confirmed by a skin biopsy of early lesion
which shows the characteristic leukocyto
clastic reaction and destruction of sma
blood vessels in the dermis. The skin biops
is essential in the diagnosis of vasculitis. I
is often necessary to biopsy two or three di
ferent lesions in order to establish the diag
nosis. It is also important that the biopsy b
deep and that the specimen have good sut
cutaneous fat and even muscle.[14] Excisio
biopsy is the preferable technique.

CLINICAL PICTURE

What is germane to our theme—and cei
tainly of clinical significance—is that cuta
neous lesions of the vasculitides show a dis
tribution mainly confined to the lower area
of the legs and thighs. Hydrostatic pressur
is the major factor resulting in localizatio
of immune complex disease of the skin to th
feet, ankles, and legs.

The clinical features of the numerous ne
crotizing angiitides are extremely protean
The vasculitis seen in the skin may presen
as a variety of reaction patterns in one perso
at the same time even though the basic path
ogenic mechanism may be similar in al
cases. Typically, necrotizing vasculitis pre
sents as a polymorphous eruption which in
cludes erythematous maculopapular lesion
subsequently evolving to form urticarial pa
pules, raised purpuric lesions (palpable pui
pura), hemorrahgic vesicles and bullae, an
ultimately necrosis with gross ulceration
The most common clinical feature is palpa
ble petechiae with necrosis of the overlyin
epidermis and subsequent ulceration. Th
salient clinical feature of the sequential ulce
is the intensely hemorrhagic necrotizing re
action. Pain usually accompanies the ulcei
ation. By and large, the eruption is bilatera
and symmetrical: It tends to occur in crops
the episodes may recur, and it usually start
on the legs and ankles. Subsequently, it cai
spread to involve other skin surfaces an
internal organs such as joints, gastrointes
tinal tract, lungs, heart, kidney, and centra
nervous system. In essence, cutaneous vas

vasculitides are not discrete disease entities and are not confined to the skin but rather are often manifestations of one or several systemic diseases. A search for the presence of systemic disease is required.

THE SPECTRUM OF CUTANEOUS VASCULITIS

Figures 3-11, 3-12, and 3-13 (see also Figs. 7-3 and 7-4) illustrate the various clinical features of cutaneous vasculitis.

TREATMENT

Methods of proper therapy, like the problems of etiology and classification, remain unsettled.

Evaluation to detect the presence of systemic disease and removal of suspected etiologic agents (drugs, underlying streptococcal or other infectious chemical agents) are primary.

Bed rest with leg elevation is indicated.

Drug therapy is a controversial issue. Supposedly once the patient is properly classified, therapy can be tailored to individual requirements. Some authors advocate prompt and vigorous administration of systemic steroids, while others believe that such therapy is of no value.[11] Indeed, there is some evidence that preceding steroid therapy has, upon occasion, given rise to necrotizing vasculitis.[10,13] Winkelmann advocates steroid or ACTH therapy for fulminating acute vasculitis, but he thinks that it is not indicated in the more subacute or chronic cases.[21] If systemic involvement in leukocytoclastic vasculitis is sufficiently severe, Sams recommends corticosteroids, although there is no definite evidence that they are effective. If they are to be used at all, the dose should be more than 80 mg of prednisone daily and must often be as high as 200 mg.[15] Antimetabolites are being used for resistant vasculitis or immune complex disease, but there is as yet insufficient experience regarding their efficacy.

Dapsone or sulfapyridine has been recommended for Schönlein-Henoch purpura, dapsone for erythema elevatum diutinum, and nicotinic acid for livedoid vasculitis.[8,22]

ATROPHIE BLANCHE

Milian,, in 1929, described atrophie blanche.[5] The features he emphasized were smooth ivory-white sclerotic plaques stippled with prominent telangiectasia and surrounded by erythema, petechiae, and hyperpigmentation. The eruption has a predilection for the legs and ankles of otherwise healthy middle-aged women without obvious venous or arterial disease. Atrophie blanche is usually asymptomatic, but in about 30% of patients slow-healing, small, punched-out, crust-covered ulcers develop within the erythematous or purpuric macules. Characteristically, the pain and tenderness associated with the ulcers are out of proportion to the extent of the cutaneous changes. The sclerotic white plaques are relatively avascular scars with thinned epidermis and sclerodermoid changes in the dermis (Fig. 3-14).[4] The erythematous and purpuric lesions show V-shaped areas of necrosis involving the epidermis and superficial dermis. The blood vessels in the papillary and upper reticular dermis, within this segmental infarct, show endothelial proliferation and fibrin deposition. Extravasated red blood cells and hemosideria are often present, but inflammatory cells are scarce. The telangiectic areas show nests of proliferating and tortuous capillaries. Vessel and blood fibrinolytic activity is decreased.[1,2]

Recently, patchy reticulated erythema, purpura, hyperpigmentation, deep linear slightly inflammatory nodules, hemorrhagic bullae, and polyangular or stellate eschar-covered ulcers which heal into sclerotic white plaques have been added to the original constellation of findings in atrophie blanche.[8] Although segmental hyalinizing vasculitis with a minimal inflammatory infiltrate was found, the involved vessels in this disease were in the mid and deep dermis. Immunoglobulins and complement components were found in the involved blood vessel walls, and several of the reported patients had associated connective tissue disease. Winkelmann and associates consider atrophie blanche as a separate disease entity with clinical and pathologic findings identical to the end stage or healing stage (or both) of livedoid vasculitis.[9]

Similar sclerotic white plaques stippled with telangiectasia and surrounded by erythema, petechiae, and hyperpigmentation have been observed in healed venous ulcers on the lower extremities, in the scars resulting from surgery or trauma, and in a variety of systemic diseases.[6,7] Atrophic lichen planus can also mimic atrophic blanche. In these cases, the sclerotic white plaque appears to be the end result of diverse traumatic insults, both local and systemic.

The term "atrophic blanche" should be reserved for the idiopathic condition described by Milian.

TREATMENT

Local treatment includes application of compresses, silver nitrate cautery of ulcers, silver sulfadiazine cream, and compression bandages. Intralesional Xylocaine and triamcinolone are used.

Systemic therapy: Phenformin hydrochloride 50 mg b.i.d. and ethylestranol hydrochloride 2 mg b.i.d.[3] Low-molecular-weight dextran is given intravenously; nicotinic acid, 300–500 mg/day, is also administered.[9]

REFERENCES

ERYTHEMA AB IGNE "TOASTED SKIN" SYNDROME

1. **Arrington JH III, Lockman DS:** Thermal keratoses and squamous cell carcinoma in situ associated with erythema ab igne. Arch Dermatol 115:1226, 1979
2. **Shahrad P, Marks R:** The wages of warmth: Changes in erythema ab igne. Brit J Dermatol 97:179, 1977
3. **Smith JG Jr:** Increased elastic tissue in the dermis; the dermal elastosis. Bull NY Acad Med 43:173, 1967

THE STASIS LEG STASIS DERMATITIS

1. **Haeger KHM:** Stasis dermatitis. Dermatol Dig Nov, 1977
2. **Menendez CV:** Ulcers of the Leg. Springfield, Ill, Charles C Thomas, 1967
3. **Ormsby OS, Montgomery H:** Diseases of the Skin, 8th ed. Philadelphia, Lea & Febiger, 1954

PIGMENTED PURPURIC DERMATOSES

1. **Barker LP, Sachs PM:** Angioma serpiginosum. Arch Dermatol 92:613, 1965
2. **Doucas C, Kapetanakis J:** Eczematid-like purpura. Dermatologica 106:86, 1953
3. **Freedman R, Hirsch P, Becker SW:** Treatment of two cases of itching purpura. Arch Dermatol 87:740, 1963
4. **Goltz, RW, Good RA:** Benign hyperglobulinemic purpura. Arch Dermatol 83:26, 1961
5. **Hambrick GW Jr:** Dysproteinemic purpura of the hypergammaglobulinemic type. Arch Dermatol 77:23, 1958
6. **Lever WF:** Histopathology of the Skin, 3rd ed, p 164. Philadelphia, JB Lippincott, 1961
7. **Loewenthal LJA:** Itching purpura. Brit J Dermatol 66:95, 1954
8. **Osment LS, et al:** Transitory pigmented purpuric eruption of the lower extremities. Arch Dermatol 81:591, 1960
9. **Randall SJ, Kierland RR, Montgomery H:** Pigmented purpuric eruptions. Arch Derm Syph 64:177, 1951
10. **Rogers WR, Welch JD:** Purpura hyperglobulinemica terminating in multiple myeloma. Arch Intern Med 100:478, 1957
11. **Savin RC:** Hyperglobulinemic purpura terminating in myeloma, hyperlipemia and xanthomatosis. Arch Dermatol 92:679, 1965
12. **Seiden GE, Wurzel HA:** Idiopathic benign hyperglobulinemic purpura. N Engl J Med 255:170, 1956
13. **Taylor FE, Battle JD Jr:** Benign hyperglobulinemic purpura: case report. Ann Intern Med 40:350, 1954

THE HUNTING REACTION

1. **Dana A Jr, Rex JH Jr, Samitz MH:** The hunting reaction. Arch Dermatol 99:441, 1969

LIVEDO RETICULARIS

1. **Bard JW, Winkelmann RK:** Livedo vasculitis Segmental hyalinizing vasculitis of the dermis. Arch Dermatol 96:489, 1967
2. **Brody JI, Samitz MH:** Cutaneous signs of cryoparaproteinemia control with burst alkeran and prednisone. Am J Med 55:211, 1973
3. **Champion RH:** Livedo reticularis: a review Brit J Dermatol 77:167, 1965
4. **Champion RH, Rook A:** Idiopathic thrombocythemia. Arch Dermatol 87:302, 1963
5. **Copeman PWM:** Livedo reticularis—a clinical sign not a disease. Brit J Dermatol 9 (Suppl 10): 1974

6. **Copeman PWM:** Livedo reticularis. Signs in the skin of disturbance of blood viscosity and of blood flow. Brit J Dermatol 93:519, 1975
7. **Davis RA, Odom RB:** Syphilitic livedo reticularis. J Assoc Mil Dermatologists 2:29, 1976
8. **Kempozinski RF:** Lower-extremity arterial emboli from ulcerating atherosclerotic placques. JAMA 241:807, 1979
9. **Lazorik FC, Friedman A, Leyden JJ:** Xerographic observations in four patients with chronic renal disease. Arch Dermatol (In press.)
10. **Marion DF, Terrien CM Jr:** Photosensitive livedo reticularis. Arch Dermatol 108:100, 1973
11. **Sigmund WJ, Shelley WB:** Cutaneous manifestations of acute pancreatitis, with special reference to livedo reticularis. N Engl J Med 251:851, Nov 1954
12. **Winkelmann RK, Keating FR Jr:** Cutaneous vascular calcification, gangrene and hyperparathyroidism. Brit J Dermatol 83:263, 1970

VASCULITIDES

1. **Braverman IM, Yen A:** Demonstration of immune complexes in spontaneous and histamine-induced lesions and in normal skin of patients with leukocytoclastic angiitis. J Inv Dermatol 64:105, 1975
2. **Citron BP, et al:** Necrotizing angiitis associated with drug abuse. N Engl J Med 283:1003, 1970
3. **Copeman PWM:** Cutaneous angiitis. J R Coll Phys 9:103, 1975
4. **Copeman PWM, Ryan TJ:** The problems of classification of cutaneous angiitis with reference to histopathology and pathogenesis. Brit J Dermatol 82:2, Suppl No 5, 1970
5. **Dahl MV, Ullman S, Goltz RW:** Vasculitis in granuloma annulare. Arch Dermatol 113:464, 1977
6. **Dodman B, Cunliffe WJ, Roberts BE:** Observations on tissue fibrinolytic activity in patients with cutaneous vasculitis. Brit J Dermatol 88:231, 1973
7. **Fauci AS, Haynes BF, Katz P:** The spectrum of vasculitis—clinical, pathologic, immunologic, and therapeutic considerations. Ann Intern Med 89(1):660, 1978
8. **Fort SL, Rodman OG:** Erythema elevatum diutinum. Arch Dermatol 113:819, 1977
9. **Handel DW, Roenig HH Jr, Shainoff J, et al:** Necrotizing vasculitis. Arch Dermatol 111:847, 1975
10. **Johnson RL, et al:** Steroid therapy and vascular lesions in rheumatoid arthritis. Arthritis Rheum 2:224, 1959
11. **McCombs RP:** Systemic "allergic" vasculitis. JAMA 194:1059, 1965
12. **Millikan LE, Duvall JM:** Cutaneous vasculitis. Cutis, 21:819, 1978
13. **O'Quinn SE, Kennedy CB, Baker DeWT:** Peripheral vascular lesions in rheumatoid arthritis. Arch Dermatol 92:489, 1965
14. **Roenigk HH Jr:** Paper read at Symposium on Internal Medicine in Dermatology, 33rd Meeting, Amer Acad Derm, San Francisco, 1978
15. **Sams WM Jr:** Leukocytoclastic vasculitis. Dermatol News, March, 1975 from First Annual Winter Skin Seminar at Given Institute of Pathobiology.
16. **Sams WM, Jr, Claman HN, Kohler PF, et al:** Human necrotizing vasculitis: Immunoglobulins and complement in vessel walls of cutaneous lesions and normal skin. J Inv Dermatol 64:441, 1975
17. **Sams WM Jr, Thorne EG, Small P, et al:** Leukocytoclastic vasculitis. Arch Dermatol 112:219, 1976
18. **Soter NA, Austen KF, Gigli I:** The complement system in necrotizing angiitis of the skin. Analysis of complement component activities in serum of patients with concomitant collagen vascular diseases. J Inv Dermatol 63:219, 1974
19. **Soter NA, Austen KF, Gigli I:** Urticaria and arthralgias as manifestations of necrotizing angiitis (vasculitis). J Inv Dermatol 63:485, 1974
20. **Soter NA, Mihm MC Jr, Gigli I, et al:** Two distinct cellular patterns in cutaneous necrotizing angiitis. J Inv Dermatol 60:344, 1976
21. **Winkelmann RK:** Diagnosis and treatment of allergic angiitis (anaphylactoid purpura). Postgrad Med 27:437, 1960
22. **Winkelmann RK, Schroeter AL, Kierland RR, et al:** Clinical studies of livedoid vasculitis. Mayo Clin Proc 49:746, 1974
23. **Zeek PM:** Periarteritis nodosa and other forms of necrotizing angiitis. N Engl J Med 248:764, 1953

ATROPHIE BLANCHE

1. **Cunliffe WJ, Menon IS:** The association between cutaneous vasculitis and decreased blood fibrinolytic activity. Brit J Dermatol 84:99, 197
2. **Dodman B, Cunliffe WJ, Roberts BE:** Observations on tissue fibrinolytic activity in patients with cutaneous vasculitis. Brit J Dermatol 88:231, 1973
3. **Gilliam JH, Herndon JH, Prystowsky SD:**

Fibrinolytic activity for vasculitis of atrophie blanche. Arch Dermatol 109:664, 1974

4. **Gray HR, Graham JH, Johnson W, Burgoon CF:** Atrophie blanche: periodic painful ulcers of lower extremities. Arch Dermatol 93:187, 1966

5. **Milian G:** Les atrophies cutanees syphilitiques. Bull Soc Franc Dermatol Syphiligr 36:865, 1929

6. **Potter B, Haeberlin JB Jr:** Infarctions due to thrombosis (atrophie blanche). Arch Dermatol 88:145, 1963

7. **Ryan TJ:** Microvascular injury, p 330. London, WB Saunders Company, Ltd, 1976

8. **Schroeter AL, Diaz-Perez JE, Winkelmann RK, Jordan RE:** Livido vasculitis (the vasculitis of atrophie blanche). Arch Dermatol 111:188, 1975

9. **Winkelmann RK, Schroeter AL, Kierland RR, Ryan TM:** Clinical studies of livedoid vasculitis (segmental hyalinizing vasculitis). Mayo Clin Proc 49:746, 1974

4 NODOSE LESIONS

While it is always useful to arrange a group of diseases in a logical manner to facilitate understanding, we believe that such systemization is not possible with the nodose lesions of the leg. Therefore, we will simply list the clinical syndromes and discuss each one in turn.

1. Erythema nodosum
2. Erythema induratum
3. Nodular vasculitis
4. Subacute nodular migratory panniculitis
5. Weber-Christian disease
6. Lipogranulomatosis of Rothmann-Makai
7. Subcutaneous nodular fat necrosis in association with pancreatic diseases
8. Polyarteritis nodosa; cutaneous periarteritis nodosa.

ERYTHEMA NODOSUM

Erythema nodosum is a skin reaction which can be elicited by a wide variety of stimuli and can have several causes. It is regarded as a hypersensitivity reaction to bacterial, fungal, viral, and drug antigenic sources and autoantigens. It is not unusual for erythema nodosum to be the only manifestation of an occult systemic disease. Proper recognition of the possible significance of the eruption can lead to comprehensive study of the patient and an etiologic diagnosis.[4] The incidence of various etiologic agents varies according to age, sex, and geographic location.

In children younger than 15 years, erythema nodosum is most frequently associated with streptococcic infections such as tonsillitis, pharyngitis, or dental abscess. Diagnosis is established by finding positive results of throat cultures and rising ASO titers. It may also be an indicator of early incubating tuberculosis. Erythema nodosum is the most common extracolonic complication in children with ulcerative colitis; occasionally it appears with Crohn's disease.[19]

The highest incidence of erythema nodosum occurs in the 20- to 30-year-old age group. Females are affected more than males, approximately 4:1.

In Africa, Asia, the Philippines, and Mexico, leprosy is the major basic disease. Erythema nodosum leprosum should be regarded as a manifestation of leprosy, not as a complication of its therapy.[18] Endemic deep fungal infections play a role in its occurrence on the west coast of the United States (coccidioidomycosis) and in the Mississippi and Ohio River valleys (histoplasmosis).

The association of erythema nodosum with benign bilateral hilar adenopathy, a negative-to-weak tuberculin reaction, and a positive Kveim test result usually denotes sarcoidosis. Other diseases that may underlie the eruption are syphilis, lymphogranuloma venereum, cat scratch disease, and lymphoblastomas.

Erythema nodosum may also be a manifestation of drug sensitivity, especially to sulfonamides, salicylates, barbiturates, penicillin, iodides, and bromides. Recently, oral contraceptive pills (probably the progestational factor) have been reported as a causative factor.[1,3,8]

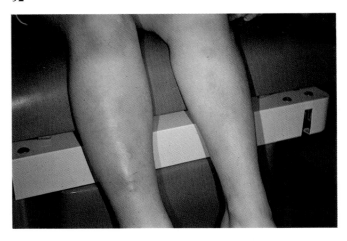

Fig. 4-1. Erythema nodosum. Patient had streptococcal infection of the throat.

The clinical picture is characteristic: The lesions consist of red, tender, painful nodules, usually on the pretibial portions of the lower legs (Fig. 4-1), infrequently developing on the arms of elsewhere. The nodules tend to appear in crops, with each episode associated with mild systemic symptoms of fever, malaise, and joint or muscle pain. The lesions never ulcerate, except in leprosy, and undergo spontaneous slow involution over a period of several weeks.

The idiopathic form of erythema nodosum usually has an abrupt onset accompanied by fever and arthralgias. The nodose lesions are relatively few in number, are almost all of the same age, and evolve through a series of color changes closely mimicking an absorbing hematoma.[12]

Symptomatic or secondary erythema nodosum displays lesions that are not as uniform in appearance as in idiopathic erythema nodosum, and their course is more variable. Recurrences are common if the provoking drug is administered or the disease state reappears.

Patients with erythema nodosum should undergo a thorough investigation, including a biopsy. The punch biopsy should not be used because it is frequently insufficient and because healing on the anterior tibial surface is always a problem. An adequate narrow and deep incisional biopsy is the advisable technique for use in erythema nodosum as well as for all other nodules on the legs discussed later in this chapter.

On histologic examination, a scattered infiltrate extending along the septa between fat cells in the upper subcutaneous tissue is seen. Abscess formation or necrosis does not occur. The walls of the blood vessels, particularly the larger veins, may show invasion by an inflammatory infiltrate and marked endothelial proliferation.[11] The histologic features of erythema nodosum, although distinctive, are not those of the underlying disease. Histopathologic studies done by Winkelmann and Forstrom have defined erythema nodosum as a panniculus response based on a delayed hypersensitivity reaction to an antigen stimulus.[25] As we see it, the limited localization must be attributed to some local conditions peculiar to this region.

Therapy should not be directed toward the erythema nodosum itself. If a drug sensitivity is suspected, the possible culprit drug should be withdrawn. If study reveals one of the underlying diseases known to incite erythema nodosum, the basic disease should be treated appropriately. For symptomatic relief, bed rest with elevation of the legs is helpful. Recently, Schulz and Whiting reported excellent results with potassium iodide in the symptomatic treatment of erythema nodosum ascribed to a variety of conditions such as tonsillitis, influenza, sarcoidosis, oral contraceptive use, and dental sepsis.[22] A dose of 900 mg given daily for 2 to 4 weeks was effective in ameliorating the pain and swelling in most cases. Idiopathic

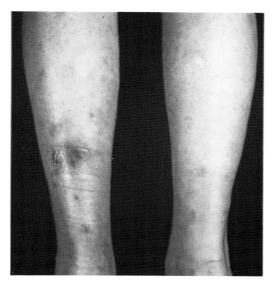

Fig. 4-2. Erythema induratum.

Fig. 4-3. Erythema induratum with severe ulcerations.

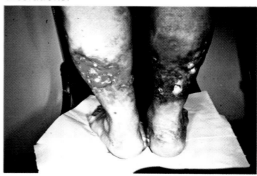

erythema nodosum is a self-limiting disease which resolves spontaneously.

ERYTHEMA INDURATUM

Lengthy debate has revolved around the use of the term "erythema induratum." The dilemma centers on those cases of erythema induratum that are classical on clinical and histologic examination, but in which no acid-fast bacilli can be found in the biopsy specimens, nor can active internal tuberculosis be demonstrated. Some authors believe that the term "erythema induratum" denotes a tuberculous id, and an internal mycobacterial infection must be assumed even if it cannot be found.[5] Irgang pointed out, however, that a histologically proved tuberculid requires adequate antituberculous therapy to eradicate the internal infection even if it cannot be located.

Other investigators think that erythema induratum is a descriptive term only and does not imply a specific etiology.[22] There is no question that nontuberculous disorders may precisely simulate erythema induratum on clinical examination. The differential diagnosis includes erythema nodosum, nodu-lar allergic vasculitis, gummatous syphilid, nodose lesions secondary to iodides and bromides, panniculitis, and thrombophlebitis.

Thus, erythema induratum "may well be a syndrome having a number of causes as yet undetermined."[17]

Classical erythema induratum, also known as Bazin's disease and tuberculosis cutis indurativa, is a notoriously chronic, recurrent syndrome predominant among young adult women. The lesions begin as deep subcutaneous nodules on indistinct infiltrated areas and gradually come nearer to the surface, forming bluish-red nodules or plaques (Fig. 4-2). Necrosis develops, often leading to the formation of ulcers (Fig. 4-3); however, the nodose lesions may resorb without the appearance of ulcers. In either case, atrophic scarring is the ultimate result.

The lesions are usually bilateral and tend to be symmetric. The nodules evolve through various stages. The nodules, plaques, and ulcers most often occur on the calves of the legs, but rarely appear on the thighs and arms. Though most authors report that sensory symptoms are usually insignificant, Feiwel and Munro described significant pain associated with the nodose lesions and increased discomfort when ulcers appeared.[5]

On histopathologic study, erythema induratum shows tuberculoid structures, caseation necrosis, and extensive infiltration and thickening of the larger arteries and veins. The changes are limited to the lower dermis and subcutis in the earlier lesions, but necrosis in older lesions may extend to the epidermis and lead to ulceration. Compared with erythema nodosum, erythema induratum has caseation necrosis and extensive tuberculoid and abscess formation, none of which occurs in erythema nodosum. The infiltrate of Bazin's disease is also more extensive and massive.[11]

It is generally agreed that the preferred antituberculous chemotherapeutic agent is isoniazid (INH), administered in daily doses of 300 mg for 9 to 12 months. Occasionally para-aminosalicylic acid (PAS) is also given, but only as an adjunct to INH. A dose of PAS 12.5 g combined with INH 200 to 260 mg daily for 9 months or more has been reported as yielding excellent results.[5]

Interestingly, Feiwel and Munro also noted that many patients who did not have systemic symptoms of tuberculosis improved and gained weight on antituberculous therapy.

NODULAR VASCULITIS

In a series of articles published during the first decade of this century, Whitfield dissociated a group of nontuberculous conditions from erythema induratum. One of these conditions, initially described by Whitfield under the name of "nontuberculous erythema induratum," is now recognized as being nodular vasculitis. This term was introduced in 1945 by Montgomery, O'Leary, and Barker to describe a chronic, painful, usually non-ulcerative, nodular eruption on the legs of middle-aged or older women.[13] The lesions often coalesced to form plaques, and on occasion, a plaque was the initial lesion. The nodules often simulate erythema nodosum or erythema induratum but usually are sufficiently distinct for clinical differentiation (Fig. 4-4).

On histologic examination, nodular vasculitis resembles the late stage of erythema nodosum, but exhibits a greater degree of vascular involvement, including vessels of a large diameter.

The cause of nodular vasculitis remains unknown at the present time. However, several factors suggest that an immune mechanism may be operative, and a recent study has lent further support to this possibility by demonstrating immune globulins at the sites of fibrinoid necrosis of vessels.[23]

An immunosuppressive effect mediated by heparin was suggested as the mode of action of potassium iodide, which has been found very effective in the symptomatic treatment of nodular vasculitis.[22] The dose schedule is similar to that recommended for erythema nodosum.

SUBACUTE NODULAR MIGRATORY PANNICULITIS

In 1956, Vilanova and Aguade described subacute nodular migratory panniculitis. Perry and Winkelmann reviewed 14 cases diagnosed as migratory panniculitis on histologic study.[16] The syndrome occurs most commonly in middle-aged women who develop discrete nontender nodules, usually on the anterolateral aspect of the leg. The lesions usually affect only one leg initially and enlarge rapidly in 1 to 3 weeks to attain a diameter of 10 to 20 cm.

The outer, extending margin of the lesion is bright red, while the resolving portion has a yellowish tint. The plaques usually become quite indurated, at times almost scleroderma-like, with a mottled consistency, and they persist for months or several years (Fig. 4-5). The erythrocyte sedimentation rate is elevated in most cases. Ulceration of the lesions is rare.

The histologic picture is characteristic, but not specific. The pathologic changes are limited to the septa between fat lobules, but there is no involvement of the fat lobules themselves or of the blood vessels. In the septa are numerous histiocytes with giant cells and a mild lymphocytic inflammatory reaction. Occasionally, hemorrhage is also present. Although Vilanova and Aguade described a capillaritis, Perry and Winkelmann believe that the picture seen is more compatible with a proliferative reaction of vessels than with an inflammatory reaction.

The lesions of subacute nodular migratory panniculitis respond quite readily to systemic iodide administration for reasons that are not clear. The cause of this interesting condition is unknown.

Perry and Winkelmann point out that on clinical examination the plaque of subacute nodular migratory panniculitis may mimic any of the other chronic inflammatory lesions of the legs. However, the characteristic history of "an asymptomatic unilateral indurated red plaque of the leg that has developed in a woman by peripheral growth in all directions from a single initial nodule, but at the same time shows central resolution" should suggest the diagnosis.

WEBER-CHRISTIAN DISEASE

Also known as "relapsing febrile nodular nonsuppurative panniculitis," or simply as nodular panniculitis, Weber-Christian disease as an entity is rapidly being replaced by better-described disease processes: Factitial panniculitis, traumatic panniculitis, panniculitis and enzyme changes, and connective-tissue-disease panniculitis are new syndromes that were once called "Weber-Christian disease."[7] This disease state consists of crops of tender, painful subcutaneous nodules, usually on the thigh or buttocks but possibly at any subcutaneous location. The nodules are of variable size and present as inflammatory lesions with overlying erythematous skin (Fig. 4-6). The disease occurs much more often in women than men and is particularly frequent in obese women between 20 and 40 years of age.

During an acute attack, the patient often has fever, and each attack of nodular panniculitis may last a month or more. By and large, the nodules do not break down or ulcerate. The fat necrosis which occurs during the acute episodes leaves the affected skin sites depressed and pigmented after the inflammatory changes regress.

The cause of this condition is unknown. On histologic study, Weber-Christian nodular panniculitis shows a nonspecific fat necrosis with numerous lymphocytes throughout the fat. Secondary vascular inflammatory involvement is common.

The clinical differential diagnosis includes erythema nodosum, erythema induratum, thrombophlebitis, nodular vasculitis, nonspecific traumatic fat necrosis, subcutaneous rheumatic nodules, dermatomyositis, leukemic infiltrates, and insulin lipodystrophy.

There is no effective therapy for this disease, not even corticosteroids. Occasionally, sulfapyridine and chloroquine have seemed efficacious, but iodides may cause an exacerbation of the eruption.

LIPOGRANULOMATOSIS OF ROTHMANN-MAKAI

This disorder is a form of circumscribed panniculitis, presenting as a relatively few subcutaneous nodules and plaques occurring on the lower extremities and trunk, occasionally on the arms and face. The lesions are firm or elastic and often are mildly tender on pressure. The overlying skin may be either hyperemic or normal. The nodules may disappear after a few days or weeks but usually persist 6 to 12 months. The majority of cases occur in children, and there are no systemic symptoms. No effective treatment for the condition has been reported, except for a case with a good response to tetracycline.[2] On histologic examination, lipogranulomatosis resembles Weber-Christian disease so closely as to make differentiation often impossible. However, on clinical study the lack of fever and other systemic symptoms in Rothmann-Makai syndrome and the fact that the lesions do not occur in crops, all of which are prominent in Weber-Christian, distinguish the two conditions.

SUBCUTANEOUS FAT NECROSIS ASSOCIATED WITH PANCREATIC DISEASES

Although there had been rare reports of nodular subcutaneous fat necrosis in relation to pancreatitis since 1889, Szymanski and Bluefarb in 1961 first clearly delineated the entity and pointed out the diagnostic histologic changes found on biopsy.[24] They reported five cases, four with acute hemorrhagic pancreatitis and one with adenocarcinoma of the pancreas, in which raised erythematous nodules (1 or 2 cm) of the legs occurred. In two of the cases, the cutaneous lesions proceded the onset of abdominal symptoms.

On clinical examination, the nodules were not diagnostic, and they simulated either erythema nodosum, allergic vasculitis, or a drug eruption. However, the histologic picture was characteristic. Except for an extension of the inflammatory reaction upward from the subcutis, there is usually no involvement of the epidermis or dermis. In the subcutis, foci of fat necrosis with "ghost cells" having thick "shadowy" walls and no nuclei, basophilic granular material representing calcium deposits, a wide variety of acute and chronic inflammatory cells around the necrotic areas, and some hemorrhage are seen. This histologic picture does not occur in any other disease of the cutaneous fat tissue.

The authors postulate that trypsin liberated from the inflamed pancreas alters the vessel walls. Circulating lipase then leaks into the tissues and produces the fat necrosis and nodules. An elevated serum amylase level was present in four cases. Serum lipases were not determined.

Schrier and coworkers reviewed 13 reported cases of subcutaneous fat necrosis in association with pancreatitis.[21] The lesions usually occurred on the legs but on occasion appeared on the abdomen, chect, buttocks, and arms. The nodules were red, raised, and tender, persisted for days or a few weeks, and then regressed without scarring (Fig. 4-7). The authors stated that the pathogenesis of the lesions was not clear. Hughes *et al* summarized from the literature 36 cases of pancreatitis and 17 cases of carcinoma of the pancreas associated with subcutaneous fat necrosis.[9] The cutaneous marker associated with pancreatitis occurred in younger patients (mean age, 46 years) than did that related to carcinoma of the pancreas (mean age, 62 years). There was a male preponderance in both types, but this was more striking in the latter. Joint manifestations were prominent in both groups, and ankle pain was common. Alcoholism was a significant associated disorder. Eosinophilia was a common finding.

An unusual association of subcutaneous fat necrosis with gout has also been reported.[14]

DISCUSSION

As mentioned in the initial paragraph of this section, the nodose lesions of the legs do not readily lend themselves to a logical classification, and therefore, we have simply listed and discussed them one by one. Attempts have been made to classify the various entities, but the criteria employed, whether clinical or histologic, have not met with universal acceptance. Some authors have championed the distinctive nature of each disorder, while others have maintained that such divisions are artificial and misleading.

Fine and Meltzer have presented the view that erythema nodosum, subacute nodular migratory panniculitis, nodular vasculitis, and even erythema induratum do not differ significantly enough clinically, histologically, or in response to therapy to warrant their separation into distinct entities.[6] These authors prefer to group them under the term "chronic erythema nodosum," in which the major histologic finding is a septitis secondary to vasculitis. They do separate as distinct entities the primary panniculitides such as Weber-Christian disease, lipogranulomatosis of Rothmann and Makai, and subcutaneous fat necrosis in pancreatic disease, since their histology is that of primary fat necrosis. Whether such drastic grouping into two categories is correct or is as artificial as having too many disease entities must await further study.

In similar manner, attempts have been made to clarify the picture of panniculitis. Niemi *et al* in their study (clinical, histologic, and immunohistologic) of 82 cases of nodular panniculitis of the legs divided the cases into 4 groups: typical erythema nodosum (35 cases), erythema nodosum migrans (11 cases), erythema induratum (11 cases), and the remaining 25 cases, not consistent with the others, as "nondefinite panniculitis."[15] In the clinical and histopathologic study of 34 cases of acute panniculitis reported by Förström and Winkelmann, 15 had clinical findings of erythema nodosum; six had infectious lesions; and five had Weber-Christian-like conditions with recurrent febrile or

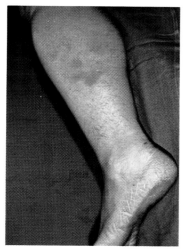

Fig. 4-4. Nodular vasculitis.

Fig. 4-5. Subacute nodular migratory panniculitis.

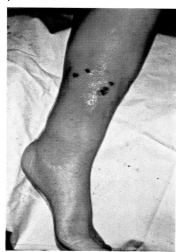

Fig. 4-6. Weber-Christian disease.

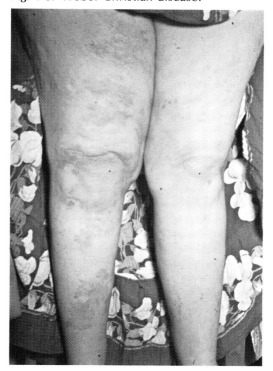

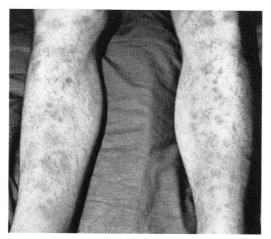

Fig. 4-7. Subcutaneous fat necrosis associated with pancreatitis. (Courtesy of Dr. L. F. Fenster)

nonsuppurative nodular eruptions; three of the five had amylase and lipase enzyme abnormalities with or without pancreatic disease.[7] Five additional patients had acute panniculitis that would be termed "erythema induratum" or "nodular vasculitis." These authors conclude that the most common relationship is with erythema nodosum in its most acute forms.

The interpretations of these studies have been confusing because of the different clinical and histologic diagnostic criteria used. Precise classification of this interesting group of nodular disorders of the legs requires further elucidation of their pathogenesis.

POLYARTERITIS NODOSA; CUTANEOUS PERIARTERITIS NODOSA

This disorder is grouped separately in this chapter but could have been reviewed in the section on vasculitis as well.

Polyarteritis nodosa is a focal transmural (panarteritis) and contiguous periadventitial inflammation involving chiefly medium-sized and small arteries and arterioles, frequently with circumferential involvement of the vessel.[1-8] There are two types: (1) Systemic polyarteritis nodosa and (2) cutaneous polyarteritis nodosa without systemic involvement.

The lower extremities are frequently the preferred site for cutaneous involvement in these diseases, which might imply an immune-complex or toxic progenitor of circulatory source.

Cutaneous manifestations of systemic polyarteritis nodosa are toxic erythemas with or without urtication or purpura, or both, vesicular lesions developing after a vascular reaction, livedo reticularis, subcutaneous nodules, and cutaneous infarction with necrosis and ulceration. Most skin lesions are not specific, and, as a corollary, the most common lesions on the skin are not nodose.

The most frequent findings in cutaneous polyarteritis (periarteritis) nodosa without systemic involvement are painful nodules which frequently precede ulceration of the ankles and lower legs, and livedo reticularis. Diagnosis is best made with full-thickness excision biopsy through the skin, since the arteries involved will be in the panniculus, usually with sparing of the dermal vessels. In essence, most skin lesions are specific, and the most common lesions are nodose.

It can be concluded that a positive skin biopsy result is strongly suggestive of the benign type of polyarteritis nodosa, especially if the lesion was a subcutaneous nodule.

Both types may be acute, subacute, chronic, or relapsing diseases. Constitutional illness is a hallmark with the systemic form; constitutional syndrome is less pronounced or even absent in the benign cutaneous form.

Treatment is with systemic corticosteroids—intense with the systemic disease, and in lower dosage for the cutaneous form.

Biopsy of a specific lesion reveals arterial inflammation involving, in different stages and different degrees, all coats of the medium-sized and small arteries with perivascular inflammation. The infiltrate in acute lesions is one of polymorphonuclear leukocytes, lymphocytes, and eosinophils. Aneurysm formation and thrombosis may occur to produce hemorrhagic, gangrenous, or ischemic changes. Arterial lesions in any and all stages of activity may be present at the same time, i.e., acute inflammation to fibrosis.

Prognosis for the systemic form is guarded since the disease may be rapidly fatal. The cutaneous form has a benign course.

There is no conclusive evidence that this is an immune-complex disease, although immunologic or toxic causes are the most speculative. Immune complexes are progenitors of inflammation and are destroyed in the process that they create, i.e., negative immunofluorescence does not preclude an immunologic pathogenesis.

One should include polyarteritis nodosa, especially the benign form, in the differential diagnosis of inflammatory nodose lesions of the legs, inflammatory edema of the lower extremities, leg ulcers, and livedo reticularis.

REFERENCES

NODOSE LESIONS

1. **Baden HP, Holcomb FD:** Erythema nodosum from oral contraceptives. Arch Dermatol 98:634, 1968
2. **Chan HL:** Panniculitis (Rothman-Makai), with good response to tetracycline. Brit J Dermatol 92:351, 1975
3. **Darlington LG:** Erythema nodosum and oral contraceptives. Brit J Dermatol 90:209, 1974
4. **Editorial:** "Nodules-on-the-leg" syndrome. N Engl J Med 274:463, 1966
5. **Feiwel M, Munro DD:** Diagnosis and treatment of erythema induratum (Bazin). Brit Med J 1:1109, Apr. 24, 1965
6. **Fine RM, Meltzer HD:** Chronic erythema nodosum. Arch Dermatol 100:33, July, 1969
7. **Förström L, Winkelmann RK:** Acute panniculitis. Arch Dermatol 113:909, 1977
8. **Holcomb FD:** Erythema nodosum associated with the use of an oral contraceptive: report of a case. Obstet Gynecol, 25:156, 1965
9. **Hughes PSH, Apisarnthanarax P, Mullins JF:** Subcutaneous fat necrosis associated with pancreatic disease. Arch Dermatol 111:506, 1975
10. **Irgang S:** Nodose erythema induratum (Bazin's disease). NY State J Med 64:2580, 1964
11. **Lever WF:** Histopathology of the Skin, pp 117–118, Philadelphia, JB Lippincott, 1961
12. **Michelson HE:** Inflammatory nodose lesions of the lower leg. Arch Dermatol Syph, 66:327, 1952
13. **Montgomery H, O'Leary PA, Barker NW:** Nodular vascular disease of the legs: erythema induratum and allied conditions. JAMA 128–335, 1945
14. **Niemi KM:** Panniculitis of the legs with urate crystal deposition. Arch Dermatol 113:655, 1977
15. **Niemi KM, Förström L, Hannuksela M, et al:** Nodules on the legs. Acta Dermatovener (Stockholm) 57:145, 1977
16. **Perry HO, Winkelmann RK:** Subacute nodular migratory panniculitis. Arch Dermatol 89:170, 1964
17. **Pillsbury DM, Shelley WB, Kligman AM:** Dermatology, p. 527. Philadelphia, WB Saunders, 1956
18. **Rea TH, Levan NE:** Erythema nodosum leprosum in a general hospital. Arch Dermatol 111:1575, 1975
19. **Samitz MH:** Cutaneous vasculitis in association with ulcerative colitis. Cutis 2:383, 1966
20. **Sandberg DH, Adams JM:** Erythema induratum and streptococcosis. J Pediatr 61:880, 1962
21. **Schrier RW, Melmon KL, Fenster LF:** Subcutaneous nodular fat necrosis in pancreatitis. Arch Intern Med 116:832, 1965
22. **Schulz EJ, Whiting DA:** Treatment of erythema nodosum and nodular vasculitis with potassium iodide. Brit J Dermatol 94:75, 1976
23. **Stringa SG, Bianchi C, Zingale SB:** Nodular vasculitis: immunofluorescent study. 7S gamma-globulin and complement (Ble-globulin) in lesions of nodular vasculitis, J Invest Dermatol 46:1, 1966
24. **Szymanski FJ, Bluefarb SM:** Nodular fat necrosis and pancreatic diseases. Arch Dermatol 83:224, 1961.
25. **Winkelmann RK, Frostrom L:** New observations in the histopathology of erythema nodosum. J Invest Dermatol 65:441, 1975

POLYARTERITIS NODOSA; CUTANEOUS PERIARTERITIS NODOSA

1. **Allen EV, Barker NW, Hines EA:** Peripheral vascular diseases, 4th ed, pp 351–361. Philadelphia, WB Saunders Co, 1974
2. **Borrie P:** Cutaneous polyarteritis nodosa. Brit J Dermatol 87:87, 1972
3. **Cohen RD, Conn DL, Ilstrup DM:** Clinical features, prognosis, and response to treatment in polyarteritis. Mayo Clin Proc 55:146, 1980
4. **Diaz-Perez JL, Schroeter AL, Winkelmann RR:** Cutaneous periarteritis nodosa. Immunofluorescence studies. Arch Dermatol 116:56, 1980
5. **Diaz-Perez JL, Winkelmann RR:** Cutaneous periarteritis nodosa. Arch Dermatol 110:407–414, 1974
6. **Frohnert PL, Sheps SG:** Long-term follow-up study of periarteritis nodosa. Amer J Med 43:8, 1967
7. **Golding DN:** Polyarteritis nodosa presenting with leg pains. Brit Med J: 1:277, 1970
8. **Lyell A, Church R:** The cutaneous manifestations of polyarteritis nodosa. Brit J Dermatol 66:335, 1954

5 METABOLIC DISORDERS

Diabetes—The lower extremities are by far the most commonly affected skin areas in diabetes.

Pretibial Myxedema (PTM)—Enhanced sensitivity in fibroblasts from the lower extremities may explain why PTM is restricted primarily to that area.

Lichen Amyloidosus (LA)—There is no histologic or histochemical difference between lichen amyloidosus (with a predilection for the lower extremities) and generalized systemic amyloidosis, but immunoglobulins and complement are not found in the benign local skin variant. Can we hypothesize that the lower extremity skin is genetically coded to behave differently?

Hyperlipoproteinemias—Tendinous and tuberous xanthomas show a predilection for the lower extremities.

Gout—The great toe is affected in classic gout.

DIABETES

There are no pathognomonic skin signs of diabetes, although some of the changes are sufficiently typical to alert the physician. The lower extremities are by far the most commonly affected skin areas in diabetes, and foot lesions can be well established early in the disease. A maxim to follow for patients suspected of having diabetes: Have the patient take off his shoes and examine his feet.

Cutaneous disorders complicating diabetes include pruritus, bacterial and fungal infections, dermal changes secondary to vascular disease and neurotrophic disorders, and pigmentations as follows:

Cutaneous Lesions Associated With Diabetes Mellitus (With a Predilection for the Lower Extremities)

Pruritus
Infections
    Bacterial: pyodermas, erythrasma
    Fungal: candidiasis, dermatophytosis
Vascular Lesions
    Obliterative arteriosclerosis—ischemia: toe and heel gangrene
    Microangiopathy:
        Diabetic dermatopathy
        Necrobiosis lipoidica diabeticorum
        Trophic ulcers
    Idiopathic bullae
Neuropathy—calluses, ulcers, gangrene
Pigmentations (in association with metabolic disorders)
    Carotenosis
    Xanthoma diabeticorum
Treatment complications
    Sulfonylurea drugs—drug eruptions, photosensitivity
    Insulin—lipodystrophy

Most diabetic foot lesions occur as a combination of ischemia, neuropathy, and infection.

PRURITUS

Pruritus is the most common symptom affecting the skin of the diabetic. While it may be generalized, it is most commonly localized to the legs. The most frequent cause is dryness or asteatosis of the skin, which is promoted by excess washing with hot water and soap or by a decrease in the humidity, as occurs in winter. Decreased perspiration resulting from impairment of cutaneous nerves may be an additional factor. Therapy consists of hydrating the skin. One should bathe the skin in lukewarm water for 15 to 30 minutes and then apply a lubricating cream or ointment such as 40% aqua in aquaphor (Eucerin), hydrophilic petrolatum, lactic acid and urea-containing, emollients, Vaseline, or a hydrogenated vegetable oil (Crisco, Spry) over the wet skin. Increasing the water content of the air with a humidifier is also important. Use of hot water and soap should be minimized.

CUTANEOUS INFECTIONS

Is the diabetic prone to infection? Experimental and clinical studies in this area are confusing or controversial, and there is no explicit answer.[13] However, most clinicians think that diabetes mellitus increases the susceptibility of the skin to infection, but the mechanism responsible is unclear.[6] Dehydration, abnormal cellular nutrition, and an altered immunologic capacity are now considered causative factors rather than elevated tissue glucose levels.

Bacterial Infections

Infection usually involves staphylococcus, proteus, pseudomonas, or streptococcus. It is usually thought that the incidence of pyoderma is greater in diabetics than in the general population.[6] There is no question that bacterial infections are much more serious in the diabetic. Such infections increase the insulin requirement and may precipitate diabetic acidisos. Diminished circulation and peripheral cutaneous diabetic neuropathy may also contribute to the severity of bacterial infections of the feet. The edema associated with infection further compromises an already impaired circulation, resulting in gangrene. Therapy consists of control of the diabetes, local soaks or compresses, systemic antibiotics, and proper foot care. For progressive lesions, aggressive therapy such as debridement, wide incision, and dependent drainage is indicated. Gram-stained smears, culture, and sensitivity studies of the organism should be done to aid in selecting the proper antibiotic. If gram-negative infection is suspected, one should avoid soaks and compresses because gram-negative organisms fluorish in a moist environment.

Infections in a diabetic foot often start with an abrasion of the skin. Careful attention to cleanliness and hygiene is essential to prevent infection. The prophylactic use of a topical antibiotic for all cuts and abrasions is recommended: Bacitracin is effective against staphylococcus and Group A streptococcus, the most common causes of foot infections in diabetics. Resistance of gram-positive organisms does not develop after prolonged use, and it is virtually nonsensitizing. If gram-negative organisms are suspected, polymyxin B sulfate should be used locally—polymyxin is effective against gram-negative organisms except for proteus and serratia. Polysporin ointment contains both antibiotics.

Erythrasma is especially common in diabetes; Montes *et al* noted unusually extensive cases in association with diabetes, and in some patients it was the presenting feature of the diabetes.[10,15] The toe web is the most common site for erythrasma. The diagnosis and treatment of this condition are reviewed in Chapter 2.

Fungal Infections

Candidiasis (Moniliasis). Recurrent or persistent cutaneous candidiasis may occasionally be the first sign or symptom of diabetes and should alert the clinician to investigate this possibility. Candidiasis is most likely to occur in the patient whose hyperglycemia is poorly controlled. Clinically, candidiasis presents as erythematous patches, often surrounded by scattered peripheral pustules, occurring primarily in intertriginous areas such as the perineum, medial aspects of the thighs, under the breasts, in the axillae, or between folds of skin. It also occurs in the toe webs resulting in a macerated fissured pruritic eruption often misdiagnosed as ringworm. Moniliasis may also involve the toenails and paronychial tissues.

The clinical diagnosis is confirmed by observing budding yeasts and filaments in KOH mounts and by culturing the organism on Saboraud's agar.

Treatment consists of proper control of the diabetes; maintaining a dry, well-ventilated skin surface through the wearing of sandals, open shoes, or shoes made of lightweight materials; use of an absorbent powder; and by wearing absorbent cotton socks rather than stretch socks of nylon or other synthetic fibers. Compresses or soaks (Burow's solution, potassium permanganate) should be used in the acute phase. Specific anticandidal topical agents such as nystatin, chlotrimazole, miconazole, or amphotericin B should be applied sparingly but frequently. Although gentian violet is also effective, it is very messy, often hinders proper clinical evaluation because of its deep purple color, and may occasionally irritate the involved skin.

Tinea Pedis

While the incidence of dermatophyte infections of the feet is probably no greater in diabetics than in nondiabetics, the disorder assumes much greater significance in the diabetic patient. Untreated or improperly treated, tinea pedis may lead to extensive secondary bacterial infection with cellulitis and the occasional case of septicemia, or to gangrene, which may necessitate amputation.

Scrupulous care of the skin of the feet, maintaining ventilation and dryness, the use of absorbent socks and powder, and the wearing of ventilated shoes or sandals are mandatory.

The clinical and laboratory diagnosis of tinea pedis and its therapy are described in Chapter 2.

VASCULAR LESIONS

Skin Changes Due to Obliterative Arteriosclerosis. Ischemia

Arteriosclerotic changes of the blood vessels of the lower extremity occur more commonly, are more severe, and have their onset earlier in diabetics. The signs and symptoms produced are due to the effects of tissue ischemia and may consist of pain after exercise or at rest, coldness of the feet, numbness, tingling or decreased tactile sensation, and atrophy of the skin and appendages (lack of hair and lack of sweating). A waxy pallor of the foot on elevation, with mottled bluish-red discoloration on lowering, accompanied by a delayed return of the color are virtually pathognomonic for occlusive arterial disease. If the pallor persists when the leg is dependent, even more severe arterial disease is indicated.

A hallmark of the ischemic foot is dry, scaly skin that cracks easily, thus providing a portal of entry of bacteria (Fig. 5-1). Most commonly, ischemic lesions develop on the tips of the toes and can be recognized by the pale, nongranulating base, surrounded by callus formation. Toenails are thickened, yellow, and brittle.

Large callosities or corns may form on the feet because of increased dryness of the skin due to atrophy of the skin and sweat glands and poor blood supply. Deep perforating ulcers (mal perforans) may develop beneath the calluses, especially on the ball of the foot (Figs. 5-2; 5-3).

Ulceration and gangrene often occur, usually beginning over the ankles, heels, or toes, precipitated by trauma and infection (Fig. 5-4).

Therapy is generally unsatisfactory. Conservative topical therapy, good foot care, and careful control of the diabetes are essential.

Diabetic Dermopathy

Melin in 1964 and Binkley shortly thereafter described multiple discrete atrophic pigmented macular lesions occurring on the shins (Fig. 5-5).[3,4,9] The lesions are usually asymptomatic and are incidental findings on physical examination. Binkley suggested the term "diabetic dermopathy"; Bauer *et al* in 1966 coined the term "pigmented pretibial patches,"but Binkley's term has currency.[2] The lesions occur most commonly in males older than 30 years of age. Bauer *et al* noted such lesions in 17% of adults with diabetes and 3% of adults without diabetes. In our experience in geriatric health care centers, such lesions would not be uncommon in older patients, but in diabetics, the lesions occur at a much earlier age. Binkley relates the lesions to pathologic changes in the cutaneous blood vessels analogous to those in neuropathy, nephropathy, and retinopathy. The lesions are probably the result of minor trauma occurring in areas of cutaneous small-vessel disease and may therefore not be specifically related to diabetes mellitus. No therapy is necessary.

Necrobiosis Lipoidica Diabeticorum

Necrobiosis Lipoidica diabeticorum (NLD) was once thought to be a pathognomonic,

although rare, sign of diabetes. It is now recognized that some persons with NLD have no clinical diabetes, although there is often the possibility that they will eventually develop the disease. Glucose tolerance tests results after ACTH administration may show a prediabetic pattern. Why is it that a significant number of patients with NLD never develop diabetes? Could a genetic factor be the explanation?

Necrobiosis lipoidica diabeticorum is a rare manifestation of diabetes, occurring in approximately 0.3% of patients.[12] Its precise pathogenesis is unknown, but an immune-complex vasculitis may be involved. The presence of IgM, IgA, and C3 in blood vessel walls suggests that an antibody-mediated vasculitis might be an initial event inducing blood vessel changes.[16] On histopathologic study, NLD is similar to granuloma annulare and rheumatoid nodules. The condition is clearly not related to the hyperglycemia or severity of the diabetes. Control of the diabetes has little effect on the skin lesions.

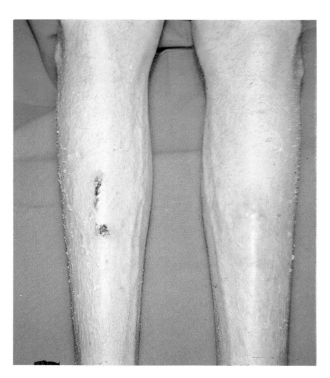

Fig. 5-1. Dry, scaly skin. This is the hallmark of the ischemic foot in diabetes.

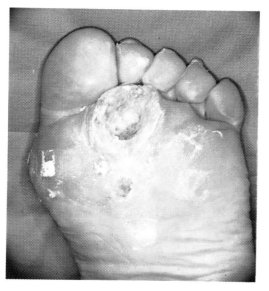

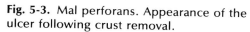

Fig. 5-2. Mal perforans in a diabetic can be especially serious. The absence of the pain sensation leads to neglect, carelessness, and infection.

Fig. 5-3. Mal perforans. Appearance of the ulcer following crust removal.

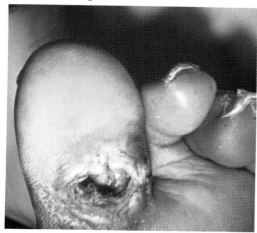

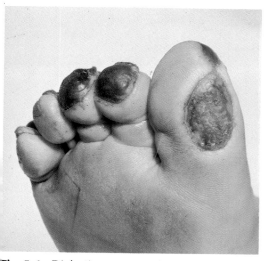

Fig. 5-4. Diabetic gangrene in a patient with peripheral vascular disease. An x-ray film showed calcification in the small blood vessels. *(Courtesy of Dr. S. Lebouitz)*

Fig. 5-5. Diabetic dermopathy. The lesions shown are discrete atrophic pigmented macules.

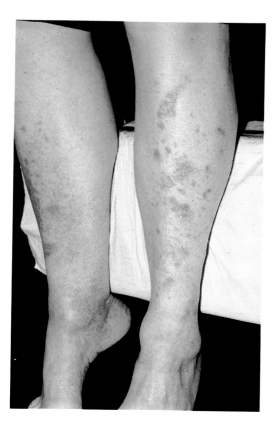

The lesions of NLD are atrophic, yellowish, depressed areas with telangiectatic blood vessels coursing through them (Fig. 5-6). They vary in number from one to several and are usually located on the shins, although uncommonly they may occur on the trunk, arms, or face. Patients of any age may be affected, but the majority are adults, women more often than men.

While NLD is usually asymptomatic, some itching may occur. In most instances, the lesions are primarily a cosmetic problem, but approximately one-third do develop ulcers within the sclerotic atrophic plaques, which can be painful and slow to heal (Fig. 5-7).

Therapy is not particularly successful, but steroids with occlusion can be beneficial. Some authors have reported improvement in about half the cases treated with intralesional steroid injections into the active borders. Excision of the lesion and grafting of normal skin usually fail because of recurrence in and around grafts.[11]

Idiopathic Bullae in Diabetics (Bullosis Diabeticorum)

Asymptomatic bullae occurring atraumatically on the dorsal surfaces of the feet of diabetics, which healed slowly without scarring, have been described.[5] The lesions resemble blisters resulting from burns, are several millimeters to several centimeters in size, contain clear fluid, and are not surrounded by erythema (Fig. 5-8). The bullae frequently occur in long-term diabetics who have peripheral neuropathy, but a definitive cause has not been established.[1]

NEUROPATHY

Awareness of the signs of peripheral neuropathy and ischemia is essential in understanding diabetic foot problems. In contrast to the ischemic foot, the neuropathic foot is usually warm and has extensive callus formation on the weight-bearing areas. Diagnosis of neuropathy is readily confirmed by evaluating the vibratory sensory threshold of the sole of the foot, plus deep-tendon patella and ankle reflexes. The foot can be brushed or pricked lightly to test for sensation. Clinically, the foot with neuropathy is especially prone to develop troubles; many times, the presence of neuropathy in the older patient can be the first indication of diabetes.[7] The phenomenon is not necessarily confined to the elderly but is quite important at all ages over forty, as reported in a syndrome described by Walsh *et al.*[17]

Neuropathy is responsible for insensitive skin: an absence of pain, no feeling, no sweating. Diabetic neuropathy produces a fairly distinct sequence of events. First there is a phase of acute neuritis with diminished skin sensation, and later, as the disease progresses, deep tendon reflexes are absent. Trauma produces hematomas, bullae, and necrosis with no pain. Walking barefoot and improper shoe fit are the chief offenders. New shoes frequently cause rubbing between the toes and formation of calluses, which may go undetected.[8] Pressure and trauma on the metatarsal heads form a callus which, if neglected, provides as ideal setting for infection of soft tissue and bone (see Figs. 5-2 and 5-3). The sequela is an ulcer. Charcot joint changes can develop frequently with great deformity. Another major complication associated with neuropathy is gangrene (Fig. 5-9).

PIGMENTATIONS

Carotenosis

Carotenosis is a harmless yellowish discoloration of the skin seen occasionally in diabetics. It is caused by the presence of excess amounts of the pigment, carotene, which is contained in such foods as carrots and squash. The discoloration is most striking on the palms and soles and over bony prominences. The precise mechanism responsible for the development of carotenemia is not known, but the condition is innocent and improves upon dietary reduction of carotenes.

Xanthoma Diabeticorum

A rare complication of diabetes, occurring in approximately 0.1% of diabetics, xanthoma diabeticorum presents as crops of papules and modules appearing rather acutely over the trunk, buttocks, elbows, knees, oral mucous membranes, palms, and soles. The papules are usually yellowish but may be erythematous and may show a surrounding inflammatory halo, thereby simulating pustules. The lesions may be tender and pruritic. Hypertriglyceridemia (Type IV) is a characteristic finding. With regulation of the diabetes and reduction of the blood lipid levels, the lesions disappear usually leaving no residue, although rarely some atrophy and pigmentation occur.

THERAPY OF LEG LESIONS ASSOCIATED WITH DIABETES

Foot Care

It is of utmost importance that the diabetic patient care for his feet with never-ending concern. A decreased blood supply to the lower leg and foot is a common accompaniment of diabetes. This underlies the development of cutaneous complications. Cutaneous fungal and bacterial infections may quickly be transformed from minor annoyances to major, occasionally fatal, complications. Minor trauma—whether mechanical as from ill-fitting shoes, thermal as from hot water bottles, or chemical as from the injudicious use of topical home remedies—can result in chronic ulcerations with great potential for secondary infection and cellulitis. In addition, infection may precipitate diabetic acidosis and coma in a previously well-controlled diabetic patient. Thus, the importance of proper prophylactic foot care and correct therapeutic measures for specific problems cannot be overemphasized.

Prophylactic foot care consists of wearing correctly fitting shoes and absorbent cotton socks and using a bland, absorbent foot powder. Lamb's wool between the toes reduces rubbing. Shoes are extremely important—the shoe should be accommodated to the foot. Special shoes with molded plastic to protect the foot from trauma and to redistribute weight help prevent ulcers.[8] The use of podiatric appliances in patients with diabetic neuropathy is described succinctly by Seder.[14] Keeping the feet dry and ventilated and avoiding going barefoot will reduce the incidence of bacterial and fungal infections.

Generally, palliative care is required for life.

When a cutaneous infection occurs, the patient should immediately be put on bed rest. Gram-stained smears, appropriate bacterial cultures, and antibiotic sensitivity studies should be done. If the involved area is oozing, compresses should be employed. Specific systemic or topical antibacterial or antifungal agents should be utilized to eradicate the infection.

When ulcerations occur, presumably related to trauma to an area of skin which has compromised vascularity, the same basic therapeutic measures of bed rest and bacterial studies should be carried out. For ischemic ulcers, the head of the bed should be raised. Often, bland compresses (saline), bed rest, and patience will result in healing of the ulcer. When debris is considerable, an enzymatic ointment could be used to clear the ulcer base but then should be discontinued, since these agents do not contribute to further healing. Hydrogen peroxide soaks followed by Gelfoam-powder packing daily is often helpful in healing an ulcer. (For detailed treatment of ulcers refer to Chapter 14.) When necessary, skin grafts may be indicated. However, in our experience such attempts at grafting are often undertaken prematurely without an adequate trial of conservative medical therapy and at times without due consideration of the decreased vascular supply to the area.

It is vital that the diabetes be maintained under good control. (See also diabetes in association with the Geriatric Foot, Chapter 9.)

THYROID DISEASE, PRETIBIAL MYXEDEMA, AND ACROPACHY

The skin of the lower extremities is especially prone to the effects of excess or deficiency of thyroid hormone and other factors associated with thyroid disease. Skin changes associated with thyroid disease are useful clinical markers, since they may precede other clinical or laboratory evidence of disease. These changes are discussed in relation to the effect of thyroid hormone on their production.[6]

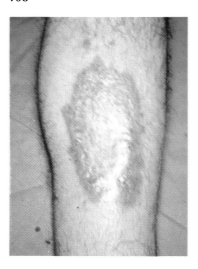

Fig. 5-6. Necrobiosis lipoidica diabeticorum. The yellowish, depressed, atrophic lesion is characteristic of this dermatosis.

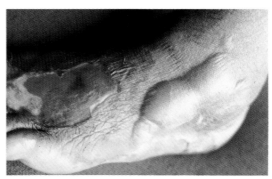

Fig. 5-8. Idiopathic bullae in diabetic patient. *(Courtesy R.I. Patel, Nairobi, Kenya)*

Fig. 5-7. Painful and slow healing ulcer in lesion of necrobiosis lipoidica diabeticorum. *(Courtesy Dr. J. Witkowski)*

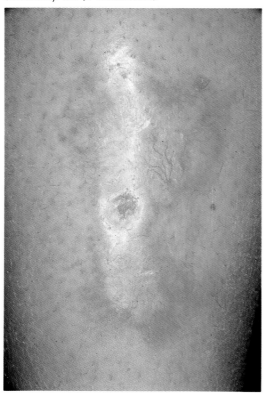

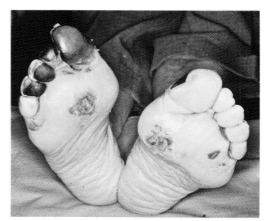

Fig. 5-9. Diabetic gangrene following application of hot water bottle in uncontrolled diabetic patient with neuropathy.

LACK OF THYROID HORMONE

The skin of cretins is pale, cool, and rough with a mottled appearance suggesting livedo reticularis. Mucin deposits, vasoconstriction, and associated anemia make the skin of adolescent and adult patients feel cold and appear pale with boggy nonpitting edema (diffuse myxedema).[3] The often-associated aberration in carotene metabolism results in yellowing of the soles. Decreased sweating and serum excretion causes dryness and superficial fissuring of the skin. Eczema craquelé is often seen. The nails grow more slowly and are thin and striated. Increased capillary fragility often results in easy bruising. Poor wound healing is a common associated finding. Tendon and eruptive xanthomas are seen occasionally if there is an associated lipid derangement.

EXCESS OF THYROID HORMONE

The skin is soft and has a velvety feel. Increased sweating on the soles is often noted. The nails grow faster and are shiny and friable. Distal onycholysis is occasionally seen.[11]

INDEPENDENT OF THYROID HORMONE

Localized myxedema or pretibial myxedema (PTM) is characterized by focal accumulation of ground substance; it is most commonly limited to the pretibial region. The association of thyrotoxicosis, exophthalmos, and PTM has become a well-recognized syndrome. Within recent years, the syndrome has been enlarged to include a fourth, related condition, acropachy.[4,9]

Pretibial myxedema occurs in about 3% of patients with toxic diffuse goiter.[13] In approximately 50% of patients, the lesions appear during the active hyperthyroid state; in the remainder they develop following treatment for the hyperthyroidism, or they occur in euthyroid patients, patients with idiopathic hypothyroidism or Hashimoto's thyroiditis.[8] Women are more often affected than men.

The characteristic lesions are firm, nonpitting, irregular swellings, nodules, or plaques which may be flesh-colored or pink to yellow and waxy. The overlying epidermis is thin and stretched; the follicles are prominent, imparting a "pigskin" appearance. The lesions appear bilaterally on the pretibial areas (Fig. 5-10), but they may be seen on the dorsa of the feet, the thighs, and, rarely, the abdomen. They may extend around the legs forming shinguard-like, thick heavy masses of uneven contour.[10] The hair in these lesions is often increased in amount, coarse, and dry. The skin temperature is decreased.

Acropachy occurs in less than 1 percent of patients with hyperthyroidism. Although it is most often associated with a past history of thyrotoxicosis, exophthalmos, and PTM, it may occur without thyroid disease.[10] It often continues to progress while the other manifestations of the syndrome persist unchanged or improve. Acropachy literally means thickening of the extremities. The syndrome consists of clubbing of the digits; thickening of the hands, feet, and digits; and subperiosteal new-bone formation of the diaphyses of the distal short and long bones.[10] Elevated growth hormone levels, prognathism, abnormal sella turcica, and lack of clubbing differentiate acromegaly from acropachy. Pachydermoperiostosis is associated with thickening of the facial and scalp skin with folding of the skin on the scalp (cutis verticis gyrata).

The histopathology of pretibial myxedema is characterized by localized proliferation of fibroblasts with an increase in amounts of dermal collagen and acid mucopolysaccharides, mainly hyaluronic acid. In the dermis, particularly the lower portion, it occurs not only as individual threads and granules, but also as extensive deposits, causing wide separation of collagen bundles. In some areas, there may be degeneration of collagen fibers, and in others there is new collagen formation with an increase in the number of fibroblasts.[7] The latter are the source of hyaluronic acid.

The pathogenesis of pretibial myxedema is now being clarified. Since the condition occurs in association with hyperthyroidism and exophthalmos, it was originally postulated that thyroid stimulating hormone (TSH) was mediating the disorder. Subse-

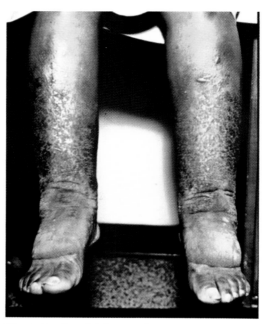

Fig. 5-10. Pretibial myxedema.

quent research showed no correlation between TSH levels and hyperthyroidism and the presence or absence of exophthalmos or pretibial myxedema.[1] Also, studies have shown that the long-acting thyroid stimulator (LATS) level is almost invariably elevated in patients with PTM. LATS is quite distinct from TSH, and is not produced by the anterior pituitary, but by antibody-producing cells. It has been suggested that this globulin is involved in the production of PTM lesions, but there is no convincing evidence that PTM is the result of an immunologic process.[12]

Recent findings by Cheung *et al* may be the first to shed light on the reasons for the localization of edematous lesions seen in patients with PTM.[2] In their culture studies, fibroblasts from the pretibial area synthesized 2 to 3 times more hyaluronic acid when incubated with PTM sera than when incubated in normal human serum. Fibroblasts cultured from the skin of the back or prepuce did not respond to PTM sera. The enhanced sensitivity to PTM sera exhibited by fibroblasts from the lower extremities may explain why the lesions in this disease are restricted primarily to that area. (Are pretibial fibroblasts coded differently?) Jolliffee *et al* hypothesized that the fibroblast-stimulating factor in sera is somatomedin and that its presence in increased amounts in thyroid disease may lead to PTM.[5]

TREATMENT

It has been reported that PTM can disappear spontaneously, but involution is highly unpredictable.

Local injection of triamcinolone suspension often produces resolution. In more widespread cases, fluorinated corticosteroid creams under occlusion often improve the condition. Local injection of hyaluronidase has no effect. Surgical excision is followed by recurrence in a few months.

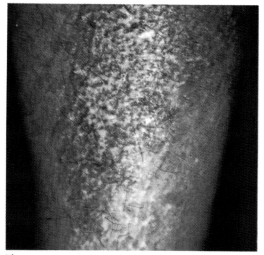

Fig. 5-11. Lichen amyloidosus. Patient's major complaint was intense pruritus.

CUTANEOUS AMYLOIDOSES

Cutaneous amyloidoses show a predilection for the skin of the lower extremities. There are three types: lichen amyloidosus, its macular variant, and amyloid tumors (tumefactive form).[3] All varieties occur predominantly in middle-aged or older persons.

LICHEN AMYLOIDOSUS

This local form of amyloidosis is characterized by an eruption of discrete, firm papules which vary in color from red to reddish-brown and occasionally are translucent. The papules may coalesce to form well-defined plaques. The eruption most frequently involves the lower extremities, usually localized on the shins, but may occur on the forearms, thighs, and back (Fig. 5-11). Pruritus is usually a prominent symptom, and because of the clinical appearance of the lesions and associated pruritus, lichen amyloidosus must be differentiated from lichen planus and lichen simplex chronicus. The diagnosis is established with histologic and histochemical studies. The lesions of lichen amyloidosus tend to persist indefinitely.

Lichen amyloidosus is the most commonly recognized form of cutaneous amyloidosis. There is a high incidence of the disease among orientals; familiar cases have also been reported.[5,7]

MACULAR AMYLOIDOSIS

In macular amyloidosis, one sees poorly delineated, oval, grayish-brown patches or well-defined macules interspersed with normal-appearing skin, creating a ripple pattern. The eruption is usually pruritic. The lower extremities are the common location. Both the papular and the macular lesions can occur in the same patient.

Lichen amyloidosus and its macular variant are strictly local conditions; amyloid is not found other than in the affected skin. These localized forms do not show skin manifestations of purpura (readily evoked by the "pinch" test) and alopecia, which are features of primary systemic amyloidosis. When the localized cutaneous forms are diagnosed, investigation for amyloid deposits in internal organs is not indicated.

Lichen amyloidosus and macular amyloidosis are characterized by the presence of

Fig. 5-12. Tendon xanthoma. The achille's tendon is most frequently involved.

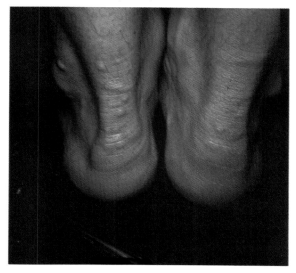

amyloid in the papillary dermis and the lack of involvement of blood vessels and dermal appendages. The papular nature of lichen amyloidosus is thought to be due to secondary epidermal changes and not to the volume of amyloid deposited.[2]

TUMEFACTIVE AMYLOIDOSIS

The amyloid tumors occur on the extremities, trunk, genitals, and face. They can be single or multiple, asymptomatic, soft-to-firm nodules, plaques, or pedunculated lesions.[3] The overlying skin is atrophic, is shiny, and may show telangiectasias. The lesions often resemble large bullae; the color varies from flesh to yellow-brown to purple. Deposits of amyloid in these lesions appear in both the dermis and the subcutis; the blood vessels and adnexal structures are infiltrated. Some of the patients with this form of cutaneous amyloidosis subsequently developed systemic disease.

Amyloid is a proteinaceous substance deposited extracellularly in a variety of conditions.[4] More than 95% of amyloid consists of fine rigid nonbranching fibrils, with a unique ultrastructure, chemical composition, and crystallographic pattern. Two types of fibrils have been identified: one similar to a portion of immunoglobulin light-chains, the other similar to the serum A-related protein. The remaining 5% of amyloid consists of a P-component or doughnut, so named because of its distinctive morphologic appearance. This substance is antigenically related to an alpha 1 serum glycoprotein. The amyloid of lichen amyloidosus has been shown to have the same characteristics as amyloid in other forms of the disease.

The origin of amyloid is still under investigation. Its similarity to serum proteins suggests that it arises as a result of an aberration of synthesis or degradation. The deposits of amyloid in the localized cutaneous forms are thought to be related to degenerating epidermal cells or to be the secretory products of dermal fibroblasts.[1,2] Direct immunofluorescent studies of lichen amyloidosus failed to detect immunoglobulins or C_3 in amyloid deposits, thus ruling out an immune pathogenesis in this disorder.[6]

Staining reactions are essentially those of acid or neutral mucopolysaccharides, which comprise 1.5% of amyloid material. In sections stained with hematoxylin and eosin, the material is observed to be an amorphous pink substance. On histochemical study, amyloid stains red (metachromatically) with crystal violet and methyl violet. It stains orange red with congo red; sections exhibit bifringence when examined under the polarizing microscope. In routine sections, amyloid can be demonstrated by staining with the thioflavine-T because amyloid develops a fluorescence which can be observed when examined with a fluorescent microscope.

TREATMENT

Topical steroids under occlusion or local steroid infiltration has been helpful.

HYPERLIPOPROTEINEMIAS

Tendinous and tuberous xanthomas are the visible and palpable stigmata of lipid deposits, with a predilection for the lower extremities. Although the cutaneous xanthomas suggest a systemic lipid abnormality, a definitive diagnosis of the type of hyperlipoproteinemia can be made only on determination of serum lipoprotein patterns and analysis of the plasma for its various lipid components. The classification of five types of hyperlipoproteinemias proposed by Fredrickson et al has gained wide acceptance, but recent genetic studies of primary hyperlipoproteinemias have suggested modification in the classification.[1-6]

Each of the hyperlipoproteinemias has its own clinicopathologic–chemical features. It has been pointed out that the appearance of the skin lesions may be the first sign of the disorder and that the kind of xanthomas observed may lead to type classification before laboratory studies are available.

The clinical features of xanthomas are

characteristic. Diagnosis is readily confirmed by histologic examination showing
typical foam cells, which are histiocytes that
accumulate lipid material in their cytoplasm.

Xanthomas appear as plaquelike infiltrations, papules, or nodules that range in size
from one millimeter to several centimeters.
The lesions are firm and usually nontender.
They are readily identified by their distinctive yellow or orange hue; however, at times
they may be pink to red or even brown. Eruptive xanthomas are small reddish-to-yellow
papules with an erythematous base. They
appear in crops; favored locations include
the buttocks, the backs of the thighs, and the
body folds. The oral mucous membranes may
also be affected. Tuberous xanthomas develop slowly as fleshy-to-firm papular, mod-
ular, or pedunculated lesions. Color ranges
from flesh to yellow to brown. They occur
characteristically over extensor surfaces
such as the elbows, knees, and buttocks. Tuberous xanthomas differ from the tendinous
type in being located in the dermis and subcutaneous layer, and they are not attached
to underlying structures. Tuberous xanthomas suggest elevated cholesterol levels, but
they may also be seen with triglyceride elevation.

Tendon xanthomas are firm subcutaneous
infiltrations of the tendon sheaths. They have
a predilection for the extensor tendons of the
hands and feet, elbows, and knees; the
Achilles tendon is the most frequently involved (Fig. 5-12). In these locations, they can
be confused with rheumatoid nodules or
gouty tophi. Tendinous xanthomas are usually associated with elevated plasma cholesterol levels and an underlying disturbance
in lipoprotein metabolism.

Most patients presenting with xanthomas
have primary hyperlipoproteinemia, especially type II. The lesions can also occur with
the secondary hyperlipoproteinemias, which
are associated with disorders that affect cholesterol metabolism such as uncontrolled
diabetes, myxedema, nephrosis, myeloma,
and glycogen storage diseases.

Xanthomas can persist for years. In some

types, regression can occur as a result of
therapy.

GOUT

Gout is an inborn error of metabolism which
results in hyperuricemia, deposits of urates
in articular cartilages and the skin, and attacks of acute arthritis. Uric acid deposits
give rise to tophi of the ears, bursae of the
elbow and knees, tendons of the fingers,
wrists, toes, and ankles, as well as to lumpy
deposits in the skin over joints.

Primary gout may be transmitted as an
autosomal dominant characteristic; a positive family history is found in about 25% of
cases. Secondary gout is an occasional complication of hematopoietic and myeloproliferative disorders attributed to an increased
turnover of nucleic acids and an overproduction of uric acid.

Gout occurs primarily in males until age
40, after which a significant number are
women, although males still predominate.
Manifestations on the lower extremities include acute gouty arthritis, gouty tophi, and
ulcers.

In classical acute attacks of gouty arthritis,
the great toe—especially the metatarsophalangeal joint—ankle, or foot is involved by a
painful, deep red, hot swelling which is
tender to the touch (Fig. 5-13). A bacterial
cellulitis may be mistakenly diagnosed. Attacks usually occur in the early morning
hours; they may follow minor local trauma,
dietary or alcohol indiscretion, drugs, mild
illnesses, or other factors, but often there is
no precipitating cause.[2]

Urate deposits tend to occur in relatively
avascular tissue such as tendons and carti-
lage. Tophi can vary in size from 1.0 mm to
several centimeters (Fig. 5-14). The overlying
skin is usually thin, shiny, and orange in
color. Ulcers occur when subcutaneous tophi
are injured (Fig. 5-15).

The diagnosis is made based on the clinical
features, an elevated serum uric acid level,
and the identification of typical needle-like
monosodium urate crystals on microscopic

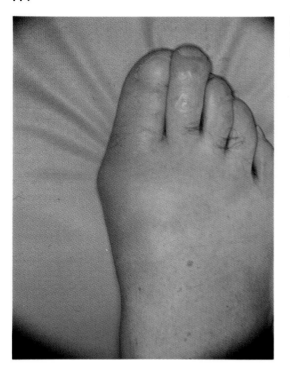

Fig. 5-13. Red and swollen metatarsophalangeal joint characteristic of gout.

Fig. 5-15. Tophus ulcer. The base is filled with a thick creamy substance that showed needlelike crystals on microscopic examination.

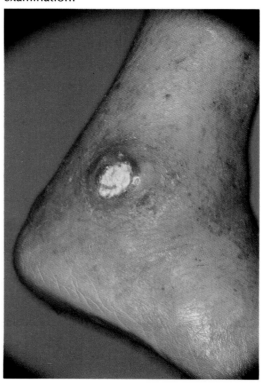

Fig. 5-14. Typical tophus of gout.

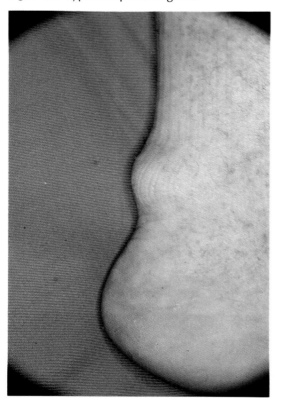

examination of synovial fluid leukocytes and ulcer discharge.

Treatment of acute gout includes immobilization of the affected joints and the use of anti-inflammatory drugs such as colchicine, phenylbutazone, indomethacin, or corticosteroids. After the acute attack subsides, an uricosuric agent or xanthine oxidase inhibitor (allopurinol) is used.[1]

REFERENCES

DIABETES

1. **Allen GE, Hadden DR:** Bullous lesions of the skin in diabetes (bullosis diabeticorum). Brit J Dermatol 82:216, 1970
2. **Bauer MF, et al:** Pigmented pretibial patches. Arch Dermatol 93:232, 1966
3. **Binkley GW:** Dermopathy in diabetes mellitus, transactions of the Cleveland Dermatological Society, September 1964. Arch Dermatol 92:106, 1965
4. **Binkley GW:** Dermopathy in the diabetic syndrome. Arch Dermatol 92:625, 1965
5. **Cantwell AR Jr, Martz W:** Idiopathic bullae in diabetics. Arch Dermatol 96:42, 1967
6. **Fitzpatrick TB:** Dermatologic lesions and diseases associated with diabetes. In Williams RH: Diabetes: With a Chapter on Hypoglycemia, pp 623–641. New York, Paul B Hoeber, 1960
7. **Goldstein H:** Foot care: Basic steps held essential to avert dangers. Diabetes Outlook 10:1, 1975
8. **McGregor RR:** Foot care: Basic steps held essential to avert dangers. Diabetes Outlook 10:2, 1975
9. **Melin H:** An atrophic circumscribed skin lesion in the lower extremities of diabetics. Acta Med Scand 176 [Suppl]:423, 1964
10. **Montes LF, Dobson H, Dodge BG, Knowles JR:** Erythrasma and diabetes mellitus. Arch Dermatol 99:674, 1969
11. **Muller SA:** Dermatologic disorders associated with diabetes mellitus. Mayo Clin Proc 41:689, 1966
12. **Muller SA, Winkelmann RK:** Necrobiosis lipoidica diabeticorum: a clinical and pathological investigation of 171 cases. Arch Dermatol 93:272, 1966
13. **Savin JA:** Bacterial infections in diabetes mellitus. Brit J Dermatol 91:481, 1974
14. **Seder JI:** Management of foot problems in diabetics. J Dermatol Surg Oncol 4:708, 1978
15. **Somerville DA, Lancaster-Smith J:** The aerobic cutaneous micro-flora of diabetic subjects. Brit J Dermatol 89:395, 1973
16. **Ullman S, Dahl MV:** Necrobiosis lipoidica. An immunofluorescence study. Arch Dermatol 113:1671, 1977
17. **Walsh CH, Fitzgerald MG, Soler NG, Malins JM:** Association of foot lesions with retinopathy in patients with newly diagnosed diabetes. Lancet 1:878, 1975

THYROID DISEASE, PRETIBIAL MYXEDEMA, AND ACROPACHY

1. **Bluefarb SM, Adams LA:** Hyperthyroidism, exophthalmos, pretibial myxedema, and early clubbing. Transactions of the Chicago Dermatological Society, May, 1966. Arch Dermatol 95:433, 1967
2. **Cheung HS, Nicoloff MD, Kamiel MB, et al:** Stimulation of fibroblast biosynthetic activity by serum of patients with pretibial myxedema. J Invest Dermatol 71:12, 1978
3. **Freinkel RK, Freinkel N:** Dermatologic manifestations of endocrine disorders. In Fitzpatrick TB, et al (eds): Dermatology in General Practice, 2nd ed, p. 1252. New York, McGraw-Hill, 1979
4. **Gimlette TMD:** Thyroid acropachy. Lancet 1:22, Jan. 2, 1960
5. **Jolliffe DS, Gaylarde PM, Brock AP, et al:** Pretibial myxedema: Stimulation of mucopolysaccharide production of fibroblasts by serum. Brit J Dermatol 100:557, 1979
6. **Lang PG:** Cutaneous manifestations of thyroid disease. Cutis 21:862, 1978
7. **Lever WF, Schaumberg-Lever G:** Histopathology of the skin, 5th ed, p. 404. Philadelphia, JB Lippincott, 1975
8. **Lynch PG, Maize JC, Sisson JC:** Pretibial myxedema and nonthyrotoxic thyroid disease. Arch Dermatol 107:107, 1973
9. **Malkinson FD:** Hyperthyroidism, pretibial myxedema, and clubbing. Arch Dermatol 88:303, Sept., 1963
10. **Nixon DW, Samuls E:** Acral changes associated with thyroid diseases. JAMA 212:175, 1970
11. **Samman PO:** The Nails in Disease, p. 114. London, Wm Kleinemann, 1978
12. **Schermer DR, Roenigk HH Jr, Schumacker OP, McKenzie JM:** Relationship of long-acting thyroid stimulator to pretibial myxedema. Arch Dermatol 102:62, 1970
13. **Trotter WR, Eden KC:** Localized pretibial myxedema in association with toxic goitre. Q J Med 11:229, Oct., 1942

CUTANEOUS AMYLOIDOSIS

1. **Black MM:** The role of the epidermis in the histopathogenesis of lichen amyloidosus. Brit J Dermatol 85:524, 1971
2. **Brownstein MH, Hashimoto K:** Macular amyloidosis. Arch Dermatol 106:50, 1972

3. **Brownstein MH, Helwig EB:** The cutaneous amyloidoses. Arch Dermatol 102:8, 1970
4. **Franklin EC:** Amyloid and amyloidosis of the skin. J Invest Dermatol 67:451, 1976
5. **Rajagopalan K, Tay CH:** Familial lichen amyloidosis: Report of 19 cases in 4 generations of a Chinese family in Malaysia. Brit J Dermatol 87:33, 1972
6. **Stringa SG, Bianchi C, Casala A, et al:** Immunoglobulins and complement C_3 in lichen amyloidosus. Arch Dermatol 105:541, 1972
7. **Wong C-K:** Lichen amyloidosus. Arch Dermatol 110:438, 1974

HYPERLIPOPROTEINEMIAS

1. **Brown MS, Goldstein JL:** Familial hypercholesterolemia: A genetic defect in the low-density lipoprotein receptor. N Engl J Med 294:1386, 1976
2. **Fisher WR, Truitt DH:** The common hyperlipoproteinemias. Ann Intern Med 85:497, 1976
3. **Fredrickson DS, Levy RI, Lees RS:** Fat transport in lipoproteins—an integrated approach to mechanisms and disorders (five parts). N Engl J Med 276:32, 94, 148, 215 and 273, 1967
4. **Goldstein JT, Brown MS:** Familial hypercholesterolemia: Identification of a defect in the regulation of 3-hydroxy-3 methylglutanyl coenzyme. A reductase activity associated with overproduction of cholesterol. Proc Natl Acad Sci USA 70:2804, 1973
5. **Motulsky AG:** The genetic hyperlipidemias. N Engl J Med 294:823, 1976
6. **Parker F:** Section 12-1. In Demis DJ, Dobson RL, McGuire J (eds): Xanthomas in Clinical Dermatology. Hagerstown, Maryland, Harper and Row, 1977

GOUT

1. **Fox TH, Kelley WN:** Management of gout. JAMA 242:361, 1979
2. **Simkin PA:** The pathogenesis of podagra. Ann Intern Med 86:230, 1977

6 NUTRITIONAL DEFICIENCIES

Avitaminosis
  Pellagra
  Scurvy
Zinc Deficiencies

AVITAMINOSIS (PELLAGRA, SCURVY)

The classic vitamin deficiency syndromes, such as beriberi, rickets, pellagra, and scurvy, are now rarely encountered in the United States. However, in those parts of the world where poverty and malnutrition remain endemic, these diseases are common. More often, multiple deficiencies are involved. Not infrequently, skin changes associated with different deficiencies are so similar that they cannot be differentiated.

Vitamin deficiency states result from many factors: improper diet, impaired absorption from the alimentary tract, failure of utilization by the tissues, and inadequate storage. Increased metabolism due to a variety of conditions (*e.g.*, hyperthyroidism, infectious diseases, pregnancy, and lactation) may predispose to the development of clinical deficiency states. In recent years, as part of the environmental conditioning and social customs of our times, new influences leading to nutritional failure have developed. Instead of the inability to obtain food, such problems today are often related to alcoholism, drug addiction, food faddism, and chronic weight reduction. Furthermore, new deficiency states have been induced by chemotherapeutic agents.

The vitamins are divisible into two major groups: the fat-soluble vitamins (A, D, E, and K) and the water-soluble (B-complex and C). Vitamin B and C deficiencies cause pellagra and scurvy, and characteristic skin lesions of these disorders often present on the lower extremities.

PELLAGRA

Pellagra is a clinical syndrome affecting the skin, the alimentary tract, and the central nervous system. Symptoms include glossitis, stomatitis, anorexia, weakness, irritability, abdominal pain, burning sensations in various parts of the body, numbness, forgetfullness, insomnia, morbid fears, and vertigo.

The skin eruption associated with pellagra may appear on any part of the body, but most often it occurs on the exposed areas, particularly over sites of injury. Trauma, pressure, heat, and sun exposure predispose to such skin manifestations. The skin eruption is at first bright red, and it is usually restricted to the areas exposed to the sun: The dorsa of the hands, for instance, are most often involved. Characteristically, there is a fine line of demarcation between the dermatitis and the adjacent healthy skin. Not uncommonly, the face is involved, especially in women and children, and shows a characteristic sparing of narrow bands of skin along the hairline and around the mouth. Involvement across the pellagrin nose and malar areas presents as greasy scaling and follicular plugging, simulating seborrheic dermatitis. Another

117

typical site is a ring (of varying width) around the entire neck (Casal's necklace or collar) or a V-shaped area anteriorly. This necklace with its pendant and the facial skin lesions are often accompanied by a facial expression that reveals the mental depression commonly affecting pellagrins.

In those parts of the world where poverty and malnutrition remain endemic, pellagra is commonly seen on the lower extremities. Following the initial erythema—resembling sunburn with redness, heat, burning, and some edema—the areas take on a dusky, reddish brown color. At this time a fine, thin desquamation appears, later becoming scaly and roughened. An acute eczematous reaction may occur, with subsequent development of fissures and exfoliations (Fig. 6-1). The intensity of pigmentation and thickening increases with each attack. The skin may become either permanently hyperpigmented and thickened, or thin and atrophic with a parchmentlike consistency.

Treatment with nicotinic acid is specific. However, it should be borne in mind that pellagrins are prone to be deficient in other vitamins besides nicotinic acid and that they may not recover until these, along with a good balanced diet, are supplied. In advanced cases, general hospital care may be necessary.

SCURVY

Scurvy is a generalized deficiency syndrome involving the vascular system. Although it is now relatively rare, less severe subclinical forms are not uncommon. Early in the development of the deficiency, lassitude, weakness, irritability, and muscle and joint pains are present, but no skin changes may be noted. The first cutaneous lesions may be manifested as hyperkeratotic papules on the buttocks and calves, closely resembling the cutaneous lesions ascribed to vitamin A deficiency. Hair in these areas takes on a broken "corkscrew" or "pigtail" appearance. Later, the characteristic hermorrhagic phenomena develop in the skin, oral cavity, and internal organs.

Cutaneous bleeding associated with scurvy

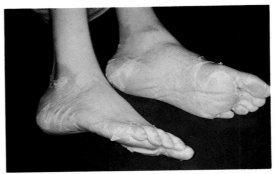

Fig. 6-1. Pellagra due to malabsorption in a postoperative patient with Crohn's disease.

Fig. 6-2. Scurvy. Perifollicular hemorrhages are most common on the lower extremities.

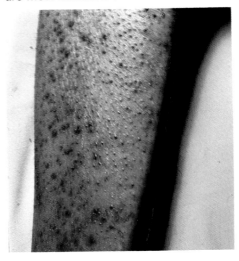

follows several patterns. Perifollicular hemorrhages are most common on the lower extremities (Fig. 6-2), extending later over the abdomen and elsewhere. Ecchymoses or large subcutaneous extravasations are not uncommon. In infants, common findings are subperiosteal hemorrhages, separation of the epiphyses of the long bones, and petechiae.

Determination of vitamin C concentration in the blood and urine, a vitamin C saturation test, and capillary resistance aid in the diagnosis. Although it takes many months for a diet deficient in vitamin C to result in clinical symptoms, administration of the vitamin affects the condition favorably within a few days.

ZINC DEFICIENCY (ACRODERMATITIS ENTEROPATHICA)

Nutritional deficiency of zinc has received much attention in the past two decades, but the unique role of zinc in bringing about improvement remains uncertain.[6] Other than the conclusive evidence that zinc is effective in acrodermatitis enteropathica, which is a manifestation of human zinc deficiency, the use of zinc for a variety of unrelated conditions for which it has been advanced remains to be determined.

Goolamali and Comaish have reviewed the particular effects of zinc and zinc deficiency on the skin.[2] For didactic purposes, those disorders that present with skin lesions on the lower extremities are divided as follows:

1. Nutritional diseases
   a. Inborn errors of metaobolism: e.g., acrodermatitis enteropathica.
   b. Acquired: e.g., kwashiorkor, in alcoholics with malabsorption and zinc deficiency after hyperalimentation.
2. Wound healing, particularly in the use of oral zinc in the treatment of chronic leg ulcers.

NUTRITIONAL DISEASES

The average serum level of zinc is 60 μg/dl. Low serum levels can result from decreased absorption (acrodermatitis enteropathica), increased loss (diarrhea, hyperzincuria), or inadequate intake (long-term intravenous feeding, phytates in food). The skin manifestations of zinc deficiencies resemble acrodermatitis enteropathica.

ACRODERMATITIS ENTEROPATHICA

Acrodermatitis enteropathica is a rare inherited human zinc-deficiency disorder characterized by gastrointestinal disturbances and severe skin lesions on the extremities and around body openings. The systemic disease usually affects infants and children, but it has been reported in adults.

The primary focus of the disease is the gastrointestinal tact. Moynahan proposed the hypothesis that acrodermatitis enteropathica is due to an enzyme (oligopeptidase) defect in the intestinal mucosa, and he suggested that this defect could be related to an inborn error in the absorption of zinc from food.[4]

The skin picture is distinctive. The eruption consists of well-defined vesiculopapulobullous and erythematosquamous patches located around body orifices and on distal parts of the extremities (Fig. 6-3). The perioral area is reportedly affected in all cases. Secondary impetiginization and moniliasis are common. During the resolution of some patches, a psoriasiform appearance becomes manifest. Other common features are nail changes, such as severe paronychia and dystrophy; mucosal changes, consisting of a white coating on the tongue and buccal mucosa in association with marked halitosis; alopecia; retarded body growth; and personality alterations resembling schizophrenia. Chronic diarrhea without evidence of malabsorption syndrome is usually, but not always, present.

Treatment at one time consisted of diio-

Fig. 6-3. Acrodermatitis enteropathica. Erythematosquamous patches on the distal parts of the extremities are a distinctive feature.

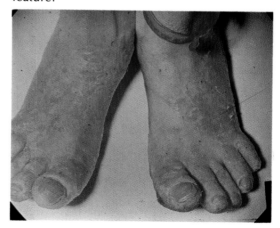

dohydroxyquinolone (Diodoquin) by mouth. However, various investigators have reported reversal of the signs of the disease with use of oral zinc therapy, with dramatic clearing of the skin lesions, restoration of normal bowel function, and rapid increase in the rate of hair growth.

KWASHIORKOR

Kwashiorkor is an example of protein malnutrition, mainly found in children, in which there is a deficiency of almost all the essential elements and vitamins besides protein. Prasad and Oberleas have alluded to the possibly unrecognized zinc deficiency or chronic zinc deficiency states in these children.[5]

Skin lesions in kwashiorkor are characteristic. Hair changes are striking. The skin eruption appears in stages: The first change is an erythema that is soon followed by development of small purple patches. The patches are scattered over the body but are most numerous over the legs, thighs, buttocks, and abdomen. The original florid color changes to dark brown, reddish brown, or black. The patches become dry, hard, scaly, and distinctly raised (enamel paint areas), and they finally desquamate.

ALCOHOLICS WITH MALABSORPTION

A chronic zinc deficiency state can occur in alcoholics with malabsorption. The patients show chronic scaling acrodermatitis, diffuse hair loss, and a pronounced, widespread eczema craquelé.[8]

ZINC DEFICIENCY AFTER HYPERALIMENTATION

This is an iatrogenic disorder due to zinc depletion in patients receiving long-term intravenous feeding.[1,3] An erosive and exudative dermatitis can occur on the feet. The disorder shows a remarkable response to zinc supplementation.

The diagnosis of zinc deficiency is based on the skin manifestations, a low serum zinc level, and response to therapy. Care must be taken in obtaining blood samples, since zinc is a universal contaminant. Specially prepared glassware is essential.

Treatment of zinc deficiency involves correction of the underlying abnormal physiologic state and administration of zinc sulfate, 220 mg t.i.d.

WOUND HEALING

Wound healing is delayed in patients with zinc deficiency; it can be restored to normal with administration of zinc. The use of oral zinc in the treatment of chronic leg ulcers is controversial. It can be categorically said that zinc therapy for venous leg ulcers is probably ineffective, because patients suffering from this disorder are generally not deficient in zinc.[7] This aspect is reviewed in Chapter 14.

REFERENCES

NUTRITIONAL DEFICIENCIES

1. **Bernstein B, Leyden JJ:** Zinc deficiency and acrodermatitis after intravenous hyperalimentation. Arch Dermatol 114:1070, 1978
2. **Goolamali SK, Comaish JS:** Zinc and the skin. Int J Dermatol 14:182, 1975
3. **Kay RG, Tasman-Jones C, Pybus J, et al:** A syndrome of acute zinc deficiency during total parenteral alimentation in man. Ann Surg 183:331, 1976
4. **Moynahan EJ:** Acrodermatitis enteropathica: A lethal inherited human zinc-deficiency disorder. Lancet 2:399, 1974
5. **Prasad AS, Oberleas D:** Zinc: Human nutrition and metabolic effects. Ann Intern Med 73:631, 1970
6. **Ulmer DD:** Trace elements. New Engl J Med 297:318, 1977
7. **Weismann K:** What is the use of zinc for wound healing? Int J Dermatol 17:568, 1978
8. **Weismann K, Roed-Petersen J, Hjorth N, Kopp H:** Chronic zinc deficiency symdrome in a beer drinker with a Billroth II resection. J Int Dermatol 15:757, 1976

7 CUTANEOUS MANIFESTATIONS OF SYSTEMIC DISEASES ON THE LOWER EXTREMITIES

We have noted a curious linkage between certain internal disease syndromes and skin changes on the lower extremities. The nature of the shared characters is obscure, but in view of the frequent associations it is apparent that certain distinctive characteristic lesions on the lower extremities are skin markers of a corresponding internal disease syndrome. Can we hypothesize that separate sets of anatomically specialized cells develop during embryonic life?

Lesions of connective tissue diseases such as lupus erythematosus (LE), dermatomyositis, scleroderma, and rheumatoid arthritis (RA) can occur on the lower extremities, but predilection for this region is not an essential clinical feature of these diseases.

LUPUS ERYTHEMATOSUS

Discoid lupus erythematosus (DLE) and signs of systemic lupus erythematosus (SLE) occur on the lower extremities. DLE and SLE represent different ends of one spectrum of an immunologic abnormality. All tissue damage—in the skin, in blood vessels, in the kidney—is related to the presence of DNA/anti-DNA circulating in the blood. The deposition of these antigen-antibody complexes, demonstrated by *in vitro* tests, leads to the fixation of complement, which in turn becomes activated with the release of chemotactic factors.

The cutaneous pathologic features of DLE and SLE are quite similar and is of little help in differentiating between the two forms. Far more important is the immunopathologic investigation. Immunoglobulins and complement (IgC) are demonstrated in the region of the epidermal-dermal junction both in the lesions and in the unchanged skin of patients with SLE; in DLE, fluorescence is positive in skin lesions and negative in unchanged skin. The immunofluorescent skin test is now considered the most reliable for the diagnosis of both DLE and SLE.

The diagnosis of lupus erythematosus is made on the basis of (1) clinical findings (history, type of lesion, and distribution); (2) histopathology; (3) serologic examination (elevated ESR, reversal of A/G ratio, leukopenia, thrombocytopenia, positive rheumatoid factor, biologic false-positive Wasserman [BFP], normochromic and normocytic anemia, positive LE cells, immunofluorescent antinuclear antibodies); and (4) special tests and procedures (immunofluorescent skin tests, chest x-ray).

Figure 7-1 illustrates the clinical feature of DLE: sharply outlined patches, initially erythematous, with peripheral activity and infiltration, adherent scales, and subsequent central atropic scar formation with depigmentation and telangiectasia. The discoid patch is pathognomonic of LE; it may also occur in SLE.

The most common cutaneous manifestations of SLE on the lower extremities are lesions of a generalized eruption simulating measles, scarlatina, or a toxic reaction. Diffuse erythema may cover the soles. Petechiae, purpura, and ecchymoses are also observed.

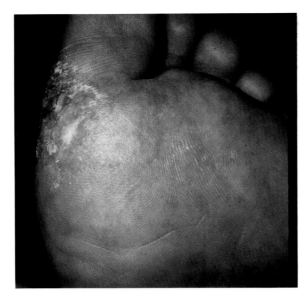

Fig. 7-1. Discoid lesions in a patient with SLE. The erythema, adherent scales, telangiectasia and atrophy are characteristic. *(Courtesy of Dr. H. Lemont)*

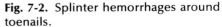

Fig. 7-2. Splinter hemorrhages around toenails.

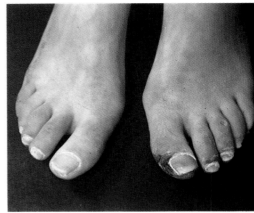

Fig. 7-3. Necrotizing vasculitis on the lower extremities is a hallmark of SLE. *(Courtesy of Dr. S. Moschella)*

Fig. 7-4. Necrotizing vasculitis of SLE.

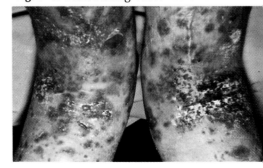

These lesions may be related to thrombocytopenia, to vasculitis, or to prolonged steroid therapy. Splinter hemorrhages around and in the toenails are of considerable importance and often tend to be indicative of the severity of the disease (Fig. 7-2). Livedo reticularis, primarily on the lower extremities and associated with leg ulcers sequential to necrotizing angiitis, is another hallmark of SLE (Figs. 7-3, 7-4). The lower extremity is the common site for necrotizing ulcers associated with SLE. Occasionally, the typical eruption of SLE may become manifest in the partially ischemic areas of the livedo pattern.

Chilblain lupus erythematosus, a chronic unremitting form of LE seen predominantly in women, has been reported by Millard and Rowell. It occurs commonly on the digits, calves, and heels and presents as a purplish-blue discoloration.[1] The chilblain lesions are the result of microvascular injury secondary to exposure to cold and possibly hyperviscosity from immunologic abnormalities. None of the usual treatments for cutaneous LE is effective for the chilblain lesions.

Fever and arthralgia are common (90% of patients); myalgia occurs in 50% and Raynaud's phenomenon in approximately 20% of patients.

TREATMENT

For treatment of connective tissue diseases (LE, dermatomyositis, scleroderma, RA), the reader is referred to general medical texts.

DERMATOMYOSITIS

Dermatomyositis is essentially a pattern of muscle inflammation producing a constellation of clinical, pathologic, electrical, and biochemical changes with a wide variety of clinical manifestations. The lower extremity shares in the general involvement of this disease. Muscle involvement (tenderness and diminution of strength) is usually prominent; in more advanced disease, the pelvic girdle and thigh muscles are usually the most severely affected.

The etiology is obscure. Muscle virus disease, upper respiratory tract infections, mesenchymal disease, malignancy, drug and immunization reactions, and sunburn have been reported as precipitating factors. Because of the coexistence of other collagen diseases—especially scleroderma, Sjögren's disease, and rheumatoid arthritis—with myositis, it has been suggested that dermatomyositis may fit under the umbrella of autoimmunity. Serologic factors that imply an immunologic disorder, however, are not always present or specific, and immunofluorescent techniques have not demonstrated localization of immunoglobulins or complement to muscle.

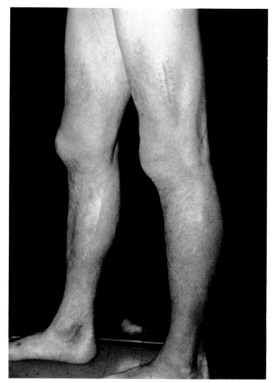

Fig. 7-5. "Salt and pepper" appearance of poikiloderma in dermatomyositis.

The diagnosis of typical dermatomyositis is made on the basis of: (1) clinical findings: history, type of lesions, distribution, and potential for malignancy; (2) histopathology: skin biopsy resembles subacute LE and is not pathognomonic, but muscle biopsy revealing degenerative changes is definite; (3) serum enzyme measurements: elevated SGOT, SGPT, LDH, CPK, and aldolase levels reveal muscle fiber destruction; and (4) special tests and procedures: electromyography to delineate a myopathic process and soft-tissue x-rays to demonstrate calcinosis.

The characteristic skin manifestations on the face (a heliotropic appearance, violaceous color, narrowing of the palpebral fissures, and edema of the eyelids), and the dusky red, poikilodermic patches over bony prominences such as the knuckles and proximal interphalangeal joints (Gottron's papules), elbows, and knees are sufficiently typical to permit a presumptive diagnosis;

however, a deep muscle biopsy is essential to confirm it. Estimation of serum enzyme levels facilitates the diagnosis, determination of the activity of the disease, and its response to therapy. Other features of the disease are Raynaud's phenomenon and minimal or moderate transitory arthralgia. The association of malignancy with dermatomyositis has been well documented: The incidence is approximately five to seven times greater than in the general population. The most common tumor sites are the breast, lung (bronchogenic), ovary, stomach, colon, and uterus.

Winkelmann *et al* described two peaks in the age of distribution, one in the first decade of life and the other in the fifth and sixth decades.[7] The sex ratio was two females to one male. The onset of childhood dermatomyositis is insidious but can be acute or fulminating. Calcinosis cutis, with subsequent physical disability and contractures, is a predominant feature. It is three times more common in children than in adults, and it constitutes a favorable prognostic sign of survival. Raynaud's phenomenon is rare, and malignancies are not associated.

Typical skin lesions on the lower extremities are dusky red, poikilodermic patches over bony prominences; older lesions show more advanced poikilodermic atrophy and pigmentation, giving rise at times to a "salt and pepper" appearance (Fig. 7-5).[4] Cuticular changes of the fingers are a consistent finding; the alterations result from circulatory stasis, yet ironically, they are not observed on the toe cuticles where one would expect stasis to be more formidable because of dependency.[3] Dermatomyositis can cause indolent, ulcerating undermined skin lesions, especially over the malleoli.

SCLERODERMA

Scleroderma has been defined as a disease complex composed of vascular changes, fibrosis, and inflammation that to varying degrees involves skin and visceral organs.[6] Clinically, scleroderma appears in two forms, localized and generalized or systemic.

Acrosclerosis accounts for 95% of all cases of scleroderma. Acrosclerosis involves predominantly the skin of the face, the upper part of the chest, the hands, the forearms, and, occasionally, the feet. Vasospastic phenomena of the hands with arthralgia are prominent and may precede the earliest cutaneous changes. Varying degrees of systemic involvement may occur, the gastrointestinal, pulmonary, and cardiorenal systems being most frequently affected. The course of the disease is usually episodic, with variable periods of arrest and exacerbation.

In contrast to the other "collagen" diseases, scleroderma is characterized by a lack of significant laboratory changes; immunoglobulin levels are not of predictive or diagnostic value. The cutaneous changes evolve through three clinical phases: the edematous, the indurative, and the atrophic. The lower extremity also shares in the general involvement in this disease. The skin is firm and waxy; diffuse or mottled melanosis or depigmentation, and obliteration of normal cutaneous lines, are characteristic (Fig. 7-6). Multiple telangiectasia and calcinosis cutis, frequently seen in scleroderma, are not uncommon on the legs. Atrophic changes as well as necrotic ulcerations and even gangrene can develop on the feet. Lower-leg ulcers have been reported in 40% of cases. The ulcers are of the ischemic type, resulting from small-blood-vessel disease. They are usually sharply demarcated in appearance and cause severe pain.

Eosinophilic fasciitis (fasciitis with eosinophilia) is a variant of scleroderma which frequently presents with signs on the lower extremities.[1,2] The syndrome was described by Shulman in 1974.[4a]

Eosinophilic fasciitis occurs more often in males and frequently follows strenuous exertion or trauma to the limbs. The disease is characterized by a rapid evolution of pain, tenderness, and sclerosis symmetrically involving the subcutaneous tissue of the arms and legs. A solid edema can also be part of the picture. The overlying skin may present a cobblestone appearance and may feel irregularly nodular. A transient eosinophilia up to 30%, elevated erythrocyte sedimentation rate, and hyperglobulinemia are characteristic of the syndrome. Diagnosis is confirmed with excision biopsy, which shows histologic features of subcutaneous scleroderma. Immunohistologic studies demonstrate IgG and C_3 in the deep fascia and muscle septa.[2] Although rapid improvement following administration of systemic corticosteroids is often obtained, some cases have involuted spontaneously.[1] Long-term follow-up has revealed that some patients eventually develop scleroderma; thus, eosinophilic fasciitis may be just another variant of the scleroderma syndrome.[5]

RHEUMATOID ARTHRITIS

On the basis of our clinical experiences and a review of recent pertinent literature, we will simply list the cutaneous manifestations of rheumatoid arthritis (RA) occurring on the lower extremities.[1–8]

1. Rheumatoid vasculitis
   a. Obliterative intimal proliferation of the digital arteries leading to digital ischemia and microinfarctions, usually around the nails. These are usually transitory and painless.
   b. Subacute lesions in the small vessels of the skin.
   c. Fulminant, widespread necrotizing arteritis indistinguishable at times from systemic polyarteritis nodosa.
   Cutaneous signs of (b) and (c) include bullae, purpura, ulceration, and gangrene. Vasculitis usually occurs in severe, chronic RA with high-titer rheumatoid factor and prominent rheumatoid nodules, often in a patient who is being treated or has been treated with systemic corticosteroids.
2. Raynaud's phenomenon
3. Pyoderma gangrenosum
4. Subcutaneous nodules—especially on areas subjected to pressure
5. Inflammatory edema with lower extremity swelling due to inflammatory synovitis or rheumatoid vasculitis
6. Cutaneous atrophy and bronzing, including nail plate atrophy
7. Coldness of the feet with or without hyperhidrosis
8. Cutaneous signs of cryoglobulinemia, which may be present as leg ulcers, urticaria, purpura, livedo reticularis, and Raynaud's phenomenon
9. Dysproteinemic purpura of the hypergammaglobulinemic type—dependent and nonpalpable
10. Leg ulcers
    a. Ischemia—localized vascular ischemia is frequently a precursor of areas of ulceration, which are usually shallow and well demarcated. The ulcers are usually painful and heal very slowly, especially if infected.
    b. Rheumatoid vasculitis—ulcers may or may not be steroid-induced. The most frequent cause of necrotic skin lesions in patients with RA is vasculitis, of the leukocytoclastic or polyarteritis type (Fig. 7-7).
    c. Felty's syndrome—leg ulcers are said to be more common in this syndrome of rheumatoid arthritis, splenomegaly, and leukopenia.
    d. Post-traumatic—skin is often atrophic, and this may be accentuated with iatrogenic Cushing's syndrome produced by systemic steroids.
    e. Neuropathic ulcer—due to peripheral neuropathy, which may be seen in rheumatoid arthritis.
    f. Leg ulcers associated with cryoglobulinemia.
    g. Decubitus ulcers associated with the immobilization due to this disease—especially on malleoli, heels, sides of feet, and knees.
11. Livedo reticularis—may be seen with rheumatoid vasculitis and cryoglobulinemia
12. Psoriasis (???)—if we consider psoriatic arthritis a variant of rheumatoid arthritis
13. Pedal edema is sometimes seen in the absence of cardiac, renal, hepatic, or nutritional disease and is probably physiologic (gravitational or orthostatic) in nature

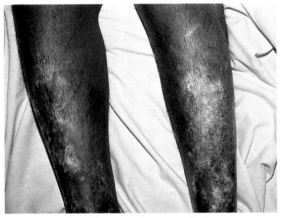

Fig. 7-6. Scleroderma. Note mottled melanosis and depigmentation; the skin has a waxy appearance.

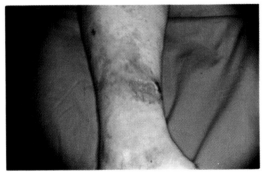

Fig. 7-7. Ulcer complicating rheumatoid arthritis.

PYODERMA GANGRENOSUM

Pyoderma gangrenosum (PG), a rare clinical lesion, is a morphologic description of an inflammatory response presenting as a reaction pattern in the skin. The distinctive features of PG are listed in Table 7-1.

Pyoderma gangrenosum was traditionally linked with ulcerative colitis, but new findings have expanded the association to other systemic diseases. About 50% of all patients with PG have ulcerative colitis, but PG can be associated with other bowel diseases such

Table 7-1. PYODERMA GANGRENOSUM (PG)

The lesions usually present on the lower extremities; also on trunk, upper extremities, face, and mouth

Lesions include papules, pustules, and plaques that can evolve and resolve without passing through an ulcerative stage (Fig. 7-8).

Aspiration from lesions of PG before ulceration shows no bacterial growth. The role of bacteria cultured from ulcerated lesions is that of secondary invaders or colonizers.

Salient clinical feature of PG is the rapid development of a necrotizing ulceration.

Phagedenic ulcerations are characteristic: painful, the borders are undermined and boggy and surrounded by a bluish-red areola. Ulcers heal with cribriform type of scar (Fig. 7-9; Fig. 7-10).

Diagnosis clinical: histopathology is characteristic but not pathognomonic; no specific laboratory changes.

as Crohn's disease, active chronic hepatitis, carcinoid, and diverticulitis. It also can be an important cutaneous manifestation of a variety of different systemic diseases in association with myeloproliferative disorders, polyarthritis and rheumatoid arthritis, paraproteinemia (including multiple myeloma), drug reactions, and delayed altered hypersensitivity. In some patients with PG, no associated systemic disease can be demonstrated.

In our studies of PG, systemic associations were defined in 18 patients in a series of 240 cases of ulcerative colitis, and in 6 in a series of 210 patients with Crohn's disease; two cases were associated with polyarthritis—one patient with leukemia and one with drug hypersensitivity.[15] In six other patients with PG, no associated systemic disease was found.

Various theories concerning the cause of PG have been considered. In our studies of PG, in association with ulcerative colitis and Crohn's disease, vasculitis was an important finding, and a defect in the cellular or humoral immune mechanism was hypothesized.[12–14,16,17] Support of this concept can be elucidated from the study of Lazarus *et al*, although the patients with PG in their study had no related colonic disease.[6] Other theories proposed include a localized Shwartzman reaction, intravascular coagulation, altered immunoglobulins, and skin-graft rejection reactions.[2,3,5,11,16,19] Because the lesions occur predominantly on the legs, one must consider that the relative venous hy-

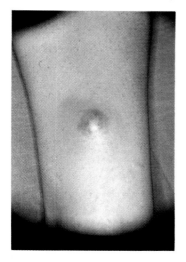

Fig. 7-8. Close-up of an early inflammatory lesion (24 hours old) of pyoderma gangrenosum. The pronounced bluish red areola is characteristic.

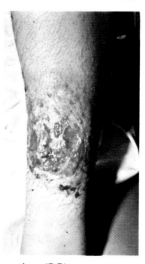

Fig. 7-10. Necrotizing ulceration (PG) complicating Crohn's disease in a 19-year-old girl.

Fig. 7-9. Severe phagedenic ulceration in patient with pyoderma gangrenosum in association with ulcerative colitis.

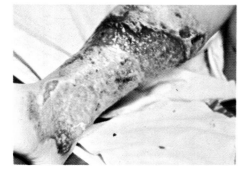

1. Infections
   a. Bacterial pyoderma
   b. Atypical mycobacteria
   c. Deep fungi
   d. Insect bites
2. Necrotizing vasculitis
3. Collagen diseases: LE, RA
4. Bromoderma and iododerma
5. Syphilis
6. Factitial

In order to establish an etiologic diagnosis, the following studies are suggested:

1. Biopsy—2 sections
   a. Histology
   b. Culture (atypical mycobacteria, fungi)
2. Complete GI evaluation
3. CBC and bone marrow, if indicated
4. RF, ANA, LE prep.
5. Serum protein electrophoresis, cryoglobulins
6. VDRL
7. Serum bromide
8. Evaluation of delayed hypersensitivy (purified protein derivative, mumps, candidiasis, and so forth; DNCB patch test)

pertension of the lower extremities may be conducive to the extravasation of a circulating agent through the venule walls with subsequent sequestration in the interstices of the skin.

The mechanism by which PG and systemic disease are related is still obscure. Further studies are necessary to provide a better understanding of this unusual skin reaction.

Skin lesions due to local factors or associated with a variety of different systemic diseases can present with features resembling PG. The conditions to be considered in the differential diagnosis include:

Many forms of treatment have been proposed for PG. No form of treatment is effective unless the underlying disease process is controlled; for the bowel association, treatment is a synthesis of skin and gut care. We have observed that medical or surgical control of the ulcerative colitis or Crohn's disease often results in simultaneous improvement in the skin complication, but this correlation may not always be the case.[4]

Treatment regimens for PG–bowel diseases are listed next.

1. Cooperation with gastroenterologist in managing the patient
   a. Restoration of normal state of nutrition
   b. Salicylazosulfapyridine (Azulfidine), prednisone, immunosuppresives (Azathioprine)
2. Other systemic therapy: Clofazimine (Lamprene), minocycline (HCl), dapsone[1,7,8,20]
3. Local care of the ulcer
   a. Gentian violet, compresses, and debridement
   b. Intralesional steroids[9]
   c. Hyperbaric oxygen[18]
   d. H_2O_2 compresses and Gelfoam packing
   e. Benzoyl peroxide[10]

In our experience, treatment of the ulcer with hydrogen peroxide compresses followed by Gelfoam packing or the application of benzoyl peroxide paste was the measure of choice in the local management of PG. Benzoyl peroxide has shown a unique ability to stimulate epithelial cell proliferation and the production of granulation tissue.

In those cases in which GI associations are not revealed, variations of this regimen will depend on the existing underlying systemic disease.

GLUCAGONOMA SYNDROME

The glucagonoma syndrome (GS) is a rare clinical condition characterized by a distinctive cutaneous eruption associated with a glucagon-secreting alpha-cell tumor of the pancreas.[2] The disorder has also been described as "necrolytic migratory erythema" presenting as chronic desquamating lesions with pseudobulla formation affecting particularly the groins, perineum, and limbs.[5] This syndrome appears to be predominantly a disease of women.

The feet and legs are commonly affected. There is a predilection for lesions to occur in sites of cutaneous trauma. The eruption is both characteristic and bizarre. Early in the clinical course, it often resembles asteatotic eczema; subsequently; annular and circinate lesions and plaques with central erythema, collapsed blisters, oozing, crusting, erosions, and hyperpigmentation appear.[1,3,4] Besides skin lesions, other symptoms are glossitis, weight loss, abnormal glucose tolerance, and anemia. On histologic examination, the most specific features include necrolysis of the upper epidermis with liquefaction necrosis of the granular cell layer and subcorneal clefting or blister formation. Elevated serum glucagon levels help define the origin of the tumor.

MIGRATORY THROMBOPHLEBITIS

Migratory thrombophlebitis (MT) can be an important diagnostic clue to cancer of the pancreas and lung. More than 40% of the cases of MT were attributed to pancreatic cancers; other studies suggest that carcinoma of the lung is the most common associated neoplasm.[1–6]

The lesions of thrombophlebitis migrans are usually multiple and may involve any part of the trunk or extremities. They are reddened, intensely inflamed, tender, and frequently fulminant. They appear, gradually subside within a few weeks, and then recur along the course of the same or a neighboring vein. Fever and leukocytosis accompany each flare-up. It has been speculated that since the condition occurs predominantly with cancer of the pancreas, mucolytic and other proteolytic enzymes may affect clotting; another theory presupposes the elaboration of a substance by the tumor cells that alters the clotting mechanism. From the clinical view, cryptic cancer, particularly in the pancreas or in the lung, should be suspected when a patient older than 40 years of age has apparently spontaneous thrombophlebitis with a discernible cause.

Subcutaneous nodular fat necrosis, a skin marker of pancreatic disease, also may present with carcinoma of the pancreas. This syndrome is discussed in Chapter 4.

BULLOUS ERUPTIONS

Bullous lesions that connote systemic disease and tend to localize on the lower extremities are not uncommon. Representative disorders are listed next.

Congenital, hereditary: epidermolysis bullosa, simple and dystrophic types

Endocrine and metabolic: idiopathic bullous diabeticorum; porphyria cutanea tarda; bullous dermatosis of chronic renal failure

Toxic: toxic epidermal necrolysis

Infectious: vesicobullous syphilis (soles of infants)

Neurologic: coma from any cause

Vascular: intravascular-coagulation-fibrinolysis syndrome (hemorrhagic bullae)

Idiopathic: chronic bullous dermatosis of childhood; bullous pyoderma gangrenosum (with myeloproliferative disease)

These bullous dermadromes must be differentiated from diseases such as erythema multiforme, pemphigus vulgaris, bullous pemphigoid, and dermatitis herpetiformis that can occur on the legs and feet as a part of a widespread eruption; from infectious diseases such as bullous herpes zoster, bullous impetigo and erysipelas, bullous arthropod bites, bullous scabies, and inflammatory dermatophyte infections, especially *T. mentagrophytes;* and from localized bullous reactions caused by friction, chemical- or thermal-induced blisters, self-induced blisters (factitious), and bullous reactions of contact allergic dermatitis.

DRUG REACTIONS

One must always be alert to the fact that presenting skin lesions may be due to drugs, and drug reactions can mimic almost any type of skin eruption. With the ever-increasing use of drugs (self-medications, patent medicines, as well as prescribed medications), more adverse reactions are constantly noted. Skin rashes are probably the most common manifestations of adverse drug reactions and may also be accompanied by visceral reactions. The lower extremities are often affected as part of a general eruption, but in some instances the topographic predilection is distinctive. In this section, we mention some characteristic drug reactions that occur mainly on the lower extremities. For detailed information on the classification and mechanisms of adverse drug reactions, the reader is referred to the many texts dealing with this important subject.

Diseases that prefer the lower extremities in which drugs can be a major causal factor or the primary cause include the following.

Erythema nodosum—sulfonamides, salicylates, barbiturates, penicillin, and so forth.

Necrotizing vasculitis—penicillin, sulfonamides, phenylbutazone, polythiouracil, chlordane, lindane. Drug abuse.

Palmo-plantar keratoderma (arsenical keratoses)—chronic inorganic arsenic poisoning.

Halogenodermas (granulomas, ulcers)—bromides.

Drug Induced Swollen Legs
(see Chap. 13)

Causes of swollen legs include these factors:

Hormones (corticosteroids, estrogen, progesterone, testosterone, aldosterone-like substances)

Antihypertensives (Ismelin, Apresoline, Rauwolfia, aldomet, monamine oxidase inhibitors)

Anti-inflammatory drugs (phenylbutazone)

Coumarin necrosis (Dicumarol and warfarin) occurs in over-anticoagulated patients taking oral anticoagulants.[2,3] The patients are usually obese females. The lesions occur in areas where subcutaneous fat is generous, *e.g.,* thigh, buttock. Initially the lesions are tender and erythematous, progressing rapidly to central blistering and gangrenous necrosis. Eschar formation and sloughing of skin and subcutaneous tissue follow, leaving deep ulcers that resemble reactions produced by application of strong escharotic chemicals.

Purple toes are deep-purple discolorations

of the toes, soles, and dorsal aspect of the feet following coumarin therapy.[1,4] This is probably a forme-fruste syndrome of coumarin necrosis.

REFERENCES

LUPUS ERYTHEMATOSUS

1. **Millard LG, Rowell NR:** Chilblain lupus erythematosus (Hutchinson). Brit J Dermatol 98:497, 1978

DERMATOMYOSITIS; SCLERODERMA

1. **Jarrett M, Bybee JD, Ramsdell W:** Eosinophilic fasciitis: An early variant of scleroderma. J Am Acad Dermatol 1:221, 1979
2. **Rodan GP, DiBartolomeo AG, Medsger TA Jr, Barnes EL Jr:** Eosinophilis fasciitis: report of 7 cases of a newly recognized scleroderma-like syndrome. Arthritis Rheum 18:422, 1975
3. **Samitz MH:** Cuticular lesions in dermatomyositis. Arch Dermatol 110:866, 1974
4. **Samitz MH:** Cutaneous lesions of the lower extremities in the diagnosis of systemic disease. J Amer Pod Assoc 65:556, 1975
4a. **Shulman LE:** Diffuse fasciitis with hypergammaglobulinemia and eosinophilia: A new syndrome. J Rheumatol 1 (suppl 1):46, 1974
5. **Torres VM, George WM:** Diffuse eosinophilic fasciitis. Arch Dermatol 113:1591, 1977
6. **Winkelmann RK:** Pathogenesis and staging of scleroderma. Acta Dermatovener (Stockholm) 56:83, 1976
7. **Winkelmann RK, Mulder DW, Lambert EH, et al:** Course of dermatomyositis-polymyositis: Comparison of untreated and cortisone treated patients. Mayo Clin Proc 43:545, 1968

RHEUMATOID ARTHRITIS

1. **Ball J:** Rheumatoid arthritis and polyarteritis nodosa. Ann Rheum Dis 13:277, 1954
2. **Cruickshank B:** The arteritis of rheumatoid arthritis. Ann Rheum Dis 13:136, 1954
3. **Hollander JL (ed):** Arthritis and Allied Conditions, A Textbook of Rheumatology, 8th ed. Philadelphia, Lea & Febiger, 1972
4. **Kemper JW, et al:** The relationship of therapy with cortisone to the incidence of vascular lesions in rheumatoid arthritis. Ann Intern Med 46:831, 1957
5. **O'Quinn SE, et al:** Peripheral vascular lesions in rheumatoid arthritis. Arch Dermatol 92:489, 1965
6. **Rodan GP (ed):** Primer on the Rheumatic Diseases. JAMA (Suppl), pp 687–700, Apr 30, 1973
7. **Schroeter AL, et al:** Immunoglobulin and complement deposition in the skin of rheumatoid arthritis and systemic lupus erythematosus patients. Rheum Dis 35:321, 1976
8. **Soderstrom CW:** Cutaneous manifestations of rheumatoid arthritis. Cutis 24:553, 1979

PYODERMA GANGRENOSUM

1. **Altman J, Mopper C:** Pyoderma gangrenosum treated with sulfone drugs. Minn Med 49:22, 1966
2. **Dantzig PI:** Pyoderma gangrenosum, N Engl J Med 292:47, 1975
3. **Delesclose J, Bast C, Achten G:** Pyoderma gangrenosum with altered cellular immunity and immunity and dermonecrotic factor. Brit Dermatol 87:529, 1972
4. **Johnson ML, Wilson HTH:** Skin lesions in ulcerative colitis. Gut 10:255, 1969
5. **Lang PI, Uesu LT:** Pyoderma gangrenosum. JAMA 187:336, 1964
6. **Lazarus GS, Goldsmith LA, Rocklin RE, et al:** Pyoderma gangrenosum, altered delayed hypersensitivity and polyarthritis. Arch Dermatol 105:46, 1972
7. **Lynch WS, Bergfeld WF:** Pyoderma gangrenosum responsive to minocycline hydrochloride. Cutis 21:535, 1978
8. **Michaelsson G, Molin L, Ohman S, et al:** Clofazamine: A new agent for the treatment of pyoderma gangrenosum. Arch Dermatol 112:344, 1976
9. **Moschella SJ:** Pyoderma gangrenosum. Arch Dermatol 95:121, 1967
10. **Nguyen LQ, Weiner J:** Treatment of pyoderma gangrenosum with benzoyl peroxide. Cutis 19:842, 1977
11. **Rostenberg A:** The Shwartzman phenomenon: A review with a consideration of some dermatological manifestations. Brit J Dermatol 65:389, 1953
12. **Samitz MH:** Cutaneous vasculitis in association with ulcerative colitis. Cutis 2:383, 1966
13. **Samitz MH:** Skin complications of ulcerative colitis and Crohn's disease (with special reference to pyoderma gangrenosum). Cutis 12:533, 1973
14. **Samitz MH:** Dermatologic-gastrointestinal relationships. Chap 166 In Bockus Gastroenterology, 3rd Ed. Philadelphia, WB Saunders Co, 1976

15. **Samitz MH:** Pyoderma gangrenosum in association with ulcerative colitis and Crohn's disease. Proc Bockus Int Soc Gastroenterol, 1978
16. **Samitz MH, Hanshaw WJ:** Pyoderma gangrenosum in association with regional enteritis and dysgammaglobulinemia. Cutis 9:57, 1972
17. **Samitz MH, Dana AS Jr, Rosenberg P:** Cutaneous vasculitis in association with Crohn's disease—Review of statistics of skin complications. Cutis 6:51, 1970
18. **Thomas CY Jr, Crouch JA, Guastello J:** Hyperbaric oxygen therapy for pyoderma gangrenosum. Arch Dermatol 110:445, 1974
19. **Thompson DM, Main RA, Beck JS, et al:** Studies on a patient with leukocytoclastic vasculitis, pyoderma gangrenosum and paraproteinemia. Brit J Dermatol 88:117, 1973
20. **Thomsen K, Rothenborg HW:** Clofazamine in the treatment of pyoderma gangrenosum. Arch Dermatol 115:851, 1979

GLUCAGONOMA SYNDROME

1. **Binnick AN, Spencer SK, Dennison WL Jr, et al:** Glucagonoma syndrome. Arch Dermatol 113:749, 1977
2. **McGavran MH, Unger RH, Recant L, et al:** A glucagon-secreting alpha-cell carcinoma of the pancreas. N Engl J Med 274:1408–1413, 1966
3. **Pedersen NB, Jonsson L, Holst JJ:** Necrolytic migratory erythema and glucagon cell tumour of the pancreas. The glucagonoma syndrome. Acta Dermatovener 56:391–395, 1976
4. **Swenson KH, Amon RB, Hanifin JB:** The glucagonoma syndrome. Arch Dermatol 114:224, 1978

5. **Wilkinson DS:** Necrolytic migrating erythema with carcinoma of the pancreas. Trans St Johns Hosp Dermatol Soc 59:244–250, 1973

MIGRATORY THROMBOPHLEBITIS

1. **Byrd RB, Divertie MB, Spittell JA:** Bronchogenic carcinoma and thromboembolic disease. JAMA 202:1019, 1967
2. **Edwards EA:** Migrating thrombophlebitis associated with carcinoma. N Engl J Med 240:1031, 1949
3. **Kenney WE:** Association of carcinoma in the body and tail of the pancreas with multiple venous thrombi. Surgery 14:600, 1943
4. **Nusbacher J:** Migratory venous thrombosis and cancer. NY State J Med 64:2166, 1964
5. **Sproul EE:** Carcinoma and venous thrombosis, the frequency of association of carcinoma in the body or tail of the pancreas with multiple venous thrombosis. Am J Cancer 34:566, 1938
6. **Wooling KR, Shick RM:** Thrombophlebitis: A possible clue to cryptic malignant lesions. Proc Staff Meet Mayo Clin 31:227, 1956

DRUG REACTIONS

1. **Feder W, Auerbach R:** "Purple toes": an uncommon sequela of oral coumarin drug therapy. Ann Intern Med 55:911, 1961
2. **Jones RR, Cunningham J:** Warfarin skin necrosis. Brit J Dermatol 100:561, 1975
3. **Lacy JP, Goodin RR:** Warfarin-induced necrosis of skin. Ann Intern Med 82:381, 1975
4. **Schleicher SM, Fricher MP:** Coumarin necrosis. Arch Dermatol 116:444, 1980

8 PEDIATRIC-DERMATOLOGIC PROBLEMS ON THE LOWER EXTREMITIES*

Cutaneous disorders that affect the lower extremities are an important aspect of pediatric dermatology. Such conditions frequently present a challenge not only to dermatologists, but to pediatricians, podiatrists, and family practitioners as well. Although there are a multiplicity of cutaneous disorders seen on the lower extremities of infants and children as well as adults, the cutaneous conditions discussed in this section include vascular disorders, shoe dermatitis, lichen striatus, frictional lichenoid dermatitis, the Gianotti-Crosti syndrome, infantile acropustulosis, scabies, Henoch-Schönlein purpura, Letterer-Siwe disease (histiocytosis X), and Kawasaki disease.

VASCULAR DISORDERS

ACROCYANOSIS

In a great number of infants, a purplish discoloration of the hands, feet, and lips occurs during periods of crying, breath-holding, or chilling. This normal phenomenon, termed "acrocyanosis," appears to be associated with an increased tone of peripheral arterioles which in turn create vasospasm, secondary dilatation, pooling of blood in the venous plexuses, and a cyanotic appearance in the involved areas. The intensity of cyanosis depends upon the degree of oxygen

*Contributed by Sidney Hurwitz, M.D., Associate Clinical Professor, Pediatrics and Dermatology, Yale University School of Medicine, New Haven, Conn.

loss and the depth, size, and fullness of the involved venous plexuses.

CUTIS MARMORATA

Cutis marmorata is a normal reticulated bluish mottling of the skin seen on the trunk and extremities of infants and young children. This phenomenon, a physiologic response to chilling with resultant dilatation of capillaries and small venules, usually disappears as the infant is rewarmed. Although a tendency to cutis marmorata may persist several weeks or months, this disorder bears no medical significance, and treatment is generally unnecessary. In some children, however, it should be noted that cutis marmorata may tend to recur until early childhood, and in patients with Down syndrome, trisomy 18, and Cornelia de Lange syndrome, this reticulated marbling pattern may persist.[7,16]

CUTIS MARMORATA TELANGIECTATICA CONGENITA

Cutis marmorata telangiectatica congenita (congenital generalized phlebectasia) is a relatively uncommon disorder of infants and children characterized by a reticulated bluish mottling of the skin which resembles an exaggerated form of cutis marmorata. Seen in males as well as females (contrary to many statements in current literature and textbooks), the disorder is seen as dilated reticulated venous and capillary channels which measure three to four millimeters or more in diameter.

In most patients the vascular pattern is distributed in a generalized manner over the trunk and extremities. In some, however, the involvement may be segmental or localized to one extremity or to a limited portion of the trunk. Ulcerations over the reticular vascular pattern have been seen in a few patients with this disorder. In general, however, cutis marmorata telangiectatica congenita has a benign course and requires no specific therapy. Since other defects have been reported in individuals with this disorder (hemangiomatous abnormalities and varicosities, patent ductus arteriosus, congenital glaucoma with mental retardation, branchial cleft cysts, and atrophy or hypertrophy of soft tissue or bone), patients should be followed carefully for the possibility of associated malformations.[1,14]

DIFFUSE PHLEBECTASIA (BROCKENHEIMER SYNDROME)

Diffuse phlebectasia is a rare hamartomatous malformation which involves the deeper venous channels of a limb or part of a limb. Characterized by gradual onset during infancy, childhood, adolescence, or early adult life, it consists of multiple, spongy, irregular venous sinusoids and dilated veins that assume bizarre patterns with tumor-like vascular swelling of the involved area. The overlying skin may be atrophic, and secondary complications consist of thromboses and phleboliths with resultant bleeding, ulceration, or infection of the affected limb.

KLIPPEL-TRENAUNAY-PARKES-WEBER SYNDROME

The Klippel-Trenaunay-Parkes-Weber syndrome (nevus vasculosus hypertophicus) is a vascular malformation characterized by local overgrowth of the bone and soft tissue of an extremity or portion of the trunk associated with phlebectasia, arteriovenous aneurysms, and cutaneous telangiectasia resembling a port-wine stain. More often an upper rather than a lower extremity, with the left rather than the right side of the body, is involved. The hypertrophy involves the

length as well as the circumference of the extremity, and boys are more frequently affected than girls.

The hemangioma may be capillary or cavernous in nature and is often complicated by arteriovenous shunts and lymphangiomatous anomalies. Treatment generally is unsatisfactory. Compression of dilated veins by support bandages has some merit, and surgery may be effective in the prevention of severe limb hypertrophy in occasional patients.

ANGIOKERATOMAS

The term "angiokeratoma" is applied to a group of disorders characterized by ectasia (dilatation of the superficial vessels of the dermis) and hyperkeratosis of the overlying epidermis. All have in common the presence of asymptomatic vascular lesions, seen as dark red to black firm papules which measure 1 to 10 mm in size, and varying degrees of secondary hyperkeratosis.

Solitary or multiple angiokeratomas represent a group of individual lesions generally seen on the lower extremities that appear to follow trauma and begin as an area of telangiectasia followed by hyperkeratosis and angiokeratoma formation. Although they may be seen in childhood, these lesions are not congenital but appear to be acquired on the basis of injury.

Angiokeratoma circumscriptum is a rare disorder usually seen as a solitary large hyperkeratotic plaque or nodule. In half the reported cases, the lesion begins in infancy or early childhood, with females reportedly affected three times as frequently as males. Usually deep red or blue-black in color, lesions are seen as localized unilateral papules, nodules, or plaques, often arranged in streaks or bands, with an uneven verrucous surface. Although they may occur on the back, forearm, and penis, the thighs, lower legs, and buttocks are the more typical areas of involvement. Small lesions may be removed with electrodesiccation and curettage; in larger lesions, extensive surgical excision appears to be the treatment of choice.

Angiokeratoma of Mibelli is a rare disorder characterized by hyperkeratotic vascular lesions that occur over the bony prominences of the extremities of children, usually girls, during late childhood or early adolescence. Lesions usually occur over the dorsal and lateral aspects of the fingers and toes, but also may involve the ears, knees, ankles, elbows, thumbs, soles, and backs of the hands and feet. Early lesions are minute reddish to purple macules or soft papules. With time they increase in size to 5 to 8 mm or more in diameter and become elevated, verrucous, and darker in color. Although often numerous and disfiguring, lesions are generally asymptomatic. Treatment of the disorder consists of cryosurgery with solid carbon dioxide or liquid nitrogen, electrocautery, or surgical excision.

Angiokeratoma corporis diffusum (Fabry syndrome) appears to be an X-linked recessive disease with complete penetrance and variable clinical expressivity in homozygous males and occasional mild penetrance in heterozygous females. The disorder is characterized by systemic intracellular accumulation of the glycosphingolipid (trihexosyl ceramide) in the skin and viscera, particularly in the cardiovascular-renal system. The cutaneous lesions characteristic of this disorder generally appear as clusters of individual punctate macular or papular dark red angiectases that do not blanch with pressure. They usually appear in the areas between the umbilicus and knees. Attacks of pain and paresthesias of the hands and feet often accompany the eruption. Although often spontaneous or elicited by exertion, they apparently are associated with vasomotor disturbances and usually occur subsequent to temperature changes. Pedal and ankle edema are present in most cases and may result in stasis ulcers. Patients with Fabry disease are often hypertensive and, with advancing age, are particularly susceptible to cerebrovascular accidents and coronary artery and renal disease. Unfortunately, there is no specific therapy to correct the biochemical defect of this disorder. Treatment, therefore, is generally supportive in nature. Replacement transfusion and periodic infusion with normal plasma have been suggested, however, in an attempt to provide ceramidetrihexosidase to patients with this inherited metabolic disease.[13]

ECZEMATOUS DISORDERS

SHOE DERMATITIS

Shoe dermatitis is an extremely common form of contact dermatitis in childhood. This disorder—all too frequently misdiagnosed as tinea pedis (a condition extremely uncommon in children prior to puberty)—usually begins over the dorsal surface of the great toe, may remain localized to that area indefinitely, and spreads by extension to the dorsal surfaces of the feet and other toes. A valuable diagnostic feature of shoe dermatitis is the fact that the interdigital spaces, except in severe cases, remain relatively normal in appearance. This is in contrast to the maceration, scaling, and occasional vesiculation of the interdigital webs, particularly those between the fourth and fifth, and, at times, the third and fourth toes of either or both feet generally associated with tinea pedis.

A variety of factors play a role in the pathogenesis of shoe dermatitis. The occlusive effect of hosiery and shoes inhibits the evaporation of moisture, which tends to "leach" out the chemicals in shoes and increases the percutaneous penetration of potentially irritating and sensitizing agents contained therein. Particularly in children, the dermatitis may become sharply localized to the dorsal aspect of the toes owing to friction and irritation of ill-fitting shoes. The diagnosis and management of shoe dermatitis is further discussed in Chapter 10.

LICHEN STRIATUS

Lichen striatus is a self-limiting, usually unilateral-linear dermatitis of unknown origin. It consists of discrete and confluent, minute, slightly raised lichenoid papules which evolve suddenly, usually on an extremity, but occasionally on the face, neck, trunk, or buttocks. It may occur early in infancy, generally affects children between the ages of 5 and 10 years, and, on occasion, has been reported in older individuals.

The eruption is asymptomatic, reaches its maximum extent within several days to a few weeks, and generally progresses spontaneously within a period of six months to a year. The involved area varies from several millimeters to one or two centimeters in width and is characterized by a linear band of small black-topped pink or flesh-colored papules, occasionally surmounted by a fine silvery scale. In dark-skinned or tanned individuals, the eruption may appear as a scaly or papular band-like area of hypopigmentation. Although the band is usually continuous, it occasionally may be interrupted or interspersed with coalescent plaques several centimeters in diameter along the area of linear band configuration.

Since lichen striatus is an asymptomatic self-limited disorder of relatively short duration, therapy is unnecessary. For those who for cosmetic reasons or otherwise prefer treatment, topical corticosteroids, steroids under occlusion, or intralesional steroids may hasten resolution of lesions.

FRICTIONAL LICHENOID DERMATITIS

Frictional lichenoid dermatitis (recurrent summertime pityriasis of the elbows and knees) is a recurring cutaneous disorder which affects children, especially boys, between 4 and 12 years of age. Most cases are seen in the spring and summer months when outdoor activities are common, and many cases are associated with playing in sand-boxes (sand-box dermatitis).

The eruption is characterized by aggregations of discrete lichenoid papules 1 or 2 mm in diameter which occur primarily on the elbows, knees, and back of hands of children in whom such areas are subject to minor frictional trauma without protection of clothing. Lesions may be hypopigmented; pruritus is occasionally but not necessarily present; and many children with this disorder appear to have a predisposition to atopy.

The management of this disorder consists of avoidance of frictional trauma to the involved areas and the use of topical corticosteroids and emollient creams with or without added urea.[3,17]

PAPULAR ACRODERMATITIS OF CHILDHOOD (GIANOTTI-CROSTI SYNDROME)

The Gianotti-Crosti syndrome is a distinctive, self-limited dermatosis of childhood characterized by the abrupt onset of non-pruritic lichenoid papules on the face and extremities which generally last about 20 days, mild constitutional symptoms, and acute, usually anicteric hepatitis. Although adults have been afflicted with this disorder, children between 3 months and 15 years of age are generally affected, with a peak incidence in the one- to six-year age group.[2,8,15]

The eruption consists of nonpruritic, generally but not necessarily symmetrical, flat-topped 1 to 10 mm flesh-colored, pale pink, or coppery red papules that appear in crops and involve the face, buttocks, extremities, palms, soles, and occasionally the upper aspect of the back (Fig. 8-1). The rash develops in a few days and lasts 15 to 20 days or more (occasionally up to 8 weeks or more). In infancy, the lesions are large (5 to 10 mm in diameter); in older children, the eruption is often micropapular and lesions generally measure 1 to 2 mm in diameter.

Constitutional symptoms and systemic manifestations include malaise, low-grade fever, mild generalized lymphadenopathy, hepatomegaly, splenomegaly, and, at times, diarrhea. Hepatitis, when present, begins at the same time as—or a week or two after the onset of—the cutaneous eruption, and the rash resolves spontaneously after a variable period of two to eight weeks (usually 15 to 20 days). Evidence of hepatitis manifested by hepatomegaly, elevated serum enzyme levels, detection of elevated serum levels of hepatitis-B surface ampigen (HBS-Ag), and virus-like particles in liver and lymph node specimens make a viral etiology of this disorder highly probably.[8,15]

Since this syndrome is benign and self-limited (with a low incidence of familial involvement), treatment other than symptomatic measures is unnecessary. Steroid creams have been used without relief and may have an adverse effect on the cutaneous eruption.[5]

INFANTILE ACROPUSTULOSIS (ACROPUSTULOSIS OF INFANCY)

Acropustulosis of infancy (infantile acropustulosis) is a recently described syndrome that is characterized by 1- to 2-mm pruritic vesiculopustules that are found primarily on the distal extremities of infants. The eruption begins between the ages of 2 and 10 months and is worse in summer. New crops of intensely pruritic vesiculopustules appear for 7 to 10 days, after which the eruption remits for two or three weeks before recurring. Lesions begin as pin-point erythematous papules and enlarge into well-circumscribed discrete pustules within 24 hours. They are concentrated on the palms and soles and appear in lesser numbers on the dorsal aspect of the hands, feet, wrists, ankles, and occasionally the scalp. The disorder persists about two years and is unresponsive to potent topical steroids and antibiotics; sulfones and erythromycin are helpful in the prevention of pustule formation, and only soporific doses of oral antihistamine appear to provide relief of symptoms.[9,10]

SCABIES

Scabies is a contagious disorder caused by an itch mite, *Sarcoptes scabiei*, which attacks infants and children as well as adults. The eruption presents as a distinctive clinical syndrome of pruritic papules, vesicles, pustules, and linear burrows. Unfortunately, most patients do not present this pure a picture, but rather a mixture of primary lesions, intermingled with or obliterated by excoriation, eczematization, crusting, or secondary infection. Primary lesions consist of burrows, papules, and vesicular lesions. In adults and older children, lesions tend to involve the webs of fingers, the axillae, flexures of the arms and wrists, the belt-line, and the areas around the nipples, genitals, and lower buttocks. In infants and young children, the distribution is altered and includes the palms, soles, head, neck, and face (Fig. 8-2). Although bullous lesions are uncommon, vesicles are often found in infants and young children owing to the predisposition for blister forming seen in this age group. The burrow, long considered a pathognomonic sign of scabies, unfortunately is demonstrable in a mere 7% to 13% of adult patients. In infants and children, this is even less convenient a clue, owing to frequent obliteration by vigorous hygiene, excoriation, and secondary eczematization, crusting, or infection.[6]

Eczematous changes, due to scratching and rubbing the involved areas or to topical therapeutic agents, is a common complication of scabies in infants and children. This is frequently aggravated by excessive bathing, overzealous attempts at hygiene, and associated dryness and pruritus. In infants, young children, and atopic individuals, this may be particularly severe and widespread.

Secondary infection, seen as pustulation, bullous impetigo, severe crusting, or ecthyma, is frequently seen as a complication of scabies in young children. Recent epidemics of nephritis suggest that scabietic lesions are particularly favorable for growth of virulent M-strains of nephritogenic streptococci. These are distinctive from the streptococcus found in the throat and have a high incidence of association with nephritis, reportedly in the neighborhood of 12%.

Therapy for scabies consists of topical application of 1.0% lindane (gamma benzene hexachloride), 10% crotamiton, 6% to 10% precipitate of sulfur in petrolatum, or a suspension of benzoyl benzoate in a 12.5% to 25% concentration. Because of possible central nervous system toxicity associated with excessive or inappropriate use of lindane, particularly in small children, 6% sulfur precipitate in petrolatum appears to be a safe, effective, and well-tolerated form of therapy for infants and small children with this disorder. Of the other available therapeutic agents, crotamiton has no reported systemic effect and may be used as a safe alternate in the treatment of pregnant women, infants, and small children.

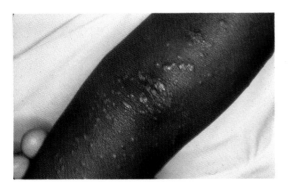

Fig. 8-1. Flat-topped lichenoid papules of Gianotti-Crosti syndrome (papular acrodermatitis of childhood). (Hurwitz S: Clinical Pediatric Dermatology—A Textbook of Skin Disorders of Childhood and Adolescence. Philadelphia, WB Saunders, 1980. *Courtesy of Ferdinando Gianotti*)

Fig. 8-2. Papules, vesicles, and a linear burrow on the foot of a 10-month-old infant with scabies. (Hurwitz S: Clinical Pediatric Dermatology—A Textbook of Skin Disorders of Childhood and Adolescence. Philadelphia, WB Saunders, 1980)

HENOCH-SCHÖNLEIN PURPURA

Henoch-Schönlein purpura is a well-defined systemic disorder of children and young adults. An inflammatory condition of multiple causes, it appears to represent a diffuse vasculitis caused by hypersensitivity to a variety of etiologic factors. The clinical picture is distinctive, and the disorder is characterized by erythematous papules followed by purpura (palpable purpura), abdominal pain, and joint symptoms.

The skin lesions of Henoch-Schönlein purpura consist of small hemorrhagic macules, papules, or urticarial lesions, or a combination of these, which appear in a symmetrical distribution over the buttocks and the extensor surfaces of the extremities (particularly the elbows and knees). Although the disease usually consists of a single episode which may last several days to several weeks, in some cases recurrent attacks occur at intervals for weeks or months. Individual lesions occur in crops, tend to fade after about five days, and eventually are replaced by areas of brownish pigmentation, purpura, or ecchymoses. New crops of lesions frequently occur over the fading lesions of a previous episode, thus creating a polymorphous appearance to the disorder.

There is no specific therapy for Henoch-Schönlein purpura. Bed rest and general supportive care are helpful. Throat cultures and appropriate antibiotics are indicated if a specific respiratory illness is identified. Since renal disease occurs frequently, and many

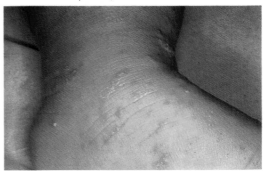

cases of chronic glomerulonephritis in adults may be related to anaphylactoid purpura during childhood, serial urinalyses are indicated. Although there is little evidence that corticosteroids influence the prognosis of this disorder, they do suppress the acute manifestations and may be justified for short periods in severe cases, particularly those with significant gastrointestinal complications.

LETTERER-SIWE DISEASE

Letterer-Siwe disease is seen at the severe fulminating end of the histiocytosis spectrum, as the acute disseminated form of the disease. It usually occurs during the first year of life and is almost exclusively limited to children younger than three years of age. The skin eruption presents in several forms. It frequently begins with a scaly, erythematous seborrhea-like eruption of the scalp, behind the ears, occasionally on the extremities, and in the axillary, inguinal, or perineal areas. On close inspection, the presence of basic lesions of histiocytosis (reddish-brown or purpuric papules) may identify the disorder.

The highest mortality is seen in patients younger than the age of six months, in particular those with widespread systemic involvement. Purpura of the palms—a finding seldom seen in skin diseases—early age of onset, and lung involvement appear to be particularly poor prognostic signs. Death, when it occurs, may be caused by pulmonary, hepatic, or splenic involvement and is frequently attributed to hemorrhage, anemia, or infection. Despite reports of long standing, the Letterer-Siwe disease bears a poor prognosis; the disease course fluctuates; and spontaneous remissions have been documented. Although in general, Letterer-Siwe disease implies a fatal outlook, therapy is often beneficial; spontaneous remissions have occurred; and at times the illness may evolve into a more chronic phase of histiocytosis X such as Hand-Schüller-Christian disease.[12]

KAWASAKI DISEASE (MUCOCUTANEOUS LYMPH NODE SYNDROME)

Mucocutaneous lymph node syndrome (MLNS) has been recognized since 1960. Although initially reported in Japan in 1967, cases have been observed in the USA, Canada, Australia, and Europe.[11] The disease occurs predominantly in infants and children younger than 9 years of age. Although the disease is generally self-limiting, 1% to 2% die during the first 3 weeks owing to coronary thrombosis.

The principal symptom is fever (101° to 104° F) which lasts 1 to 2 weeks, associated with conjunctivitis, erythema and fissuring of the lips, dryness of the oral mucosa, strawberry tongue, and swelling of the cervical lymph nodes. Three to five days later, erythema and indurative edema develop on the hands and feet, followed by a polymorphous erythema on the trunk. During the second week, desquamation occurs, beginning on the periungual areas and extending centripetally. One to two months later, most nails show Beau's lines. Other significant findings are carditis, diarrhea, arthralgia, proteinuria, leukocytosis, and an elevated ESR. MLNS must be differentiated from erythema multiforme and scarlet fever.

The cause of MLNS is unknown. Rickettsia-like bodies have been identified by electronmicroscopy on biopsy specimens from the skin and lymph nodes; however, immunologic studies with Rickettsia agents were negative.[4]

REFERENCES

1. **Feldaker M, Hines EA Jr, Kierland RR:** Livedo reticularis with summer ulcerations. Arch Dermatol 73:31–42, 1975
2. **Gianotti F:** Papular acrodermatitis of childhood, an Australian antigen disease. Arch Dis Child 48:794–799, 1973
3. **Goldman L, Kitzmiller KW, Ritchfield DF:** Summer lichenoid dermatitis of the elbows in children. Cutis 13:836–838, 1974
4. **Hamashima Y, Kishi K, Tasaka K:** Rickettsia-like bodies in infantile acute febrile mucocutaneous lymph node syndrome. Lancet 2:42, 1973
5. **Hjorth N, Kopp H, Osmundsen PE:** Gianotti-Crosti syndrome—a papular eruption of infancy. Trans St John's Hosp Derm Soc 53:46–56, 1967
6. **Hurwitz S:** Scabies in childhood. Pediatr Rev 1:91–95, 1979
7. **Hurwitz S:** Skin Disorders of Childhood and Adolescence—A textbook of clinical pediatric dermatology. Philadelphia, WB Saunders Company, 1980 (*in press*).
8. **Ishimaru Y, Ishimaru H, Toda G:** An epidemic of infantile papular acrodermatitis (Gianotti's disease) in Japan associated with hepatitis-B surface antigen subtype ayw. Lancet 1:707–709, 1976
9. **Jarratt M, Ramsdell W:** Infantile acropustulosis. Arch Dermatol 115:834–836, 1979
10. **Kahn G, Rywlin AM:** Acropustulosis of infancy. Arch Dermatol 115:831–833, 1979
11. **Kawaski T:** Acute febrile mucocutaneous syn-

drome with lymph node involvement with specific desquamation of the fingers and toes in children. Clinical observations in 50 cases. Jpn J Allergol 16:178, 1967

12. **Lahey MD:** Histiocytosis X: Analysis of prognostic factors. J Pediatr 87:184–188, 1975

13. **Mapes CA, Anderson RL, Sweeley CC:** Enzyme replacement in Fabry's disease, an inborn error of metabolism. Science 169:987–989, 1970

14. **Petrozzi JW, Rahn EK, et al:** Cutis marmorata telangiectatica congenita. Arch Dermatol 101:74–77, 1970

15. **Rubenstein D, Esterly NB, Fretzin D:** The Gianotti-Crosti syndrome. Pediatrics 61:433–437, 1978

16. **Solomon LM, Esterly NB:** Transient cutaneous lesions. In Neonatal Dermatology (Major Problems in Clinical Pediatrics, Ser Vol. 9) Philadelphia, WB Saunders Company, 1973

17. **Waisman M, Sutton RL:** Frictional lichenoid eruption in children, recurrent pityriasis of the elbows and knees. Arch Dermatol 94:592–593, 1966

9 THE GERIATRIC FOOT

Foremost cutaneous disorders on the lower extremity of the geriatric patient are seen most commonly on the foot, ankle, and lower leg (Fig. 9-1).

Problems in Association with Systemic Diseases

1. Arteriosclerosis obliterans—with or without diabetes mellitus or hypertension.
2. Diabetes mellitus—with or without clinically significant arteriosclerosis obliterans.
3. Edematous states of cardiac origin—with or without hypertensive cardiovascular disease. Malnutrition, primary renal disease, and hepatic disease may also cause or contribute to dependent edema in the aged. Lymphedematous states of advanced degree with keratoderma and lymphostatic verrucosis are also seen in the elderly, particularly in those patients with Kaposi's sarcoma and elephantiasis nostras verrucosa. (See Chapter 13.)
4. Complications seen in patients with rheumatoid arthritis. (See Chapter 7.)

Local Problems

1. Physical trauma (mechanical, chemical, thermal), especially occurring on an ischemic, edematous, neuropathic, diabetic, lipedematous, or erythrocyanoid lower extremity.
2. Decubitus ulcers on the feet and ankles as sequelae of immobilization. Examples are plegic and paretic states, crippling arthritides, organic brain syndromes, hip fractures, peripheral neuropathies, Parkinson's disease, and other chronic disabling and incurable illnesses.
3. Pruritus. Burning feet.

4. Chronic stasis dermatitis.
5. Contact dermatitis of an irritant or allergic nature, often occurring on a background of xerotic, asteatotic, and neurodermatitic eczema.
6. Drug eruptions, either iatrogenic or due to topical self-medication.
7. Corns and calluses.
8. Ingrown toenail.
9. Nail dystrophies, infectious (*e.g.,* onychomycosis, paronychia) or noninfectious (*e.g.,* onychogryposis).
10. New growths, benign and malignant.

DISCUSSION

VASCULAR DISORDERS

Acute arterial occlusion is recognized by the presence of pain, pallor, pulselessness, paresthesia, and paresis. This event commonly complicates atrial fibrillation. Patients recovering from myocardial infarction who have a mural thrombus in the left ventricle, and patients with myocarditis—often being geriatric patients—are also affected.

Chronic arteriosclerotic occlusive disease is associated with coldness of the feet, elevation pallor, dependent rubor, delay in venous filling time, ischemic ulcers, gangrenous ulcers, thin nail plates or onychomadesis or both, sparse or absent hair, atrophic skin, resting pain, and ischemic neuropathy.

Edematous states, such as congestive heart failure (with or without hypertension) and benign arteriolonephrosclerosis (with or

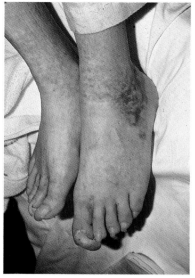

Fig. 9-1. Common manifestations of the geriatric foot: poor hygiene, xerosis, pruritus, onychogryphosis.

without hypertension) with chronic renal failure, may be involved.

Stasis disease may occur in the postphlebitic leg.

The most common cause of leg ulcers in the elderly is arteriosclerotic ulcers, stasis ulcers, and pressure-induced ulcers (from excess pressure on relatively small areas of skin).

DIABETES

Physical trauma of a mechanical, chemical, or thermal nature is a notorious source of trouble on the diabetic lower extremity, and also on the ischemic, edematous, lymphedematous, neuropathic, lipedematous, or erythrocyanoid lower limb. Corns and calluses can favor the development of underlying necrosis, soft tissue infections, and even osteomyelitis; such occurs in diabetic mal perforans, commonly seen over the plantar metatarsal heads.

Any persistent nonhealing ulcer, particularly associated with a callus, may be caused by neurotrophysm. In the diabetic patient, particularly the elderly, more thought should

be given to prophylactic measures to protec the region of the metatarsal heads. In th elderly diabetic with a neurotrophic ulcer o few months' duration, debridement of th ulcer and trimming of the callus, combinec with restriction of activity and the wearin; of adequately padded shoes, may be suffi cient to heal the ulcer and prevent furthe difficulty.

In diabetic patients, lesions of the foot du to occlusive vascular disease constitute ar entirely different problem. Infection, neuro trophic factors, and occlusive vascular dis ease can and, in some degree, usually d coexist in the diabetic patient. When occlu sive vascular disease of a moderate or markec degree is present, the foot must be treatec primarily for this. Ill-advised use of mino surgical procedures may hasten the need fo a major amputation.

Those who deal with the diabetic recogniz a clinical difference between lesions of th foot seen in diabetes and lesions of the foo seen in nondiabetic arteriosclerosis obliter ans. The diabetic differs from the patien with pure occlusive arteriosclerotic diseas in that in addition to being prone to havin; arteriosclerosis obliterans, he is liable als to have invasive and spreading infection i his diabetes is poorly controlled. In addition peripheral neuropathy with its all-too-com mon sequel, neurotrophic ulcer, may de velop. A more subtle difference is that in th patient with diabetes, an ischemic lesion re quiring amputation often develops throug| trauma to the foot; in the nondiabetic patien with arteriosclerosis obliterans, the lesio more often develops as a result of sudder arterial occlusion.

In summary, the lower extremities of th diabetic patient can be affected by three com plications, namely, occlusive arterial diseas (arteriosclerosis obliterans), peripheral neu ropathy (neurotrophic ulcer), and infection In a given situation, any one of these ma operate almost to the exclusion of the others or they can all be present in varying degree: in the same patient. Often, purely infectiou: lesions or purely neurotrophic lesions can b handled conservatively. However, in thos with manifest atherosclerosis, the problen becomes very serious, and all too often ab lative surgical treatment must be employed

Thus, the outstanding endocrine and metabolic disease seen in the geriatric foot is diabetes mellitus and its complications—ischemic and gangrenous and neurotrophic ulcers, pyodermas and deeper soft-tissue infections, onychomycosis and tinea pedis (which may create a portal of entry for infection, *e.g.*, the "fissure ulcer" in the lateral toe web), arteriosclerosis obliterans, and occasionally idiopathic bullous diabeticorum.

TRAUMATIC DISORDERS

Traumatic disorders include *decubitus ulcers* seen on the heels, malleoli, and other pressure points on bedridden or relatively immobilized patients. The most important part of treatment is to prevent sustained pressure on the skin, which comes from lying in one position. A foam rubber pad shaped in the form of a donut is helpful (for local measures in treating ulcers, see Chapter 14). Malnutrition is occasionally seen in these patients, especially those in nursing homes, and may often be due to unwillingness to eat. Hypoalbuminemia can result and may contribute to dependent edema, which can initiate or perpetuate the ulcer. Measures to correct these deficits should be instituted.

Examples of trauma which can cause havoc in the geriatric foot are toenail manipulations, callus and corn treatments, tight-fitting shoes or shoes that rub, hot water soaks, hot water bottles, hot packs, submersion in hot water, cold weather exposure or frostbite, or both, incising and probing blisters and calluses, a tight cast or splint, and chemicals such as corn cures, iodine preparations, carbolic acid, merthiolate, strong disinfectants, and so forth.

Patients should be instructed to avoid crushing, bruising, scratching, cutting, skin cracks, blisters, burns, and frostbite on the feet and toes. They should wear comfortable shoes that do not rub or bind. One should always test the bath water with the hand before putting feet in to make sure that the water is not too hot. Excessive soap and scrubbing should be avoided.

Pruritus without primary disease and without demonstrable systemic cause is not uncommon, especially in the elderly, and the lower extremities are commonly involved.

Pruritus in diabetics, especially on the legs, is well known (see Chapter 5); it is also seen in patients with polycythemia vera, lymphoma, obstructive biliary disease, and chronic renal failure—diseases often affecting the elderly. Itching that is a symptom of systemic disease is best controlled by proper management of the underlying cause.

More frequently, pruritus is associated with aging skin, and aging can often be initiated and hastened by environmental factors. Lack of moisture in the skin leads to senile pruritus, a common complaint of the elderly. The itching can occur at any time of the year but is particularly bad in the fall and winter (winter itch—pruritus hiemalis). Bathing routines, low humidity, and overheated houses are other trigger factors. The condition usually appears initially on the legs; it is worse at night shortly after undressing for bed, or after getting out of bed in the morning. Along with this extremely annoying symptom is sleeplessness and a mental reaction that the symptom is due to some disease. Occasionally, such patients present with delusions of parasitosis. Clinically, the patients show varying degrees of asteatosis and xerosis (discussed in Chapter 10).

Burning feet is discussed in Chapter 20.

Contact dermatitis of an irritant or allergic nature and drug eruptions are the main iatrogenic conditions seen on the geriatric foot, although both may occur owing to patient self-medication (topical or systemic). Drug eruptions are often more intense on the lower leg and foot, probably because of the relative increase in venous pressure. Practically all elderly individuals take medication of one sort or another, and they often take several drugs simultaneously. It is therefore necessary to consider the possibility of a drug eruption when such individuals have any type of reaction.

Corns and calluses are the most frequently encountered foot complaints in elderly patients. These conditions are discussed in Chapter 20.

The ingrown toenail, troublesome to most people, can be a serious problem to aged patients, chiefly because of the metabolic and vascular complications common to this age group. Not only can such a nail be exquisitely painful, but it can also become infected or ulcerated, and can even precipitate gangrene. Causes of this vexing problem include external pressure caused by digital deformities, improper care of the feet (*e.g.*, binding shoes), and poor stance and gait; internal pressure exerted by subungual growths, malformed phalanges, inflammatory processes and arthropathies, and numberous forms of traumatic and anatomic anomalies. Trauma is the most common cause of ingrown toenails. Conservative treatment is preferred (see Chapter 18) because of the usually associated poor circulation. Teaching the patient to cut the nails straight across and examination by a qualified podiatrist are helpful preventive measures.

For additional discussion of the ingrown toenail (as well as the pincer nail seen usually in the elderly), the reader should refer to Chapter 18.

Nail Dystrophies. The incidence of thickened and dystrophic toenails increases with age. The toenails of elderly people, because they are so frequently abnormal, provide an especially favorable substrate for the growth of fungi.[1] Onychogryposis is not uncommon on the geriatric foot, and probably most cases originate from trauma.

Proper care of the feet is important to the health of any person; in the elderly patient, it is essential.

To the elderly patient with vascular disease and to the diabetic, it is top priority. The importance of trauma as a cause of gangrene in vulnerable ischemic limbs must be emphasized. If the patient with ischemic disease of the limb is a smoker, he should be advised to stop. Hydration measures to counteract cracking of dry skin and subsequent entry of infection and initiation of gangrene must be taken. If carried out daily, this procedure allows the patient to inspect his feet carefully for minor injuries, and to obtain treatment for himself. Avoidance of exposure to cold and heat is important in the proper care of ischemic extremities. Tinea pedis can cause blistering and fissuring of the skin, and may thereby foster infection and gangrene in ischemic extremities. Prophylaxis may suppress the incidence of this problem (see Chapter 2 on tineas).

REFERENCE

1. **English MP, Atkinson R:** Onychomycosis in elderly chiropody patients. Brit J Dermatol 91:67, 1974

10 ECZEMATOUS DERMATITIDES

CONTACT DERMATITIS—ENVIRONMENTAL AND OCCUPATIONAL

Eczematous dermatitides account for a large proportion of skin diseases. The term "eczematous dermatitis" describes a morphologic-histologic picture; a qualifying adjective, for example, eczematous contact dermatitis includes an etiologic definition. Contact dermatitis is the most frequent type of eczematous dermatitis and is commonly observed on the lower extremities, especially the feet.

One has only to see the limping patient with oozing and painful eczematous contact dermatitis of the feet to know the serious nature of this disease. Not only is he susceptible to severe cellulitis, thrombophlebitis, or lymphangitis, but often he is also totally unable to carry on important daily activities. The well-trained physician can recognize the problem and successfully treat it. More important, he can discover the cause of the problem and prevent recurrence. The importance of a good history regarding onset, topical medications, types of shoes, and occupational and environmental factors cannot be overstressed.

Contact dermatitis is an inflammatory condition of the skin caused by external agents. Etiologically, it can be divided into primary irritant (toxic) and allergic contact dermatitis. The acute phase is characterized by erythema, edema, papulation, vesiculation, oozing, and scaling and is accompanied by pruritus; chronic reactions show scaling, thickening, fissuring, lichenification, and pigmentary changes. On histologic study, acute contact dermatitis shows spongiosis, intra-epidermal vesiculation, and infiltration of inflammatory cells with vascular dilation in the upper dermis. Distinction between allergic and primary irritant reactions by clinical findings is often difficult; histologic examination within several hours of the start of the dermatitis, as at patch test sites, is more informative. Allergic reactions show early perivascular accumulation of lymphocytes in the upper dermis; in irritant reactions, neutrophile predominate. Chronic contact dermatitis appears as acanthosis, hyperkeratosis with areas of parakeratosis, and a predominantly lymphocytic infiltrate in the upper dermis.

A primary irritant is a substance that is always capable of causing tissue damage when applied for sufficient time and in sufficient concentration. A contact allergen is a substance that causes a hypersensitivity reaction. Characteristically, there is an induction period between an initial sensitizing exposure and development of the capacity to react to a subsequent exposure. With most allergens, only a fraction of the population will develop contact allergy. In the irritant type, the chief variable is the substance itself; an antibody is not required (nonimmunologic mechanism). In sensitization, the chief variable is the host; the intervention of an antibody is required (immunologic mechanism). Contact sensitivity is considered to be

145

a thymus-dependent immune response. The recognition of foreign structures in the skin is carried out by lymphocytes which have two important characteristics, specificity and memory. Although much work has been directed at the immunology of the development of contact sensitivity, the underlying mechanisms are still not completely known.

The hypersensitivity is of the delayed type. Certain prerequisites must be satisfied to induce contact allergy: (1) surface contact, (2) penetration into the skin, and (3) haptene linkage with a protein carrier molecule in the skin. The antigenicity of this haptene-carrier complex sensitizes a population of thymus-derived lymphocytes, leading to a typical delayed hypersensitivity reaction upon exposure. It still remains to be proved that Langerhans cells are necessary for the development of contact dermatitis, but they do participate in the cellular reaction of delayed hypersensitivity and disappear from the epidermis as the reaction subsides.[18] There are underlying factors that determine individual susceptibility (predisposition) or resistance (protection) to the development of contact hypersensitivity.

The feet must resist the onslaught of many irritants and sensitizers under markedly adverse conditions. The feet are not often involved in irritant contact dermatitis in civilian life, but in the services, where the military must spend many hours in wet footwear, it is frequently seen. Among civilians, it occurs in those engaged in wet work where the feet are improperly protected and when footwear become soaked with water and degreasing agents. Kitchen workers may spill juices, dishwater, and chemicals on their feet; mechanics may spill greases and oils.

On the other hand, the feet are common sites of allergic eczematous contact dermatitis. Frequently, the condition is misdiagnosed as tinea or "sweaty sock" dermatitis or remains unrecognized. A variety of factors play a role in the allergic type. The occlusive state produced by stockings and shoes inhibits the evaporation of moisture and results in increased water content of the stratum corneum. This promotes percutaneous absorption by as much as 100 times. Hyperhidrosis can act as a precipitating factor. Sweating of the soles is under psychic influence and can be markedly increased in times of emotional stress. Sweat also has the capacity to leach out chemicals, such as chromium salts, from shoes.[26] Alkaline solutions damage the horny layer by breaking cross-links in keratin and thereby allowing penetration of water with subsequent swelling. Inflammatory changes in the epidermis, whether caused by irritants, sensitizers, or simple friction, further facilitate percutaneous absorption of noxious materials. Scratches and frankly denuded areas caused by friction permit unrestricted penetration.

On the feet, contact allergy is commonly caused by four major groups of materials: wearing apparel, components of shoes and stockings; applied medicaments; appliances used on feet; and substances encountered in certain occupational exposures. In particular, shoe allergens have evoked much enthusiasm for investigation among dermatologists.

SKIN DISORDERS DUE TO SHOES AND FOOT APPAREL

This classification provides a framework to identify these disorders objectively. (Problems caused by footgear used in sports are discussed in Chapter 19.)

Heritable
   Cockayne syndrome. Shoes in causation of symptoms (see Chap. 16)
   Atopic dermatitis. Effect of shoes in localized atopic dermatitis of the feet (see in the latter part of the chapter)

Acquired
   Nonallergic   Allergic
   Nonallergic
      Wide shoes—"Shoe bites"
         (linear blister on the dorsal aspect of the hallux joint of the great toe)
      Narrow shoes—Ingrown toe nails
      Loose shoes—Friction blisters (heels and toes)
      Tight shoes—"Vamp disease"
      Foreign bodies in shoes—Traumatic lesions (*e.g.,* nails in soles)
      Loose linings—Friction dermatitis
      Sneakers—Sweaty foot dermatitis
      Shoe boots—Pernio syndrome in children
      "Pantyhose"—Irritant dermatitis

Allergic Contact Dermatitis
  Shoes and sandals
  Bedroom slippers; urethane peds used
  by hospital patients
  Golashes and boots
  Liners, inner soles, arch supports
  Socks, stockings including elastic stockings
  Peds

Nonallergic Dermatitis

Vamp Disease. This entity is distinctive yet often misdiagnosed. The clinical features and biopsy findings were described by Shapiro and Gibbs: inflammatory swellings on the dorsal aspect of the base of the hallus, secondary to irritation from the edge of the vamp of a shoe.[30] In their experiences and in ours, only women were affected. The swelling is characterized by a horn-filled sinus, resembling a corn or keratinous cyst, on the surface (Fig. 10-1). The process may extend deeply to involve the extensor hallucis longus tendon. Avoiding the ill-fitting shoes is crucial and is probably the most important therapeutic measure. Warm compresses and the application of 1-2-3 Burow's paste with a fixed dressing relieve discomfort and encourage involution in the acute stage. Incision and drainage during the subacute or chronic state and possibly excision of any residuum may be necessary at a later date.

Sweaty Foot Dermatitis. Gibson described a "sweaty sock dermatitis" due to occlusive footwear that unlike contact dermatitis, involves the web areas.[15] This dermatitis is due to maceration by sweat and is seen in children whose feet perspire excessively and who wear either stockings of synthetic fibers or sneakers for prolonged periods. For treatment, the crucial factor should be avoided.

Shoe Boot Pernio. This condition was reported by Coskey and Mehregan.[8] A dermatosis with the features of acute pernio occurred on the plantar surface of only one foot in young girls, about 24 hours after exposure to a cold and wet environment. It was induced by the wearing of shoe boots, the linings of which had become wet. The dampness or wetness of this lining did not evaporate

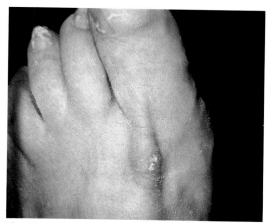

Fig. 10-1. Vamp disease—the swelling resembles a keratinous cyst. *(Courtesy Drs. Carrel, Davidson and Goldstein, Podiatric Affiliates, Buffalo, N.Y.)*

because of the waterproof outer part of the boot, causing a persistent vasospasm. The foot lesions appear as painful, tender, bluish-red nodules that last about 10 days to 2 weeks and then resolve. The histologic findings were similar to those of an early stage of chronic pernio.

"Pantyhose" Dermatitis. The wearing of pantyhose may produce a characteristic irritant dermatitis of the thighs and legs of women. Adams described the eruption as numerous acuminate, pinhead-sized or slightly larger, scaling papules occasionally pierced by a hair.[1]

Allergic Contact Dermatitis

Shoe Dermatitis. *History.* Contact dermatitis resulting from wearing of shoes is a problem that must surely date back to the first days that man strapped chemically treated materials to his feet. Yet, it was not until 1929 that Bloch first documented a case of dermatitis of the feet caused by sensitivity to shoe leather.[5] Subsequent reports were quick to follow. In 1949, Gaul and Underwood called attention to the fact that many dermatoses of the feet are misdiagnosed as fungal infections and are in reality caused by irritants and allergens.[14]

In 1952, Blank and Miller tested 24 cases of shoe dermatitis with 10 representative antioxidants and 17 accelerators.[4] They determined that the most common offenders were the rubber additives monobenzyl ether of hydroquinone, 2-mercaptobenzothiazole, and tetramethylthiuram monosulfide. Rubber additives were further emphasized by Shatin and Reisch in 1954.[31] In the 1950's and 1960's, several studies showed the importance of the tanning agents in leather as a cause of dermatitis.[11,21,29] Changing trends in shoe styles and technical developments using leather substitutes have created problems by introducing new allergens. For example, about 75% of Spanish shoes made today (and many American women's shoes are imported) are mostly "artificial leather," i.e., plastic.[16,24] Dodecyl mercaptans and resins from polyurethane (isocyanates) were the sensitizers resulting in shoe-contact dermatitis. As more artificial leather and synthetic linings are used, contact dermatitis caused by plastics in the shoe is likely to increase.

Incidence. The number of cases of contact dermatitis varies with climate and with the particular compounds used in preparing shoes. Shatin and Reisch reported that 1 in 10 cases hospitalized at a V.A. hospital in New York City because of dermatitis of the feet was diagnosed as shoe dermatitis.[31] This was 2% of the total dermatologic admissions to the hospital over a 5-year period. In a study of 213 patients with shoe dermatitis done over a 13-year period in England, the ages ranged from 3 to 80 years, with about 85% being between 12 and 60 years.[7,9] There are three times as many women as men. It has been speculated that the changing styles, colors, and materials of women's shoes cause women to be exposed to many different sensitizers.[14] Also, the fashion of not wearing hose allows more intimate contact between shoe and skin. Shoes are perhaps the most common cause of allergic contact dermatitis in children and adolescents, next to poison ivy. In Adams' series of 20 patients with dermatitis due to footwear, 16 were younger than 20 years of age, with an equal distribution of 10 males to 10 females, but 6 of the latter had sandal dermatitis.[1]

Structure of Shoes. The basic structure of all men's shoes is fairly similar regardless of style or trademark.[31] This also applies to the oxford worn by women and children. In brief, the sole usually consists of an innersole of leather, a midsole of fabric or reclaimed rubber, and an outersole of leather, plastic, or rubber. The upper portion consists of outside leather, waterproofed paper, the box toe, and the lining. Adhesives are used throughout.

The box toe is one of three general types: rubber, thermoplastic, or celastic. Linings may be dyed and may be impregnated with fungicides to prevent mildew. Women's dress shoes are of lighter construction and contain fewer materials. Often, the upper portion consists of several straps of leather or fabric lined with leather. The sole may consist of several sheets of leather only. Moccasins have neither a box toe nor a lining.

Diagnosis. The diagnosis of allergic contact dermatitis depends upon history, an eczematous eruption, and its localization. Special testing (patch test) is valuable in defining the causal agent.

A good history is essential. The time relationship between wearing a new pair of shoes and onset of the dermatitis is important. However, in many cases of bona fide shoe dermatitis, there may be no such history. Also, some patients known to be sensitive are able to wear shoes containing the offending agent successfully for months before developing a dermatitis. Often, a recurrence of the dermatitis occurs in hot weather when there is excessive sweating of the feet.

Sweat that accumulates inside shoes produces hydration of the stratum corneum, which in turn causes an increase in percutaneous absorption. Sweat leaches out chrome and other chemicals from leather, and these, plus the heat, pressure, and friction that accompany standing and movement, enhance the development of sensitivity.

Clinical Picture. In the classic case, shoe dermatitis presents as an eczematous dermatitis beginning on the dorsal aspect of the big toe with eventual extension to other toes, sparing the toe webs and soles. In those cases where hydroquinone is the sensitizing agent, the presenting lesions at these sites may be patches of leukoderma (Fig. 10-2) without features of eczematization. It is reasonable to suspect this area is the common site of involvement, because dorsal skin is thinner and contains numerous follicular openings through which materials can penetrate, and because more intimate contact of sensitizers with the dorsum of the toes often follows excessive friction and wearing away of the inner shoe linings of the box toe. The majority of cases reported by various investigators had dorsal surface involvement.[6,12,31] The soles are another common site of involvement. In a series of cases reported by Cronin, the soles were involved in 59 out of 77 patients and were the only affected sites in 28 of these patients; the dorsal toe surfaces, however, were the predominant areas of involvement.[9]

The type of shoe alters the distribution of the dermatitis. Unusual patterns can result; for instance thong sandals, many styles of which consist of only a single thong between one or more toes and a strap or two across the instep or heel, has caused a dermatitis pattern which matches the areas contacted by the straps (Fig. 10-3). Allergic contact dermatitis due to Indian buffalo-hide sandals usually presents with a marked vesiculobullous reaction.

At times, during acute exacerbations of shoe dermatitis, the patient may present "id-like" lesions on the hands or even widespread or generalized eruptions, especially following overtreatment or secondary infections. One may speculate that these distant flares represent the hematogenous dissemination of (1) bacterial products from superimposed infections, or (2) fungal products from dormant sites of tinea, or (3) altered keratin from the affected sites or from drugs used topically which have the capacity to be absorbed percutaneously and so act as drug allergens.

Causative Agents. Components of shoes. Rubber and Rubber Adhesives. The rubber in shoes today is made from either

1. Natural rubber: latex, an emulsion of isoprene in an aqueous phase;
2. Synthetic rubber: polyisoprene and butadiene polymers;

3. A combination of both natural and synthetic rubber.

Rubber appears in the soles, in the box toe, and in rubber adhesives; it contains accelerators and antioxidants to make it more serviceable. The rubber additives present in the soles are usually responsible for contact dermatitis at these areas. The rubber box toe is one of the most common causes of shoe dermatitis, the actual sensitizers being the rubber adhesives used to glue the lining to the upper leather. These are usually the rubber accelerators such as 2-mercaptobenzothiazole or tetramethylthiuram monosulfide, or antioxidants such as monobenzyl ether of hydroquinone.[11] The rubber box toe is popular because it is inexpensive.

Recently, adhesives and cements have also been examined for allergens. Adhesives contain: rubber with antioxidants and accelerators; ether as the volatile phase; plasticizers; phthalic esters that improve plasticity of rubber and facilitate vulcanization, and phenolic resins. Brandao reported that all of his 16 shoe dermatitis patients were sensitive to dilute solutions of phenolic resins supplied by shoe manufacturers.[6] A high incidence of hypersensitivity to phenolic resins has been documented by other investigators.[10,19] Suurmond and Mijnssen in the Netherlands found that 8 out of 15 patients were positive to phenolic resins and 6 out of 15 patients were positive to accelerators and antioxidants.[35]

The celastic box toe is composed of cotton flannel impregnated with pyroxylin, a cellulose nitrate, and includes in addition an inorganic fire retardant, a mold retardant, and a special solvent. The special solvent cements the lining and leather completely, negating the use of rubber cement. The celastic box toe is generally considered dermatologically harmless.[9]

The thermoplastic toe is a third form consisting of polystyrene, polyvinyl acetate, or acrylic resins. They are rarely sensitizers. Shoes made with polystyrene toe boxes, however, contain butadiene, which is a synthetic rubber.

Tanning Agents. The many compounds used in various steps of the tanning procedure have been tabulated by Brandao.[6] In his se-

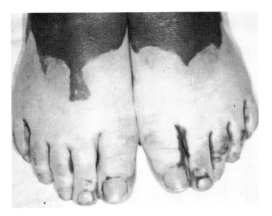

Fig. 10-2. Hydroquinone was the agent causing leukoderma. The condition was misdiagnosed as vitiligo.

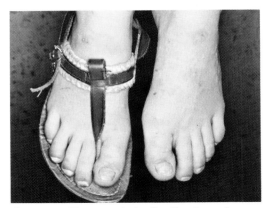

Fig. 10-3. Characteristic distribution of contact dermatitis in patient wearing thong sandals.

ries, chromates, vegetable tannins, and aldehydes are the principal materials.

There has been much controversy as to whether the hexavalent or the trivalent chromium is more significant in shoe dermatitis. The trivalent species is used to tan leather and is theoretically in close chemical combination with the hide protein. We have demonstrated that trivalent chromium is extractable from chrome-tanned leathers by human sweat. We have also shown that hexavalent chromium is present as well, and it is this form, because of its higher sensitizing potential, that is generally considered to be the more likely offender.[26,27]

The incidence of shoe dermatitis to chromium compounds varies. Scutt reported that of 67 naval ratings who returned from the tropics with dermatitis of the dorsa of the feet, 45 reacted to 0.25% potassium dichromate.[29] Fisher found that 20% of his cases of shoe dermatitis were caused by allergic reactions to the dichromates.[12] Bettt, on the other hand, found that dichromates play a rather minor role.[1] Samitz and Gross reported that of 28 workers with known sensitivity to dichromate, only one developed a shoe dermatitis, and in this case sensitivity to rubber materials in his shoes was not tested.[27] Also, in Cronin's series of 213 cases of shoe dermatitis, only 12 cases were positive to 0.5% potassium dichromate, and 3 of 13 cases tested were positive to 10% basic chromic sulfate.[9]

Vegetable tanning is generally used for processing hides to make heavy leathers. In the past, vegetable tannins have not bee considered to cause dermatitis. Recently, however, Cronin has shown that all of 12 patients tested with semichrome leather (containing vegetable tans) and East Indian vegetable-tanned leathers were consistently positive.[9]

Fig. 10-4. Contact dermatitis due to stocking dye.

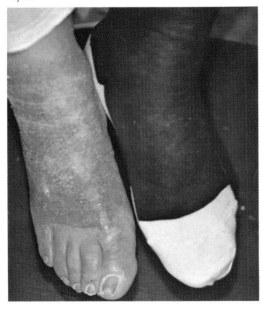

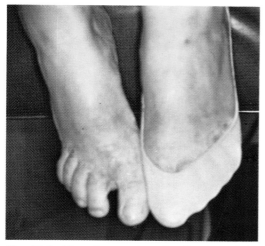

Fig. 10-5. Note interesting distribution of the eruption that follows the elastic band in the Peds. The sensitizing agent was 3-mercapto-benzothiazole.

Fig. 10-6. The rubber in garters was responsible for contact dermatitis on upper legs.

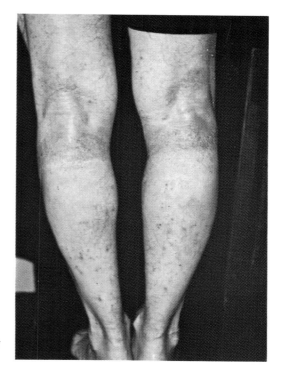

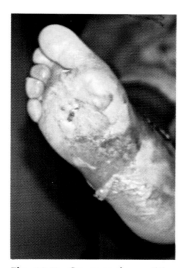

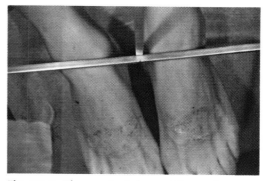

Fig. 10-8. The contact dermatitis conforms to the metal buckle on the shoe. Patient showed positive reaction to nickel on patch test.

Fig. 10-7. Contact dermatitis caused by spray used to treat "tired feet." Patch tests were positive for formaldehyde and menthol, constituents of the spray.

Fig. 10-9. Allergic contact photodermatitis. Note line of demarcation where shoes have covered toes.

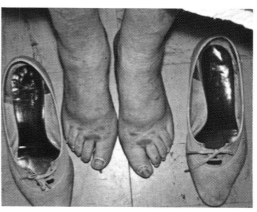

We have also observed a similar finding in an outbreak of shoe dermatitis due to a leather sandal imported from India. Cronin has determined that vegetable tans are in fact complex mixtures of chemicals, mainly polyphenolic substances of the pyrogallol and catechol type. In Cronin's opinion, it is vegetable-tanned rather than chrome-tanned leather that is now the most common cause of shoe dermatitis in England. This is an interesting new finding and emphasizes the need for up-to-date testing and analysis of ever-changing shoe materials.

Vegetable tanning currently in common use employs wattle, myrtan, spruce, chestnut, quebracho, and sumac.[1] The tanning ingredients employed in Indian buffalo hide were considered, at one time, the cause of many cases of sandal dermatitis.[20,22] Sumac was implicated, especially since the bullous reactions on the skin resembled poison ivy dermatitis (sumac and rhus are antigenically similar). However, recent studies done by Spoor suggested that in cases of dermatitis caused by Indian leather, the oil used as a softening agent was the culprit.[33]

Aldehyde tanning, as with formaldehyde, is used in white skins such as "white kids" or "bucks". A positive patch test reaction to formaldehyde in a patient with foot dermatitis is therefore significant.

Dyes. Leather dyeing is done principally with the "azoaniline" group of dyes and so well fixed to the leather in the manufacturing process that shoe dye dermatitis is extremely rare.[12] Suurmond and Mijnssen reported a series of 15 patients with 3 positive to paraphenylenediamine; however, all 3 had positive reactions to other shoe materials as well.[35] It is important to note that dyes can be more easily leached from fabric and plastic shoes and from redyed shoes than from leather. In these instances, dyes must be recognized as likely contactants.

Miscellaneous Substances. Other contactants in shoes are rare causes of dermatitis: antimildew agents, such as mercaptobenzothiazole, paranitrophenol, salicylanilide, and inorganic mercury compounds; nickel present in eyelets, buckles, ornaments, and arch supports.

Footgear other than regular shoes can also be offenders. Vinyl and unpolymerized acrylic resins, formaldehyde, antioxidants, and plasticizers used in plastic shoes can all be allergenic. As noted previously, shoes made from "artificial leather," (*i.e.*, plastic) contain the potent sensitizers dodecyl mercaptans and isocyanate resins.[16,24] Rubber overshoes, especially galoshes, bathing shoes, sneakers, special shoes used in various athletic activities, and bedroom slippers may be responsible for allergic contact dermatitis on the feet.

Stocking Dermatitis. Stocking dermatitis is often related to the dyes or to the detergents used in laundering. Although dermatitis from nylon stockings has been reported, most cases are actually caused by sensitivity to azo dyes which may cross-react with paraphenylenediamine and related rubber chemicals.

In stocking dermatitis, the shape of the stocking may be outlined on the leg (Fig. 10-4). Typical sites of involvement, however, are the feet, popliteal fossae and inner thighs. In a few instances, with localization to the feet, the eruption can be mistaken for shoe dermatitis, but is probably due to sweat and friction inside the shoe, especially on the anterior part of the foot. Slight involvement in other areas such as the popliteal fossae and inner thighs is a valuable clue but is usually overlooked by the patient. Patch testing with the stocking confirms the diagnosis.

Peds, frequently worn by women who go without stockings, may cause contact dermatitis. We have observed rubber sensitivity from the elastic band which encircles the ped. The eruption is confined to a moccasin pattern (Fig. 10-5).

Von H. Suter described 11 cases of dermatitis to polyamide stockings.[34] Without exception, dyes were incriminated, and no case of sensitization was caused by polyamide itself, by substances used in the preparation of fibers, or by antistatic materials.

The use of elastic stockings has also been responsible for contact dermatitis in patients allergic to rubber. The eruption in these patients conforms to areas covered by the special stockings. Also included under this category is contact dermatitis caused by garters.

Rubber again is the sensitizer, the eruption being localized to sites covered by the garters (Fig. 10-6).

Medication Dermatitis. One of the leading causes of dermatologic disease is overtreatment. With our preoccupation with health and the influence of television and other advertising media, feet are constantly inundated with a host of creams, lotions, powders, and ointments. We suffer from a plethora of absorbents, analgesics, antiseptics, anti-inflammatory, antibacterial and antifungal agents, and keratolytics to be applied, supposedly for our comfort.

Almost any medicament, proprietary or prescribed, applied to normal or damaged skin will sensitize some persons (Fig. 10-7), although weak sensitizers rarely do so unless used on burns or severe dermatitis. Neomycin and topical formulations containing sensitizing preservatives may play a significant role in contact dermatitis.[23,28] Patch testing of components in recommended concentrations should be carried out. Often a trial application of a suspected allergen to a small limited test area will be helpful.

Appliances Used on Feet. Included under this group are arch supports, orthopedic braces, elastic supports, athletic tape, pads, and other devices used to relieve painful foot problems. Nickel, rubber compounds, and plastics are the offenders (Fig. 10-8).

Photodermatitis of the Feet. An unusual dermatitis of the feet is the allergic contact photodermatitis, resulting from contact with photosensitizing antimycotic topical medications used to treat athlete's foot. In some patients with a long-standing allergic contact photodermatitis, hyperpigmentation and lichenification have been so striking that the affected areas resemble a chronic neurodermatitis (Fig. 10-9). Photopatch tests with the preparations used confirm the diagnosis.

Figures 10-10 to 10-18 illustrate various clinical features of shoe dermatitis.

Occupational Dermatoses. Climatic and environmental factors play a role in the development of some occupational skin diseases affecting the lower extremities. Farmers and rural workers, especially in tropical countries, often wear short pants and sandals or go barefoot. The lower extremities, thus without protection, are exposed to physical trauma from plants and thorns or occupational injuries. Some of these injuries may become the portal of entry for pathogenic organisms found in nature. The exposed extremities are also easily accessible to arthropods that bite or sting, causing local and systemic reactions, or inoculate parasites of tropical diseases. For example, mycetoma is a common occupational disease concentrated in scattered regions of the tropics and subtropics. The mode of infection is inoculation of the involved organisms through the skin, especially that of barefoot workers in rice paddies and plantations.

Bare feet exposed to trauma can cause occupational koilonychia of the toe nails in "Rickshaw boys."[3]

Chemical agents are the predominant causes of industrial dermatitides. The reactions they produce on the skin may be due to either primary irritancy or sensitization. An understanding of the work environment is important. In many industries, contact with these agents usually results from working in bare feet (as in agricultural workers), and from leakage of chemical agents spilling over the shoes and feet. An example of the latter is the herbicide allergic dermatitis of farmers, reported by Spencer.[32] In construction workers, cement can cause an irritant dermatitis due to the corrosive action of cement and/or an allergic reaction from chromates in the cement (Fig. 10-19). Another type of exposure may be due to components of especially designed work shoes and rubber boots worn in various occupations. The vagaries of rubber boot dermatitis in fishermen were described by Ross.[25]

Patch Tests. Allergic eczematous contact dermatitis on the feet may be so characteristic that it is readily recognized from history and examination. Clinical acumen and a high index of suspicion are the physician's greatest tools in diagnosing shoe dermatitis. Often, the only convincing evidence for a shoe dermatitis is the disappearance of a rash after substituting shoes with a totally different

(text continues p. 156)

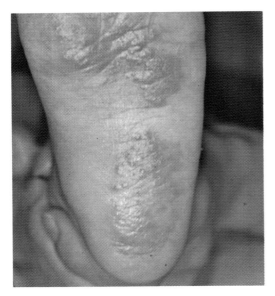

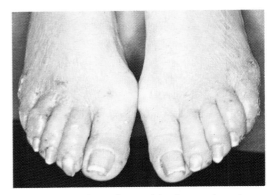

Fig. 10-10. Contact dermatitis due to components of inner sole.

Fig. 10-11. Shoe dermatitis due to box toe. Rubber adhesives used to glue the lining were sensitizers.

Fig. 10-12. Chronic shoe dermatitis. The lichenified lesions had been treated as a neurodermatitis.

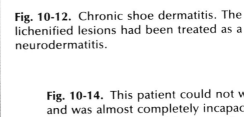

Fig. 10-14. This patient could not wear shoes and was almost completely incapacitated. She had been treated for neurodermatitis for 4 years.

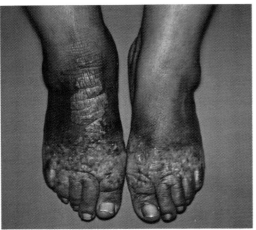

Fig. 10-13. A classical picture of box-toe dermatitis. The sensitizer was tetramethylthiuram monosulfide.

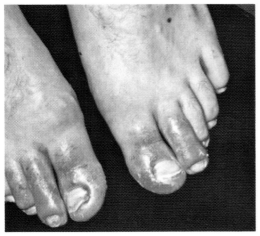

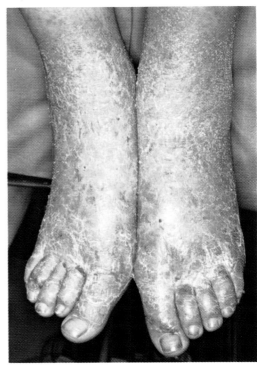

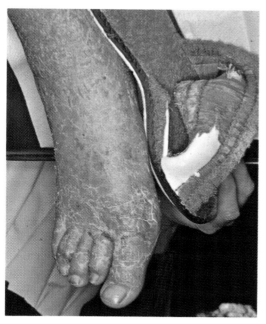

Fig. 10-15. The same patient (Fig. 10-14) could get around only in soft bedroom slippers. When the bedroom slippers were stripped, foam rubber was exposed. Patch tests confirmed a rubber sensitivity.

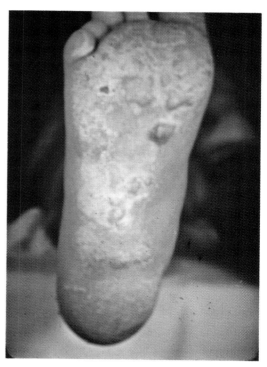

Fig. 10-16. Contact dermatitis due to rubber additives in glue used in soles. The sensitizer was 2-mercaptobenzothiazole.

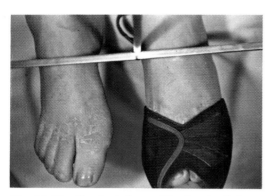

Fig. 10-17. Contact dermatitis due to lining in the slippers of the shoe.

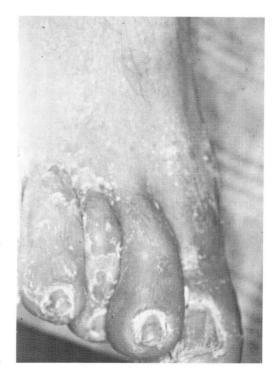

Fig. 10-18. Box-toe dermatitis with superimposed pyocyaneous infection.

construction (*e.g.*, plastic or cloth instead of leather shoes).

The patch test is the means of establishing the cause of contact dermatitis. It is a specific procedure that reproduces the patient's clinical disease in miniature and is used solely in allergic contact dermatitis and not at all in irritant dermatitis. Although patch testing may seem a simple procedure, the manner of application and the interpretation of the tests require the experience of the expert.

The test material is applied directly to the normal skin on a small square (0.5 sq cm) of white cotton cloth. The patch is covered by a larger piece of cellophane and both are kept in place with a piece of adhesive. Commercial patches are available and simple to use. The Al-Test patch with Scanpoe tape (Hollister-Stier Laboratories) is an excellent example. The material remains on the skin for 48 hours to promote penetration and allow time for the delayed reaction to develop. The upper part of the back is the preferable patch test site. The patient is instructed to remove the test material at any time from any site of burning or pain. Readings are made 30 minutes after removal of the patches and the sites are reexamined after 2 to 5 days for delayed reactions (Figs. 10-20, 10-21). Often, however, the patch test is unreliable because (1) the testing conditions do not duplicate the adverse conditions of the feet in shoes, and (2) testing materials may not include the proper allergens.

Every effort should be made to obtain patch-test evidence to confirm the diagnosis. Defining the allergen is the key in prevention.

A shoe "screening tray" is a useful adjunct for patch testing. Fisher has recommended a list of standard substances; however, revisions are needed every few years because new products are always being introduced.

Using clinical standards established by the North American Contact Dermatitis Group, the American Academy of Dermatology (AAD) has prepared patch test kits. For 1980, the AAD patch test kit has been revised and updated. Patch test instructions are included (AAD, P.O. Box 552, Evanston, IL 60204).

Diagnostic Series for Allergic Shoe Dermatitis (Fisher[13])

1. Rubber box toe material (as is).

2. 1% monobenzylether of hydroquinone in petrolatum (rubber antioxidant).
3. 1% mercaptobenzothiazole in petrolatum (rubber accelerator).
4. 1% tetramethylthiuram monosulfide in petrolatum (rubber accelerator).
5. 1% hexamethylenetetramine in petrolatum (rubber accelerator).
6. 1% phenyl beta napthylamine in petrolatum (rubber antioxidant).
7. 0.25% potassium dichromate in aqueous solution (tanning agent).
8. 5% formaldehyde in aqueous solution (tanning agent for white shoes).
9. 2% paraphenylenediamine in petrolatum (may cross-react with shoe dyes).
10. 5% nickel sulfate in aqueous solution (eyelets, buckles, tips of shoelaces).

Suggested Patch Test Substances for Shoes (Adams[1])

1. Potassium dichromate, 0.5% pet.
2. Mercaptobenzothiazole, 2% pet.
3. Tetramethyl thiuramdisulfide, 2% pet.
4. Diphenyl-p-phenylenediamine, 1% pet.
5. Paratertbutylphenol formaldehyde resin, 1% pet.
6. N-cyclohexylbenzothiazylsulfenamide, 1% pet.
7. Monobenzyl ether of hydroquinone, 1% pet.
8. 1,3 diphenylguanidine, 1% pet.
9. p-phenylenediamine, 1% pet.
10. Phenylbetamethylamine, 1% pet.
11. Isopropylaminidophenylamine, 0.1% pet.
12. Scrapings of shoe (or pieces).

In our experience, it is preferable to patch-test patients with small pieces of the components of their own shoes. Specimens are obtained easily by using a 6- to 8-mm skin biopsy punch (Fig. 10-22). This provides a satisfactory sample of all the shoe materials. The lining is separated from the leather, and the actual materials are then applied, "glue" surface face down directly on the skin. Soaking leather and lining pieces in water or sweat (artificial sweat can be used) for 10 to 15 minutes before testing will enhance percutaneous absorption.[27] Patch test samples of 2.0 to 4.0 cm are adequate; avoid sharp, rough, or thick sections.

Treatment. The first principle in the treatment of allergic eczematous contact dermatitis is to identify and eliminate the sensitizer. Cure cannot be attained unless contact with the causal agent is avoided. Thus, it is of primary importance that the patient cease wearing the shoes or type of stocking to which he has shown a positive patch test, or to avoid contact with topical medicaments and occupational sensitizers.

Management of the individual case depends upon the stage of the eruption and the severity of the inflammatory reaction.

Local Measures. For the acute stage:

1. Local rest and elevation of the affected feet according to the severity and extent of the dermatitis.
2. Interdict use of soaps.
3. Wet dressings such as Burow's solution (1:40 to 1:20) and saline solution are simple and effective. Compresses or soaks should be applied every 3 to 4 hours for 15 to 20 minutes. Clean sheeting, or muslin or a turkish towel are good dressing materials. Do not use plastic or other impervious material to prevent evaporation.

   BluBoro powder packets (Derm-Arts Laboratories), Buro-Sol (Doak Pharmacal Co., Inc.), Domeboro Tablets (Dome Laboratories) are convenient proprietaries for preparing Burow's solution.

   When the exudative or oozing phase subsides, the following may be used:
4. Simple pastes with Burow's solution applied as fixed dressings.

Burow's solution	1 part
Aquaphor	2 parts
Lassar's paste	3 parts
5. Corticosteroid creams. These anti-inflammatory agents can be applied following compressing or on the dry skin. We have found Kenalog 0.025%, Valisone 0.1%, Synalar 0.025%, Hytone 1–2.5%, Westcort 0.2%, and Cordran 0.025% creams effective agents in this stage. Topical antibiotics may be used when secondary infection is present. These are often combined in the steroid creams. Dressings should be light, comfortable, and nonocclusive.

For the dry, scaly, and thickened stages of eczematous eruptions, the following are suggested: ointments containing corticosteroids or creams and ointments containing iodochlorhydroxyquin (Vytone, Dermik Labs). Corticosteroid creams may be used under a plastic film or short periods.

With ambulation, open shoes (sandals or shoes in which the box toes have been cut away) are recommended for short periods of time until complete involution of the eruption takes place.

Systemic Measures. Occasionally, secondary infection of cutaneous lesions may require oral or parenteral administration of antibiotics. Bacterial cultures and sensitivity tests to determine the antibiotic of choice are advisable and will afford a more direct attack on the infectious process.

Oral corticosteroids may be indicated in severe disabling cases. They should be used with caution and only by practitioners experienced in their use and aware of their adverse reactions and contraindications. When such treatment is necessary, it should be for short-term use, usually 2 or 3 weeks. Initial high doses are tapered off gradually to prevent a "rebound" of the dermatitis. The following regimen is effective in most instances:

40 mg prednisone or its equivalent (10 mg qid) for 2 to 3 days;
30 mg (10 mg tid) for 2 days;
20 mg (10 mg bid) for 3 days;
15 mg (5 mg tid) for 3 days;
10 mg (5 mg bid) for 3 days; 5 mg daily for 3 days

This can be modified by an initial intramuscular injection of a long-acting steroid suspension (Kenalog IM, Aristocort Forte, Celestone Soluspan) given on the first day followed by oral therapy with corticosteroids, as shown in the above schedule.

Following recovery, it is essential that the patient be instructed in measures to help prevent recurrences. Measures to control hyperhidrosis are valuable. A noncaking dusting powder such as Zeasorb powder (Stieffel) should be dusted freely into stockings, shoes, or sneakers. The causative agent, be it shoes, stockings, topical medicament, or occupational exposure, must be avoided. The problem of stockings and topical medicaments is

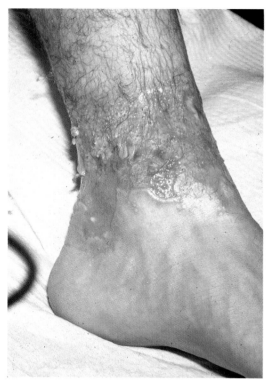

Fig. 10-19. Occupational dermatitis. Cement irritancy and chromate sensitivity.

simple to correct. Finding shoes that are free of the particular sensitizer may be more difficult. Patients should be given explicit advice as to the type of shoes to be worn and the places to purchase them. Specific examples are unlined moccasins, shoes made with canvas, cloth, and plastic uppers; shoes with celastic box toes for patients sensitive to rubber and its adhesives in rubber box toe shoes; vegetable-tanned shoes for those reacting to chrome-tanned shoes and chrome-tanned leather for the patient sensitized to vegetable tanning materials. Fisher lists manufacturers and shops where such shoes can be bought in many metropolitan centers, and Hack provides the addresses of firms which manufacture special shoes and stockings.[13,17] Foot-So-Port Shoe Co., subsidiary of Musebeck Shoe Company (Oconomowoc, Wisconsin 53066) manufactures shoes using vegetable-tanned leather and has eliminated all rubber cements in their shoes. The company is most cooperative in supplying the physician with samples of the materials used in their shoes for patch testing and a style folder which will give the patient an idea of the shoes available.

Fig. 10-20. Patch tests. Screening tray.

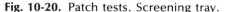

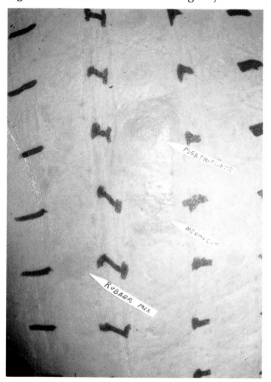

Fig. 10-21. Patch tests. Shoe leather components.

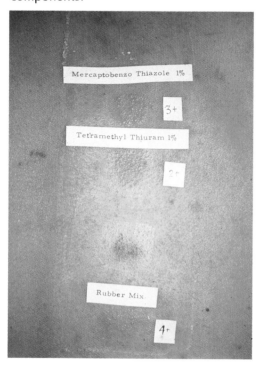

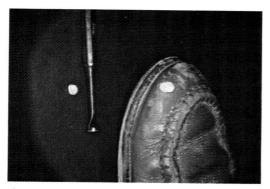

Fig. 10-22. A skin biopsy punch is used to remove leather and lining for patch testing.

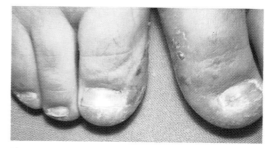

Fig. 10-23. Atopic dermatitis (juvenile type). The condition may often be misdiagnosed as a shoe box-toe dermatitis.

ATOPIC DERMATITIS

In contrast to contact allergy, which is a type of delayed hypersensitivity (cell-mediated immunity), atopic dermatitis was considered primarily to be one of the classic examples of immediate hypersensitivity (humoral immunity). This concept is now being redefined in the light of modern immunology, and several lines of evidence attest to defects also of cell-mediated immunity, associations with immunodeficient states, and altered pharmacologic activity.[1,2] Patients with atopic dermatitis have increased susceptibility to unusual severe cutaneous infections with viruses such as herpes simplex, vaccinia, and molluscum contagiosum; a decreased sensitization rate for poison ivy; and decreased response to candida and streptococcal antigens. Considerable work is being carried out to identify the primary defect responsible for the disease.

The term "atopy" was coined by Coca to describe a group of allergic diseases characterized by a strong hereditary background. The designation includes hay fever, asthma, and atopic dermatitis. Reagins which have the capacity to be transferred to nonatopic individuals by the Prausnitz-Küstner (P-K) test prove the existence of circulating antibodies. In atopic dermatitis, however, it is difficult to assign the cause solely to an an-

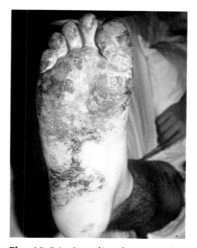

Fig. 10-24. Localized atopic dermatitis. Severe reaction due to overtreatment and secondary infection.

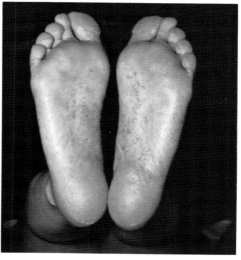

Fig. 10-25. Atopic dermatitis. The eruption was pronounced on the soles. At this site, differential diagnosis from hyperhidrosis is often difficult.

tigen-antibody reaction, because the disease depends on the interplay of numerous constitutional and precipitating factors.

Clinical studies have established the presence of high serum IgE levels in more than 80% of patients with atopic dermatitis. The levels tend to be highest in patients with atopic dermatitis and coexisting allergic respiratory disease; the degree of elevation roughly corresponds to the severity of the skin disease; and the serum IgE levels may remain high in spite of resolution of the dermatitis.[2] Yet the pathogenic significance of IgE in atopic dermatitis is unclear. The increased amount of IgE is not the sole determinant for the clinical expression of atopic dermatitis but may reflect dysfunctional control of the immunoglobulin-producing cells. As a practical test, serum IgE levels offer little aid to either diagnosis or prognosis in clinical situations.[2]

With our present knowledge, the following can be summarized:

Atopic dermatitis is a disease characterized by abnormalities related to both type 1 and type 4 immune responses, yet the skin lesions cannot be classified under either of these reaction types. The disease is difficult to define; diagnosis depends on a combination of morphologic, distributional, and historical features.[2]

Most characteristic of atopic dermatitis are its exacerbations and remissions. Factors in producing remissions may be changes in mode of life and season. Factors producing exacerbations may be heat, humidity and perspiration; exposure to certain antigens either by injection, inhalation, or ingestion; infection; greasy topical medicaments; stress; overwork; and fatigue.

Atopic dermatitis (also known as atopic eczema and neurodermatitis) is divided into infantile, childhood, and adult phases. In the infant and younger child, the lesions are more generalized than in the older child and adult. In the infantile phase, the condition is acute and subacute with erythema, edema, vesiculation, weeping, and oozing. In the childhood and adult phases, it presents subacute and chronic features with erythema, papulation, and lichenification, and a predilection for the flexural areas of the extremities. In addition, there is usually a gener-

alized dryness of the skin, a characteristic facies manifested by periorbital discoloration and eyelid folds, white dermographism (upon stroking the skin a white line appears rather than the customary red line), delayed blanch response to cholinergic agents, and poor tolerance to various stresses such as cold, heat, humidity, trauma, infections and emotional tensions.[3] Itching is a cardinal symptom. As a rule, the value of skin testing in atopic dermatitis is slight, and treatment by specific desensitization is seldom helpful and at times may cause aggravation of the skin lesions.

It is not unusual to find the eruption localized to various parts of the body. Lesions confined to the lower legs and feet are more commonly seen in childhood and adolescence. The pattern of the disease in these areas presents special problems in diagnosis. One or more of the sites (e.g., the dorsa of the toes, the ankle, or the soles) may be affected without other areas being involved. Thus, a chronic or recurrent dermatitis of the feet may be part of a more widespread dermatitis or a localized form of atopic dermatitis. It is necessary in these cases to question the patient regarding the familial background and past personal atopic history. It is also necessary to examine the patient for other atopic lesions or stigmata.

With children and adolescents, atopic dermatitis may manifest as lichenified patches around the ankles or behind the knees. With children particularly the dermatitis may become sharply localized to the dorsal aspect or to the tips of the toes (Fig. 10-23). The lesions may be confined to an area even as small as the dorsum of one toe. On the other hand, localized atopic dermatitis when complicated by injudicious treatment or overtreatment, infection, or dyshidrosis, can involve the soles (Fig. 10-24), the legs, and even become generalized. Toe involvement is usually the result of friction and irritation of ill-fitting shoes. The lesions and localization may resemble the picture of box toe dermatitis. However, reactions to patch tests with shoe materials are negative. While the soles are ordinarily not involved in atopic dermatitis, dyshidrosis frequently occurs here and causes difficulty in diagnosis (Fig. 10-25).

A syndrome recently described as juvenile plantar dermatosis found mainly in children between 3 and 14 years of age presents with redness, shiny hyperkeratosis, lamellar scaling, and painful fissure formation in the weight-bearing parts of the soles and toes.[4] External factors, occlusive socks and footwear, possibly together with an atopic constitution, are believed to be the cause of the disease, which is very difficult to treat. Also, many cases which give the appearance of nummular eczema on the legs, in reality, are atopic dermatitis and must be treated as such.

Therapy for atopic dermatitis can be difficult even for the expert. It must be remembered that this is an inherited constitutional diathesis and therapy cannot change or cure this. There are no satisfactory systemic medications. Treatment should be directed toward allaying the itch-scratch symptoms and controlling process of eczematization and superimposed pyogenic infection (see treatment under contact dermatitis). Chronic lichenified patches respond well to coal tar pastes alone or over a previous application of corticosteroid creams. We advise against continued daily use of topical steroids because they can cause undesirable side effects. In children with toe and sole involvement, avoidance of friction and irritation will remove a precipitating factor and, along with the use of properly fitting shoes, should afford considerable relief.

NUMMULAR ECZEMA

Nummular eczema presents a fairly typical clinical picture. Diagnosis depends on the characteristics of the lesions and distribution. Many hypotheses, as yet unsubstantiated, have been proposed regarding etiology. We consider the entity as a reaction pattern on a certain type of skin which is triggered by a variety of stimuli (*viz,* irritants, allergens, soap and water in association with microbial sensitization).

The lesions in nummular eczema, usually limited, are coin-shaped, varying in size from a dime to a palm-sized plaque (Fig. 10-26). They are discrete with erythematous papulovesicular features, especially at the periph-

ery. The centers often show a tendency for clearing. The vesicles are thin-walled and tend to rupture easily, thus leading to oozing and crusting. The lesions may also present as isolated, mildly red plaques which are dry and scaly with superficial fissuring. Symmetrical distribution is characteristic: the dorsa of the hands and the extensor surface of forearms and legs. Less frequently, the shoulders, buttocks, face, breasts and nipples are involved. The disorder may begin as a single patch on a lower leg, usually on the calf or anterolateral aspect.

Nummular eczema is characterized by its persistence. After clearing, recurrences appear on exactly the same sites. The eruption tends to be worse in the cold weather. It is aggravated by soap and greasy applications and is associated with itching and burning.

The treatment of nummular eczema is trying to both the patient and the physician. We have found the use of steroid creams alone or in association with a vioform-pine tar paste (3% vioform, 10% pine tar ointment in Lassar's paste), along with the administration of a broad-spectrum antibiotic such as tetracycline (250 mg qid for 3 to 5 days followed by 250 mg every morning for several weeks) to be effective.

ASTEATOTIC ECZEMA

Under this heading we include eczematous pictures manifested by a dry, scaly, or fissured state of the skin usually seen in elderly individuals. The skin usually presents a wrinkled or a "crazy-pavement" appearance (Fig. 10-27). Redness, edema, vesiculation, and oozing may follow. Thickened and fissured lesions characterize the chronic stages of the disorder, and itching is a very common complaint.

Various factors play a role in the etiology: an aging skin, the winter season, dryness of overheated homes, excessive cleansing with soaps (especially alkaline or bactericidal soaps), and friction from wearing apparel. The interplay between these factors results in an altered physiology of the skin. Soaps and cleansers may damage the epidermis and cause the production of an abnormal horny layer which cannot serve as an efficient bar-

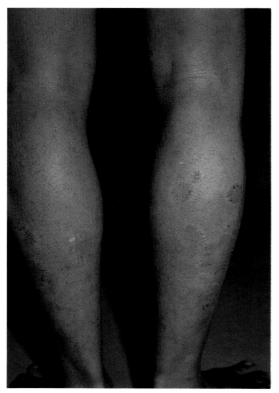

Fig. 10-26. Typical lesions of nummular eczema.

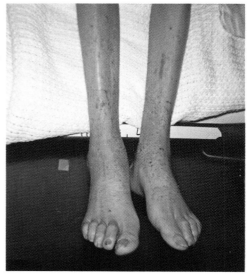

Fig. 10-27. Asteatotic eczema. The lower extremities are common sites for this problem.

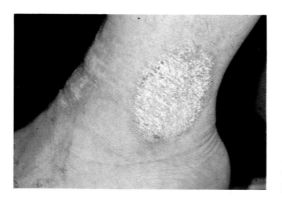

Fig. 10-28. Lichen simplex chronicus. The ankle is a common site for the itch-scratch picture.

rier and leads to dryness and chapping. The dryness is a significant factor in producing tiny fissures in the stratum corneum. If the process continues, the whole epidermis becomes involved with resultant eczematization. The lower extremities are common sites.

Treatment is simplified if the structural and functional integrity of the horny layer is restored and maintained. This is accomplished by lessening contact with irritants, the use of humidifiers, protection against exposure to cold, and the replacement of water in the skin by a hydration routine. A simple procedure is to have the patient soak the affected parts in lukewarm water for 10 to 15 minutes and, without drying the legs, apply an emollient such as white petrolatum or Eucerin, or a vegetable fat such as Crisco or Spry and allow it to remain on the skin for 30 minutes, removing the excess with a towel. Another simple measure is the salt bath: one cup of ordinary table salt is added in a tub of warm water for bathing; the salt acts as a hydrating agent. Bath oils are ineffective. If inflammatory changes are present, corticosteroid creams or ointments are preferable. The routine can be repeated once or twice daily. The hydration helps to retain the normal suppleness of the skin.

LICHEN SIMPLEX CHRONICUS

Lichen simplex chronicus, also known as circumscribed neurodermatitis, occurs as variable-sized patches in which lichenification is the distinctive feature (thickening and accentuation of the skin lines). The reaction arises on skin previously apparently normal and represents the response of the predisposed skin to repeated scratching and rubbing. External factors such as an insect bite or friction from wearing apparel may play a role in initiating the lesion. Emotions play a role in its perpetuation. The predominant symptom is intense pruritus which is often paroxysmal. Emotional events trigger the reaction. Scratching is the release mechanism. Thus, the term "itch-scratch complex" is highly descriptive.

The fully developed lesion presents as a sharply demarcated patch of thickened skin, red and edematous during its early stage and subsequently dry, scaly, excoriated, and hyperpigmented. A zone of grouped lichenoid papules surround the patch.

Lesions may occur in any area accessible to scratching. Favored sites on the lower extremity are the anterior surface of the leg, especially just below the knee and on the ankles (Fig. 10-28). The typical lesion is a solitary patch. The condition may also occur on the soles. In this area, it is often misdiagnosed as callus or psoriasis.

The objective in treatment is to break the itch-scratch cycle. The patient should be made to understand the causal relationships involved. Whatever therapy that can be directed to this end will help. We have found that discussing problems with the patient is far more useful than prescribing sedatives or tranquilizers.

Topical measures are very helpful, with steroid cream as the treatment of choice. In the acute phase, simple compresses followed by the application of a steroid cream are most effective (see under contact dermatitis).

Occlusive dressings are preferable for chronic lesions, having a double purpose: They provide a barrier to prevent scratching and permit contact of the medication for longer periods of time. Modified Unna boots can be reapplied weekly. Tar pastes held in place with stockinette (an excellent simple form of dressing for the lower extremity) can be applied daily by the patient. Steroid creams applied under an occlusive plastic dressing can be changed once or twice daily. When occlusive dressings are discontinued, a greasy base should be substituted to prevent excessive loss of moisture from the skin with its now altered barrier layer. Dusting this ointment layer lightly with talc provides an excellent dressing.

Intralesional injections of corticosteroid suspensions (hydrocortisone or triamcinolone) are often used in lichen simplex. However, we do not recommend this modality for lesions on the ankle or foot because of a variety of adverse effects which we have observed. Severe lower back pain was experienced by several patients immediately following the injection. In others, ulcers (aseptic necrosis) developed at injection sites weeks after treatment.

If secondary infection is present, a topical antibiotic or an oral broad-spectrum antibiotic may be required for a few days.

REFERENCES

CONTACT DERMATITIS

1. **Adams RM:** Dermatitis due to clothing. Cutis 10:577, 1972
2. **Bett DCG:** The potassium dichromate patch test. Trans St John's Hosp Derm Soc 40:40, 1958
3. **Bentley-Phillips B, Bayles MAH:** Occupational koilonychia of the toe nails. Brit J Dermatol 85:140, 1971
4. **Blank IH, Miller OG:** A study of rubber adhesives in shoes as the cause of dermatitis of the feet. JAMA 149:1371, 1952
5. **Bloch B:** The role of idiosyncrasy and allergy in dermatology. Arch Dermatol Syph 19:175, 1929
6. **Brandao FN:** Shoe Dermatosis. Dermat Ib Lat Am (Eng Ed) 11:29, 1967
7. **Calnan CD, Sarkany I:** Shoe dermatitis. Trans St John's Hosp Derm Soc 43:8, 1959
8. **Coskey RJ, Mehregan AH:** Shoe boot pernio. Arch Dermatol 109:56, 1974
9. **Cronin E:** Shoe dermatitis. Brit J Dermatol 78:617, 1966
10. **deVries HR:** Allergic dermatitis due to shoes. Dermatologica, Basel 128:68, 1964
11. **Fisher AA:** Some practical aspects of the diagnosis and management of shoe dermatitis. Arch Dermatol 79:267, 1959
12. **Fisher AA:** Contact Dermatitis. Philadelphia, Lea & Febiger, 1967
13. **Fisher AA:** Contact dermatitis, 2nd ed, p. 154. Philadelphia, Lea & Febiger, 1973
14. **Gaul LE, Underwood GB:** Primary irritants and sensitizers used in fabrication of footwear. Arch Dermatol Syph 60:649, 1949
15. **Gibson WB:** Sweaty sock dermatitis. Clin Pediatr 2:175, 1963
16. **Grimalt F, Romaguera C:** New resin allergens in shoe contact dermatitis. Cont Derm 1:169, 1975
17. **Hack M:** Chemical and mechanical etiology of shoe dermatitis. Cutis 6:529, 1970
18. **Hunziker N, Winkelmann RK:** Langerhans cells in contact dermatitis of the guinea pig. Arch Dermatol 114:1309, 1978
19. **Malten KE, van Aerssen GGL:** Kontaktkzeme durch Leime bei Schuhmachern and Schujtragern. Berufsdermatosen, 10:264, 1962
20. **Minkin W, Cohen WJ, Frank SB:** Contact dermatitis to East Indian sandals. Arch Dermatol 103:522, 1971
21. **Morris GE:** "Chrome" dermatitis. Arch Dermatol 78:612, 1958
22. **Pilgram RE, Fleagle GS:** Indian sandal strap dermatitis. JAMA 211:1378, 1970.
23. **Provost T, Jillson OF:** Ethylenediamine contact dermatitis. Arch Dermatol 96:231, 1967
24. **Romaguera Sagrera C, Grimalt Sancho F, Pinol Aquade J:** New allergens of the resin group related to contact dermatitis due to shoes. Med Cutanea 11:201, 1974
25. **Ross JB:** Rubber boot dermatitis in Newfoundland: A survey of 30 patients. Canad Med Ass J 100:13, 1969
26. **Samitz MH, Gross S:** Extraction by sweat of chromium from chrome-tanned leathers. J Occup Med 2:12, 1960
27. **Samitz MH, Gross S:** Effects of hexavalent and trivalent chromium compounds on the skin. Arch Dermatol 84:404, 1961
28. **Schamberg IL:** Allergic contact dermatitis to methyl and propyl paraben. Arch Dermatol 95:626, 1967
29. **Scutt RWB:** Chrome sensitivity associated with tropical footwear in the Royal Navy. Brit J Dermatol 78:337, 1966
30. **Shapiro L, Gibbs RC:** Vamp disease. Inflammation of the great toe due to pressure from women's shoes. Arch Dermatol 102:661, 1970
31. **Shatin H, Reisch M:** Dermatitis of the feet due to shoes. Arch Dermatol Syph 69:651, 1954
32. **Spencer MC:** Herbicide dermatitis. JAMA 198:1307, Dec 1966
33. **Spoor HJ:** Indian leather dermatitis. Cutis 11:805, 1973
34. **Suter VH:** Investigation of polyamide stocking eczema. Dermatologica 130:411, 1965
35. **Suurmond D, Verspijck Mijnssen GAW:** Allergic dermatitis due to shoes and a leather prothese. Dermatologica, 134:371, 1967

ATOPIC DERMATITIS

1. **Grove DI, Reid JG, Forbes IJ:** Humoral and cellular immunity in atopic eczema. Brit J Dermatol 92:611, 1975

2. **Hanifin JM, Lobitz WC Jr:** Newer concepts of atopic dermatitis. Arch Dermatol 113:663, 1977

3. **Mihm MC Jr, Soter NA, Dvorak HF, et al:** The structure of normal skin and the morphology of atopic eczema. J Inv Dermatol 67:305, 1976

4. **Neering H, VanDijk E:** Juvenile plantar dermatitis. Acta Dermatovener (Stockholm) 58:531, 1978

11 PAPULOSQUAMOUS DISEASES

PSORIASIS

Psoriasis is a common disorder which is know to be inherited as an autosomal dominant trait with irregular penetrance. Elucidation of an association between psoriasis and the histocompatibility system (HLA-12, BW 17) has opened new avenues of study.[2,4] (See Chap. 1.)

Psoriasis is characterized by its epidermal kinetics and by certain histologic features. Its clinical morphology is distinctive.

The cause of psoriasis is unknown. Endocrine, infectious, metabolic, and neurogenic factors have been considered. However, there are no conclusive scientific data to confirm these theories. The fundamental psoriatic defect is undoubtedly linked to an inherited predisposition to an abnormal biochemical sequence of events.

KINETICS

The regulation of cell division and differentiation is significantly altered in psoriatic keratinocytes. The epidermal turnover time (*i.e.*, the time required for a basal cell to reach the surface and be cast off) is reduced from the normal 28 to 30 days to 3 to 4 days (a seven-fold increase in transit time). This implies an intense metabolic activity, which has been demonstrated with various techniques. The abnormally rapid cell cycle is responsible for the pathophysiologic defect in psoriasis.

HISTOLOGY

Psoriasis includes both epidermal and dermal alterations: (1) an increased and abnormal horny layer (parakeratosis); (2) the migration of polymorphonuclear leukocytes into the horny layer which produces characteristic microabscesses (Munro's abscesses); and (3) dilatation of dermal papillary capillaries with a surrounding round cell infiltration. The clinical appearance of the psoriatic lesion is determined by the predominance of one or another of these changes.

Fig. 11-1. Psoriasis on plantar surfaces.

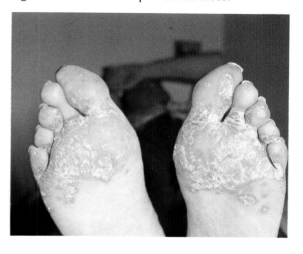

CLINICAL FINDINGS

The abnormal horny layer gives rise to the distinctive scale characteristic of the psoriatic lesion. The silvery appearance of the scale is due to air pockets in the horny layer. The microabscesses in the horny layer are not apparent on gross examination. Dilatation of the capillaries in the tips of the elongated dermal papillae give the vivid red color to the psoriatic lesion.

Two clinical hallmarks of the disease are the (1) Auspitz sign in which manual removal of scale exposes the capillaries through the thinned suprapapillary portion of the stratum malpighii and results in minute bleeding points, and the (2) Koebner phenomenon which refers to extension or aggravation of the psoriatic lesion after local trauma such as scarification or scratching. The Koebner phenomenon is not diagnostic but only suggestive evidence of psoriasis.

The forms of psoriasis are many. Those most commonly seen on the lower extremities are: (1) regular psoriasis on the legs, (2) psoriatic keratoderma on the soles, (3) interdigital psoriasis, (4) pustular psoriasis, localized to the palms and the soles, (5) psoriasis of the nails, and (6) psoriatic arthropathy.

Psoriasis en Plaque

It is rarely seen on the lower extremities but is usually part of a more extensive process involving upper extremities, trunk, and scalp. The lesions may cover the entire body, producing an erythroderma. It is manifested by well-demarcated erythematous plaques capped by white scales. Involvement tends to be symmetrical. It is particularly chronic and difficult to manage. Lesions on the lower extremities respond to therapy last and least.

Psoriatic Keratoderma

It presents as marginated hyperkeratotic plaques and is an especially protracted and rebellious form of psoriasis. This form may involve the palms as well as the soles. Palmoplantar psoriasis displays various degrees of erythema, hyperkeratosis, and fissures. It is almost always bilateral and symmetrical extending in well-defined erythematosquamous plaques and exfoliating in dry, friable lamellae. Massive yellowish or grayish keratoderma due to a greatly thickened horny layer is often seen with deep painful fissures (Fig. 11-1).

Interdigital Psoriasis

This entity, otherwise known as "white psoriasis," was described by Waisman.[3] Five percent of psoriasis patients are supposedly affected. The lesions are marked by whitish hyperkeratosis accompanied by maceration and fissuring located between the toes or at their bases (Fig. 11-2). It is usually accompanied by other localizations, but as an isolated finding it must be differentiated from interdigital dermatophytosis and erythrasma. The histology is diagnostic of psoriasis.

Pustular Psoriasis

It is a morphologic variation of psoriasis. A localized form involves the palms and soles. This type often occurs in the absence of typical psoriasis elsewhere, but may occur concomitantly. The eruption, almost always bilateral and symmetrical, usually starts on the internal aspect of the plantar arch (Fig. 11-3). Occasionally, the initial attack may be characterized by showers of pustules which are sterile. They involute slowly to form hard, brownish squamous crusts. Recurrences of pustules may be preceded by a smarting sensation. Recurrences produce scaly and parakeratotic surfaces before exfoliating. Histopathology shows changes of psoriasis and distinguishes pustular psoriasis from other chronic disorders such as pustular bacterid and forms considered to be nonspecific immunologic responses, classified under pustulosis palmaris et plantaris.

Psoriasis of the Nails

Psoriatic nail changes occur with or without skin involvement, in 10% to 60% of psoriatics. The nail changes are analogous to those of psoriasis of the skin. Biochemical changes are similar to those in psoriatic scales. Nail abnormalities range from simple stippling or punctate pitting and from a yellow, opaque discoloration with disfigurement and terminal crumbling with hyperkeratotic debris to shortening, partial destruction, and detachment of the nails (Fig. 11-4). Periungual changes, diffuse redness, swelling, and desquamation are frequent.

Differential diagnosis of psoriasis of the nails should include onychomycosis, eczematous dermatitides, lichen planus, occupational or traumatic changes, alopecia areata, and various onychodystrophies.

Psoriatic Arthropathy

The psoriatic type of arthritis is usually seen in diffuse forms of psoriasis (Fig. 11-5). The psoriasis and arthritis usually wax and wane together. Distal interphalangeal joints of the hands and feet are most commonly involved. The affliction is asymmetrical, and the deformities are unlike the classical changes in rheumatoid arthritis. Absence of rheumatoid factor differentiates the latter.

TREATMENT

Our present limited understanding of the pathogenesis of psoriasis precludes a cure. Meanwhile, a rational therapeutic approach should utilize measures to correct the known tissue abnormalities. In our experience, there is little need for systemic medication for ordinary psoriasis. Control of the psoriatic eruption is obtained with suitable topical regimens which include such measures as hydration baths, tar and ultraviolet light combinations (Goeckerman regimen), and externally applied medications fitted to the requirement of the individual patient.

Local therapy is still the safest method of treatment. Acute types of psoriasis do best with fluorinated corticosteroids applied two to three times daily. An occlusive technique (overnight or 24-hour occlusion) with plastic wrap or with flurandrenolone tape (Cordan tape) usually initiates involution in most lesions. Occlusion enhances penetration. Topical steroids are potent enough to improve about 50% of psoriatic lesions. Chronic types of psoriasis can be benefited with inunctions of tar-ammoniated mercury-salicylic acid ointments (2% to 10% crude coal tar, 3% to

5% ammoniated mercury, and 2% to 5% salicylic acid).* The Goeckerman regimen (3% to 5% crude coal tar is applied overnight and followed by exposure to ultraviolet light) has the distinct advantage of producing longer remission than do most other modalities. In patients resistant to previous therapy, the Ingram method is suggested. This uses 0.1% to 0.2% anthralin paste with salicylic acid (Lasan 1 or Lasan 2) applied with a wooden tongue blade after a coal-tar bath, then dusted with talc and covered with stockinette. In our experience, the most effective treatment for extensive psoriasis is a modified Goeckerman regimen: The Goeckerman routine in conjunction with a hydration bath uses initially a corticosteroid ointment such as Valisone or Hytone which is later replaced by petrolatum. It is best carried out as an inpatient treatment but can be continued as an outpatient treatment.

Castellani's paint may be used for fissured lesions and interdigital psoriasis.

Because of their location, psoriatic toenails do not present the cosmetic problem seen in fingernail involvement, but patients often insist on treatment. We have found 20% urea in petrolatum or aquaphor effective in removing psoriatic nails. The method consists of applying the urea ointment to the nail, covering the nail with a plastic film wrap and then with adhesive tape. The patient is instructed to keep the area completely dry, and within 5 to 10 days the nail can be removed by either lifting the entire nailplate from the nailbed and trimming it behind the proximal nail fold or by cutting the abnormal portion piece by piece. (See also Farber's method of removing nails with 40% urea ointment in Chap. 18.) Following avulsion, the patient applies a steroid cream to the affected parts.

Intralesional steroids (preferably triamcinolone in a concentration of 5.0 mg per cubic centimeter) are effective for localized lesions; however, we do not recommend their use for lesions on the ankle or foot because of adverse reactions which we have observed when used on these sites.

Ionizing radiation inhibits cellular proliferation and can be useful in controlling the

*Ung. Bossi, Doak Pharmacal Co.

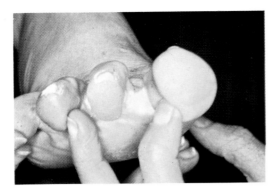

Fig. 11-2. "White psoriasis" (close-up).

Fig. 11-3. Typical lesions of pustular psoriasis of soles.

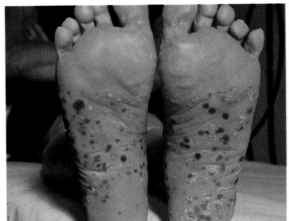

psoriatic lesion. However, the potential dangers of these ionizing rays has been well established and x-ray treatment should be used with caution in this chronic disease. We are against its use.

There are no ideal drugs that can be administered systemically for the treatment of psoriasis.[1]

Various types of systemic therapy have been proposed in the past four decades. There is no conclusive scientific data to confirm the efficacy of hormone therapy; fat-free, low-cholesterol, low-protein, low-tryptophan, or low-amino-acid taurine diets; dietary supplements such as vitamins or wheat germ; pancreatic enzymes; or anti-infective agents. There was a movement supporting the use of systemic steroids, soon followed by use of antimetabolites such as methotrexate and hydroxyurea; more recently, PUVA therapy has come in the vogue (see next section).

Many dermatologists do not favor systemic steroids for psoriasis under any circumstances. The risk of complications such as exfoliation and the likelihood of serious exacerbation on withdrawal of medication are too great. Others limit their use to severe cases of psoriatic arthritis or psoriatic erythroderma.

Methotrexate given orally or parenterally has proved effective in many cases of psoriasis resistant to other modalities of treatment. However, it is a potent antimetabolite of folic acid, and its benefits must be weighed carefully because of its toxic effects on multiple organ systems. The only existing indi-

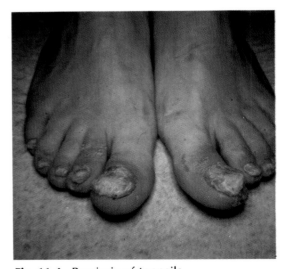

Fig. 11-4. Psoriasis of toenails.

cation for its use in psoriasis is the presence of grave emotional disability ensuing from this disease or severe disabling psoriatic arthritis. Major side effects of hydroxyurea are

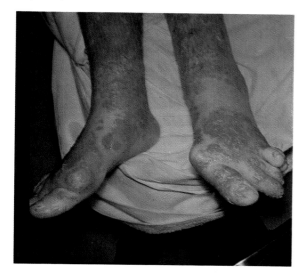

Fig. 11-5. Psoriatic arthropathy.

bone marrow suppression and megaloblastic anemia.

PUVA therapy (photochemotherapy), which combines an oral medication (Psoralen) with local exposure of the skin to ultraviolet light, has been effective in controlling the psoriatic lesions. Immediate side effects are quite tolerable and readily controlled, but the possibility of long-term damage to the skin in the form of multiple malignancies or premature cataracts must be considered. PUVA requires long-term maintenance therapy.

LICHEN PLANUS

Lichen planus is an inflammatory dermatosis of unknown origin, starting insidiously or suddenly. Recent findings have opened new avenues in understanding this disorder. Studies of histocompatibility antigen typing has shown an association between HLA-A3 and lichen planus. According to current evidence, it seems that lichen planus, whether idiopathic, drug-induced, or the product of graft-versus-host reaction after bone marrow transplantation, may be initiated by a cell-mediated response to an induced antigenic change in the skin or mucosa.[3]

CLINICAL FEATURES

Lichen planus runs a sluggish course and often is recurrent. Although the eruption may be asymptomatic, more often there is pruritus of variable degree. Characteristic lesions occur in variable patterns on both the skin and the mucous membranes. The diagnostic lesion is a small, flat-topped, polygonal, violaceous papule that later becomes brownish and may leave deep pigmentation. Other lesions of lichen planus may be annular or centrally umbilicated. The surface may show a whitish network called Wickham's striae. Papules may be arranged in patches, in linear or annular configuration, or confluent in large plaques. Common sites of involvement are the flexor aspects of the arms and the extensor surface of the lower extremity, the buccal mucosa, and the penis.

Most cases of lichen planus last 6 to 9 months; there are few forms of therapy that alter its natural course. The prospect of permanent remission in lichen planus is much better than in psoriasis.

HISTOLOGY

On histologic examination, the features of lichen planus are diagnostic regardless of the site of involvement or the clinical type. There is hyperkeratosis, a thickened stratum granulosum, irregular acanthosis, and liquefaction necrosis of the basal layer. A band of cellular infiltrate presses against the epidermis, hugging and invading it. T lymphocytes are the predominant mononuclear cells in the dermal infiltrate, and the lymphocytes carry HTLA on their surface.[1,2] Colloid bodies have also been considered as an important histologic feature.[8]

VARIATIONS OF LICHEN PLANUS ON THE LOWER EXTREMITY

The most persistent form of lichen planus is hypertrophic lichen planus that classically involves the shins and ankles. Such lesions persist for many more months and even years than does ordinary lichen planus. The lesions are thickened, warty, hypertrophic plaques covered with fine adherent scales. The patches vary in size and configuration, are reddish brown or purplish, and are characterized by their chronicity (Fig. 11-6). The lesions usually itch severely; burning and stinging are less common complaints. Careful inspection of the lesions will usually reveal a typical papule. When hypertrophic lichen planus lesions eventually involute, corresponding areas of depigmentation and some degree of atrophy may remain (Fig. 11-7). The differentiation from lichen amyloidosus and from lichen simplex chronicus may be difficult.

Lesions of lichen planus of the sole are usually situated along the sides rather than the center of the sole. Their color may range from pink to yellow. Here they present as papules or nodules (Fig. 11-8); less often because of coalescence and thickening, they resemble calluses.

Nail changes vary from longitudinal striations, ridging, splitting, and midline fissures to progressive atrophy with eventual total destruction (Fig. 11-9).[12,13] Most characteristic is the paper-like thinning of the nail plate in association with an overgrowth of the cuticle and its subsequent attachment to the nail plate (pterygium formation) (Fig. 11-10), the great toenails being most often affected in this way. The minor nail changes are temporary, but the more severe forms are often permanent. Lichen planus of the nails must be differentiated from onychomycosis, psoriasis, and nail changes due to impaired peripheral circulation or following trauma.

Permanent loss of nails due to lichen planus has been reported by Cornelius and Shelley.[5] In this unusual case, a 60-year-old woman showed permanent loss of her toenails with scaling and superficial erosion of the nail bed and matrix. The patient gave a history of recurrent, painful, superficial ulcerations occurring in the areas of the toenail, which healed without complications. Biopsy of the nail matrix of an involved toe showed the typical histology of lichen planus.

An unusual syndrome of lichen planus has been reported, characterized by bullae and ulcerations confined to the feet and toes, permanent loss of toenails, and a cicatricial alopecia of the scalp.[6,7,10] Distinctive were the chronic, painful, and disabling ulcerations of the feet which present a problem in diagnosis. The toes showed bleeding and the granulating ulcers were surrounded by atrophic depigmented skin. In a recent case report, an autoimmune mechanism was considered an etiologic factor.[14] Along with this concept are the cases reported under the legend of unusual variant of lupus erythematosus or lichen planus.[4,11] In these patients, the clinical lesions consisted of livid red to violaceous atrophic patches and plaques, most common on acral aspects of the extremities. Nails were also commonly involved, often showing anonychia. Immunofluorescent findings showed overlap features of both lupus erythematosus and lichen planus.

TREATMENT

Because the cause of lichen planus is still unknown, treatment is mainly symptomatic and often unsatisfactory.

Apart from symptom-relieving topical medications, there are no known effective therapeutic measures to prevent or combat lichen planus. Antipruritic lotions and corticosteroid creams help relieve itching. We prefer applying the latter on the wet skin. Fluorinated steroid creams under occlusive plastic films can be beneficial. Occasionally, intralesional injections of triamcinolone are useful; for nail lesions, a single local injection (0.2 ml) of triamcinolone acetonide suspension (10 mg/ml) into the affected nail matrix, preceded by a digital Xylocaine block, can be helpful.

At times, the patient requires rest and relief of tensions; thus, mild sedatives or antihistaminics are helpful. There is no indication for systemic corticosteroids in the localized forms of lichen planus on the lower extremities. Treatment with griseofulvin, topical vitamin A acid, and systemic vitamin A are hopeful possibilities. Ortonne et al reported that oral photochemotherapy (methoxypsoralen and long-wave ultraviolet radiation) was effective in lichen planus.[9] The doses required are about double those required for clearing psoriasis. The responses seem to be maintained without further treatment.

PITYRIASIS RUBRA PILARIS

Pityriasis rubra pilaris is a rare, chronic, mildly pruritic inflammatory disease, characterized by fine, acuminate, horny, follicular papules. The cause is unknown, but some feel that it is an inherited, simple autosomal, heterozygous condition. The papules may be preceded by or superimposed upon a seborrhea of the scalp and face. There is often a striking keratoderma of the palms and soles. This unusually thick keratinous, salmon-yellow scaling of the palms and soles is called the "keratodermic sandal of pityriasis rubra pilaris." There is a slow evolution of widespread areas of follicular papules involving not only extremities, but also the trunk and face. Differential diagnosis must include phrynoderma (vitamin A deficiency), psoriasis, and exfoliative erythroderma. Diagnostic are the black, horny, follicular plugs in hair follicles one sees on the dorsa of the fingers. "White islands" of uninvolved skin may be seen within red papulosquamous plaques.[5] Erythematous scaling plaques may resemble psoriasis, and in some cases there may be exfoliation. The keratodermic sandal of pityriasis rubra pilaris is often difficult to differentiate from the heritable plantar keratodermas.

HISTOLOGY

On histologic study, pityriasis rubra pilaris shows follicular and diffuse hyperkeratosis with spotty parakeratosis. The epidermis shows mild irregular acanthosis, and there is liquefactive degeneration of the basal cell layer. A mild chronic perivascular inflammatory infiltrate is found in the dermis.

TREATMENT

Approximately 50% of patients become symptom-free after an average duration of 2 to 3 years of the disease regardless of the therapy used.[3] It is therefore difficult to evaluate the effectiveness of therapy or, in fact, whether treatment is useful.

Vitamin A, 150,000 units daily orally or by intramuscular injections, proved to be favorable in some cases. Prolonged and massive doses (Aquasol A, 500,000 units daily) together with moderate doses of hydroxy-chloroquine (Plaquenil 400 mg daily) have been reported as improving the keratoderma of palms and soles, with no improvement of the rest of the body.[8]

A case report by Waldorf and Hambrick, Jr. described a patient with pityriasis rubra pilaris, myasthenia gravis, and hypovitaminosis A.[7] Among other findings, the patient had progressive yellow thickening of her palms and soles which diminished considerably after 10 weeks' therapy with water-miscible vitamin A, 200,000 units orally bid. Topical 2% vitamin A methyl ester in an emoillient base, tried previously, was unsuccessful. The serum vitamin A level rose to normal after one week of therapy.

Methotrexate, preferably in daily small doses, has brought about a marked clinical improvement which was maintained when treatment was stopped.[2] The folic acid antagonist carries with it the potential for severe side effects. Its use should be restricted to severe expressions of the disease which cannot be controlled by conventional therapy.

The keratoderma of the soles may require only keratolytic ointments and lubricating agents; much more effective has been the topical use of vitamin A acid and vitamin A alcohol.[1,4,6] We have seen a dramatic response with vitamin A acid (0.1% to 0.5%) under occlusion (Fig. 11-11).

REITER'S DISEASE

Although not generally classified among the better-known papulosquamous diseases, Reiter's disease has been included in this chapter because the cutaneous findings are often indistinguishable from psoriasis both clinically and histologically. Reiter's disease is also linked closely to the histocompatibility antigen HLA-B27 which is present with psoriatic arthritis.

Reiter's disease classically consists of urethritis, arthritis, and conjunctivitis but is also often associated with lesions of both the skin and mucous membranes.

The cause is unclear. Most cases are sporadic and usually follow sexual exposure; epidemics have occurred following dysentery. Various theories have attempted to

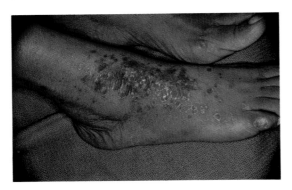

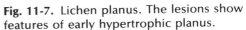
Fig. 11-6. Lichen planus. Note characteristic color of lesions.

Fig. 11-7. Lichen planus. The lesions show features of early hypertrophic planus.

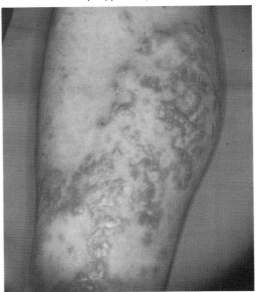

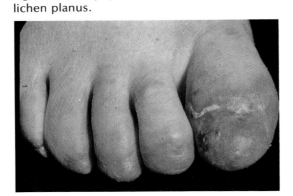
Fig. 11-8. Lichen planus of soles.

Fig. 11-9. Atrophy and destruction of nail in lichen planus.

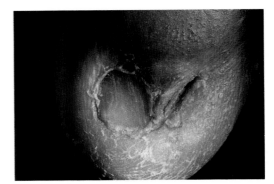
Fig. 11-10. Pterygium formation in lichen planus of nail. (*Courtesy of Dr. I.R. Patel, Nairobi*)

implicate the gonococcus, Shigella and pleuropneumonia-like organisms or an autoimmune hypersensitivity phenomenon. However, the mechanism of the complete Reiter's syndrome, as contrasted to the cause of the urethritis, remains unknown.

Most cases occur in young adult males, in whom urethritis is often the initial manifestation. The urethritis may vary from an acute, painful, hemorrhagic purulent drainage to a mild, often unnoticed, clear discharge. The remaining portions of the syndrome follow in approximately 10 to 14 days, although the mucocutaneous lesions may be delayed for 2 months or longer.

The conjunctivitis is noted in about 50% of cases and is usually bilateral, transient, and rather mild. Of the various components of the syndrome, it is the one most likely to be overlooked by history or on examination. Attacks usually last 5 to 10 days, although occasionally they may be more prolonged. Recurrences of conjunctivitis tend to be unilateral.

Iritis has been reported in about 8% of initial attacks, but in as many as 30% to 50% of recurrent protracted cases. Keratitis and ulceration of the cornea are rare. Interstitial keratitis, optic neuritis, and glaucoma have been reported.

Arthritis is the dominant feature of the syndrome and occurs in at least 90% of cases. The joints are usually bilaterally and symmetrically involved, with weight-bearing joints of the lower extremity and the sacroiliac region the areas most frequently and severely affected. Initially the joint involvement is transient, but recurrent attacks may lead to permanent deformity and may resemble ankylosing spondylitis. X-ray changes may be seen in up to 40% of patients but may also be absent, even in patients suffering repeated attacks.

Skin lesions consist of a marked keratoderma, usually of the soles but possibly other areas, and nail dystrophy. The keratoderma has in the past been termed "keratoderma blennorrhagica," but this term has been largely discarded since it implies a gonococcal etiology. The keratoderma occurs in about 8% of the venereal cases and less often in the postdysentery cases. It begins as a dull red macule which evolves to resemble a

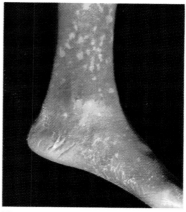

Fig. 11-11. Pityriasis rubra pilaris. The keratodermic sandal of this patient has involuted considerably with use of vitamin A under occlusion. Note the "white islands" of uninvolved skin within the red papulosquamous plaques.

Fig. 11-12. Reiter's disease. Once termed keratoderma blenorrhagic disease; the hyperkeratotic lesions resemble rupial psoriasis.

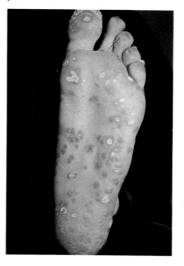

vesicle, but the lesion remains hard. The center of the lesion changes to thicken and form massive cone-shaped hyperkeratotic masses, in some instances resembling rupial psoriasis (Fig. 11-12). In moist intertriginous areas, cheesy, flaccid pustular lesions develop. Rarely, widespread psoriasiform lesions may involve the entire body.

The nail involvement begins as an erythematous swelling of the posterior nail fold; subsequently the nails become grossly distorted by massive subungual hyperkeratosis and nail plate thickening and are shed. The skin lesions involve in from 8 weeks to 10 months.

Mucous membrane lesions occur in up to 50% of venereal cases and in about 10% of postdysentery cases. A circinate painless balanitis lasting a few days to several weeks and erythematous papules, opaque vesicles, or shallow erosions of the oral mucosa are seen.

Thrombophlebitis associated with arthritis of the knee has been reported, as have myocarditis, pericarditis, aortic incompetence, heart block, pleurisy, and pulmonary infiltrations.

The prognosis is generally good, since attacks are self-limiting, lasting a few weeks to several months. However, recurrences are not rare and may lead to disabling arthritis as well as, occasionally, other complications mentioned previously.

The self-limiting nature of Reiter's disease makes therapy difficult to evaluate and should encourage the physician to be conservative in his therapeutic approaches. For the arthritic complaints, bed rest, salicylates, heat, and occasionally a short course of phenylbutazone are effective. Broad-spectrum antibiotics should be used for the urethritis. Cutaneous lesions usually respond to soaks, topical steroids, and keratolytic agents. In severe cases, systemic steroids or methotrexate have seemed helpful, but their use should be reserved for only the most severe and recalcitrant cases.

REFERENCES

PSORIASIS

1. Research Needs in 11 Major Areas in Dermatology. 1. Psoriasis. J Inv Dermatol 73 (Part II):402, 1979
2. **Russell TJ, Schultes LM, Kuban DJ:** Histocompatibility (HL-A) antigens associated with psoriasis. N Engl J Med 287:738, 1972
3. **Waisman M:** Interdigital psoriasis ("white psoriasis"). Arch Dermatol 84:733, 1961
4. **White SH, Newcomer VD, Mickey MR, Terasaki PI:** Disturbance of HL-A antigen frequency in psoriasis. N Engl J Med 287:740, 1972

LICHEN PLANUS

1. **Alario A, Ortonne JP, Schmitt D, Thivolet J:** Lichen planus: Study with anti-human T lymphocyte antigen (anti-HTLA) serum on frozen tissue sections. Brit J Dermatol 98:601, 1978
2. **Bjerke JR, Krogh HK:** Identification of mononuclear cells in situ in skin lesions of lichen planus. Brit J Dermatol 98:605, 1978
3. **Black MM:** What is going on in lichen planus. Clin Exp Dermatol 2:303, 1977
4. **Copeman MPW, Schroeter AL, Kierland RR:** An unusual variant of lupus erythematosus or lichen planus. Brit J Dermatol 83:269, 1970
5. **Cornelius III CE, Shelley WB:** Permanent anonychia due to lichen planus. Arch Dermatol 96:434, 1967
6. **Corsi H:** Lichen planus associated with atrophy of nail matrix and hair follicles on scalp. Proc R Soc Med 30:198, 1936
7. **Cram DL, Kierland RR, Winkelmann RK:** Ulcerative lichen planus of the feet. Bullous variant with hair and nail lesions. Arch Dermatol 93:692, 1966
8. **Eady RA, Cowen T:** Half-and-half cells in lichen planus: Possible clue to the origin and early formation of colloid bodies. Brit J Dermatol 98:417, 1978
9. **Ortonne JP, Thivolet J, Sannwald C:** Oral photochemotherapy in the treatment of lichen planus (LP): Clinical results, histologic and ultrastructural observations. Brit J Dermatol 99:77, 1978
10. **Pierini LE, Abulafia J, Barnatan M:** El liquen como factor de exoniquia definitiva. Arch Agent Dermatol 4:287, 1954
11. **Romero RW, Nesbit LT Jr, Reed RJ:** Unusual variant of lupus erythematosus or lichen planus. Arch Dermatol 113:741, 1977
12. **Ronchese F:** Nail in lichen planus. Arch Dermatol 91:347, 1965
13. **Samman PD:** The nails in lichen planus. Brit J Dermatol 73:288, 1961
14. **Thormann J:** Ulcerative lichen planus of the feet. Arch Dermatol 110:753, 1974

PITYRIASIS RUBRA PILARIS

1. **Beer P:** Studies on the effect of vitamin A acid. Dermatologica, 124:192, 1962

2. **Chernosky ME:** Pityriasis Rubra Pilaris: Treatment with methotrexate. Paper read at 28th Annual Meeting of Amer Acad of Derm, Bal Harbour, Florida, Dec. 11, 1969

3. **Davidson CL Jr, Winkelmann RK, Kierland RR:** Pityriasis rubra pilaris. Arch Dermatol 100:175, Aug., 1969

4. **Lamar LM, Gaethe G:** Pityriasis rubra pilaris. Arch Dermatol 89:515, 1964

5. **Sidi E, Zagula-Mally ZW, Hincky M:** Pso-riasis. Springfield, Ill, Charles C Thomas, 1968

6. **Stuttgen G:** Local treatment of keratoses with vitamin A acid. Dermatologica 124:65, 1962

7. **Waldorf DS, Hambrick GW Jr:** Vitamin A-responsive pityriasis rubra pilaris with myas-thenia gravis. Arch Dermatol 92:424, 1965

8. **Watt TL, Jillson OF:** Pityriasis rubra pilaris: penicillin and antituberculous drugs as pos-sible therapeutic agents. Arch Dermatol 92:428, 1965

12 IMMERSION INJURIES

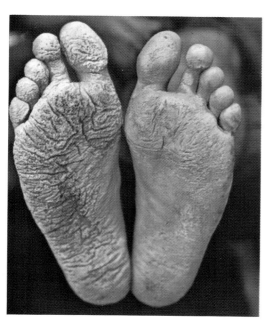

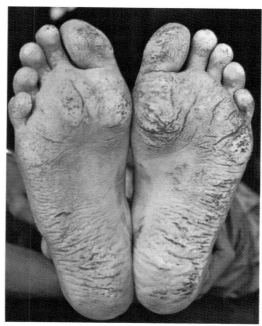

Fig. 12-1. Warm water immersion injury showing marked difference in response to the injury in one individual.

Fig. 12-2. Warm water immersion injury showing more severe response in calloused areas.

WARM WATER IMMERSION FOOT*

The name "warm water immersion injury" refers to the syndrome that has the following signs and symptoms: whitening and wrinkling of the sole with associated pain and/or altered sensation of the sole.[1] The importance of the disorder lies in the fact that it is an occupational hazard among certain military combat personnel operating in tropical areas, although it can disable any susceptible individual who is exposed to the proper environmental conditions.

There is some confusion regarding the relationship between immersion foot and

*In collaboration with G. T. Anderson, M.D.

179

warm water immersion injury. From a practical standpoint, the etiologic factors that cause both these conditions are identical except for the element of cold. Both disorders develop as a result of prolonged immersion in a wet environment. Thus, both might be more properly classified under the descriptive term "immersion injury." As classically described, immersion foot occurs when the water temperature is between 32° and 60° F and is capable of producing permanent tissue damage. On the other hand, warm water immersion injury occurs after prolonged exposure to water warmer than 60° F and is known to cause only temporary disability. It should be pointed out that the figure of 60° F is an arbitrary one; there is no exact temperature level at which one suddenly develops one disorder or the other.[7] Validation of this distinction is now possible (see tropical immersion foot discussed later in this chapter).

The initial signs of warm water immersion injury occur during the first 24 hours, when the weight-bearing surfaces of the sole begin to wrinkle and turn white. More often than not, the skin covering the lateral and dorsal aspects of the foot develops fine wrinkles and some whitening as the feet continue to be exposed to the wet environment. Within 48 to 72 hours, the individual develops symptoms related to the weight-bearing surfaces, especially under the metatarsal areas. These symptoms are variously described as burning pain, pinching, tingling, itching and pain, or aching on bearing weight. It is at this point that the individual becomes a victim of warm water immersion injury, and during combat he becomes a casualty who requires evacuation from the battlefield.

There is a wide range of susceptibility to the effects of an occluded wet environment. Many individuals develop varying degrees of whitening and wrinkling but no symptoms, and there are a few individuals who show almost no evidence of immersion injury even after several days in water. On occasion, one notes a marked inexplicable difference between the feet in the same individual. The areas of the sole with thickened stratum corneum are the first areas to develop signs of immersion injury, and persons with thick

calluses are generally those individuals who develop symptoms more quickly and to a greater degree (Figs. 12-1, 12-2). The wrinkling of the sole frequently becomes so marked that deep fissure-like grooves appear on the sole in the areas between the metatarsal heads. Severe maceration generally develops between and under all toes.

The clinical course during the postimmersion period appears directly related to the severity of the immersion injury. In those individuals who have been affected to a lesser degree, one notes that the soles have nearly regained their preimmersion appearance within 24 hours. In the moderately severe cases, one notes a mild erythema, tenderness on bearing weight, and slight edema of the weight-bearing surfaces which generally disappears gradually over the first 24 to 36 hours. In the most severe cases, the symptoms and signs can take several days to disappear. As the injured stratum corneum begins to dry and exfoliate, fissures can appear beneath the toes and may be a source of secondary pyoderma.

The cause of warm water immersion injury is not fully understood. The histology has never been reported. Clinical observations suggest, however, that the signs and symptoms of this condition are the result of the absorption of water by the stratum corneum and the edema of the underlying tissues. The absorption of water by the stratum corneum makes it thicker, opaque, and white. Fibrous attachments of the sole to the underlying fascia probably help produce the convulted and wrinkled appearance of the sole when edema appears. It seems likely that the symptom of pain, and possibly the edema, occur as the result of the simple traumatic experience of a thick water-laden wrinkled epidermis impinging upon the soft, sensitive tissues beneath.

The most effective prophylaxis for immersion injury is drying the feet for a period of 6 to 8 hours out of every 24 (e.g., sleeping without shoes). This had been shown experimentally and has been known by military commanders for years.[8] This fact possibly explains why this disorder has not been reported in people who do not wear occlusive footgear in a wet environment. The obvious treatment for warm water immersion injury is to maintain a condition of cleanliness and dryness until the skin over the feet has reverted to normal.

EROSION INJURY*

Another clinical expression of immersion injury has been noted during certain combat operations conducted over sandy, muddy terrain during periods of constant rain. This injury, begins to appear in certain individuals within 24 hours as multiple red, sharply circumscribed superficial erosions appearing much like the base of fresh bullae (Figs. 12-3, 12-4) and is generally seen independently of warm water immersion injury because the incubation period is much shorter. As the factor of time in a muddy, wet environment increases, one can see both conditions concurrently. There is a marked individual variation in the extent of this disorder, from a few bright red patches on the dorsum of the toes to extensive erosions from boot top level to the soles. Burning pain is the presenting symptom, and it frequently becomes so severe that the individual has to be evacuated from combat. All patients with this condition state that they can feel their skin being abraded by the dirt from the paddies and fine sand from the streams sifting into and through their boots. Fine particles of sand or dirt can usually be palpated on the surface of these lesions.

The developmental dynamics of erosion injury are not fully understood. Some medical officers have verbally reported that bullae are occasionally noted prior to the appearance of the erosion, but the author has never been witness to this fact. One thing is clinically apparent: walking for extended periods over sandy, wet, or muddy terrain while wearing boots, with or without socks, is common to all cases.

After removal of the patient to a dry environment, the lesions of erosion injury form a thin, dry crust and the patient experiences healing in several days. As in warm water immersion injury, secondary pyoderma can

*In collaboration with G. T. Anderson, M.D.

occur during the postimmersion period and can obviously extend the period of disability.

TROPICAL IMMERSION FOOT

Tropical immersion foot, described by Allen and Taplin, is a different disease from warm water immersion foot.[1] The syndrome was studied in US Army units in Vietnam. The principal characteristics were: temporary inability to walk due to painful swollen feet; history of protracted exposure (>72 hours) to relatively warm water (22° to 32° C); erythema, edema, and tenderness of the skin covering the ankles and dorsa of the feet; chronic inflammation and vasculitis of the upper dermis, with maceration of the stratum corneum; and pronounced variation in individual susceptibility to immersion injury. Complete healing occurred promptly after drying and elevation of the feet. Evidence suggests that tropical immersion foot is caused by an effect of water itself on the dermis, whereas warm water immersion foot is due to hyperhydration of the plantar stratum corneum.[1]

PITTED KERATOLYSIS

For completeness in discussion of immersion foot injury, one must also include a fourth entity, keratoma plantare sulcatum, which was first described in 1910 by Castellani.[3] Because of the recently intensified studies of the feet, it has become known as pitted keratolysis and is commonly associated with warm water immersion foot injury.[9] It may be seen frequently in patients who do not develop the full-blown syndrome.

Pitted keratolysis was originally distinguished in individuals under combat conditions, whose feet are continually wet for 3 days or more, but recently cases of a "forme fruste" type—because of their mild manifestations and occurrence in nontropical areas, especially in athletes (see Chapter 19)—have been described. Small shallow pits develop in the stratum corneum of the sole over the weight-bearing surfaces, particularly the heels, balls of the feet, and toe pads. The lesions begin to occur after 24 to 48 hours

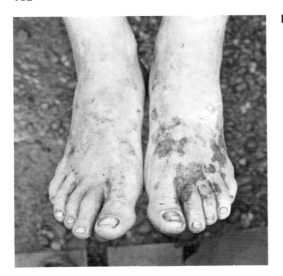

Fig. 12-3. Erosion injury.

Fig. 12-4. Erosion injury 3 days postimmersion.

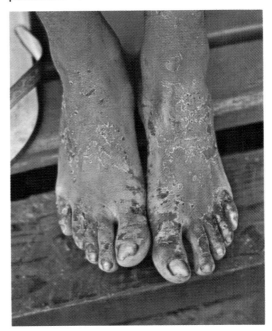

of immersion and range from 2 to 4 mm in diameter and 1 to 2 mm in depth. The number of pits ranges from 5 to more than 100. At times, individual lesions coalesce to form shallow pits 1 to 2 cm in diameter. Some of the pits have a dirty brown to black pigmentation of the crater floor and walls which cannot be removed by washing. The lesions are asymptomatic, and most are completely healed 48 to 72 hours after the patient is removed from the wet environment. The feet by then will also regain the preimmersion appearance. These findings occur more frequently in individuals with hyperhidrosis.

Biopsy of lesions reveals that the pits are confined to the stratum corneum.[4] The floor and walls contain an organism consisting of filamentous and coccal forms. The filaments are branched and are 1 to 2 microns in diameter, and the coccal forms are 2 to 3 microns in diameter. An organism identified as corynebacterium species has been cultured from lesions of pitted keratolysis. The same organism has been used to produce pitted keratolysis in human subjects.

Lamberg described symptomatic pitted keratolysis in which the usual asymptomatic pits are accompanied by plaques of reddened thinning and distinct tenderness on the soles occurring in areas of greatest pressure.[6] Pain

is sufficient to prevent walking, and as much as 14 days of bed rest may be necessary before the patient can walk without pain. Treating patients from the military, Lamberg found 40% formalin in aquaphor effective, as was 1 g erythromycin daily, given orally for one week. In "forme fruste" cases observed in nonmilitary personnel, Gordon found that the signs and symptoms were relieved by 2% buffered gluaraldehyde applied twice a day.[5]

REFERENCES

1. **Allen AM, Taplin D:** Tropical immersion foot. Lancet 2:1185, 1973
2. **Buckels LJ, Gill KA, Anderson GA:** Prophylaxis of warm-water-immersion foot. JAMA 200:681, 1967

3. **Castellani A:** Keratoma plantare sulcatum. J Ceylon Gr Brit Med Assoc 7:10, 1910
4. **Gill KA Jr, Buckels LJ:** Pitted keratolysis. Arch Dermatol 98:7, 1968
5. **Gordon HH:** Pitted keratolysis, forme fruste: A review and new therapies. Cutis 15:54, 1975
6. **Lamberg SI:** Symptomatic pitted keratolysis. Arch Dermatol 100:10, 1969
7. **Taplin D, Zaias N:** Tropical immersion foot syndrome. Mil Med 131:814, 1966
8. **Taplin D, Zaias N, Blank H:** The role of temperature in tropical immersion foot syndrome. JAMA 202:546, 1967
9. **Zaias N, Taplin D, Rebell G:** Pitted keratolysis. Arch Dermatol 92:151, 1965

13 THE SWOLLEN LEG: EDEMA

The swollen lower extremity resulting from disorders of lymphatic and venous circulation, mixed vascular anomalies, benign and malignant tumors, and lipedemas can readily be explained, but precise explanation of the predilection for the lower extremities still remains obscure in many situations.

We are indebted to Taylor and Young for an excellent schematic classification of the swollen limb.[6] We have adapted sections of this classification to fit our theme. Cutaneous clues to diagnosis and treatment are self-explanatory, and many of the disorders mentioned in the following adaptation are reviewed throughout the text.

The Swollen Leg (Edema)*

Systemic diseases
  Cardiac edema
  Renal edema
  Hepatic edema
  Nutritional edema
  Drug-induced edema
Disorders of lymphatic circulation
  Primary lymphedema—
    congenital lymphedema, lymphedema praecox
    syndromes—yellow nail syndrome
  Secondary lymphedema—
    following recurrent lymphangiitis and cellulitis
    elephantiasis nostras verrucosa
Disorders of venous circulation
  Statis dermatitis and chronic venous insufficiency

*Adapted from Taylor & Young.[6]

Thrombophlebitis
Extrinsic pressure on peripheral veins; popliteal and femoral aneurysms
Mixed vascular anomalies
  Klippel-Trenaunay-Weber syndrome
  Arteriovenous fistulae
Tumors
  Benign—cavernous hemangioma, cavernous lymphangioma
  Malignant—Kaposi's sarcoma, liposarcoma, fibrosarcoma
Trauma
  Anterior tibial compartment syndrome
  Ruptured Baker's cyst
  Ruptured gastrocnemius muscle
Miscellaneous
  Metabolic—pretibial myxedema, obesity
  Disorders of subcutaneous fat—lipedema
  Infection—mycetoma, chromoblastomycosis
  "Puffy" feet
  "Idiopathic" edema

Edema is the accumulation of an abnormal amount of water in cells, tissues, or serous cavities; usually it results from excess interstitial fluid in the tissues, which is the definition of edema that we see clinically.

Pitting edema means that finger pressure over the affected part, especially overlying a bony structure, will cause a pitlike depression which matches the contour of the finger. This develops because tissue pressure is increased locally and the interstitial fluid is squeezed into adjacent tissues. Once the pressure is released, the fluid seeps back after a few minutes, and the pit gradually disappears. Because of this characteristic, edema of subcutaneous tissues is easy to recognize. Usually, it is influenced by hydrostatic pressure, and the effects of gravity are evident in that dependent portions are more involved than others—the feet and ankles of a person who is up and about or the back of a person who is bedfast. If subcutaneous edema is localized, as in the case of a bee sting, a small amount may be readily detected. If edema is generalized, however, distributed more or less evenly over the body as often occurs in congestive heart failure and some types of renal disease, 5 or 6 liters of edema fluid may accumulate before it becomes clinically evident. For this reason, the patient's weight gain is a much better indication of generalized edema (a pound for every pint) than is inspection or palpation of tissues. Thus, a record of daily weight gain or loss is an important contribution to the study of patients with generalized edema.

Much is known of the physiologic and biochemical alterations responsible for the pitting edema associated with cardiac, renal, hepatic, nutritional, and drug disorders. For a review of the etiology and pathogenesis of these systemic-dermatologic relationships, the reader is referred to standard texts in physiology and medicine.

Several syndromes with distinctive clinical features infrequently mentioned in the literature but of sufficient importance are described here.

NUTRITIONAL EDEMA ("FAMINE EDEMA")

Hypoproteinemia with resulting decreased colloid osmotic pressure of blood is important in famine edema, but altered renal function with resulting sodium retention is probably more important.

Hypoproteinemia is an inevitable consequence of starvation, but its level varies—in part, perhaps, because of variations in blood volume. Some marasmic patients have a considerably "contracted" blood volume. The plasma protein level in the severely ema-

ciated, starved person is ordinarily 5 g/% or so, but it may fall to less than 1.0 g/%. Many persons starve to death without developing generalized edema, and curiously, when edema does develop, the amount does not bear direct relationship to the degree of hypoproteinemia. Although hypoproteinemia is surely a factor in its production, the complete pathogenesis of famine edema is not understood. The amount of salt taken in and the amount of water consumed are certainly important factors, and patients with hypoproteinemia are quite susceptible to overhydration.

Changes in capillary permeability resulting from attendant vitamin deficiency (vitamin B_1 deficiency resulting in beriberi; vitamin C deficiency resulting in scurvy) may also contribute to nutritional edema. In beriberi ("wet type"), congestive heart failure may result with its attendant edema, augmenting that which may already be present.

Decreased tissue pressure (turgor), that is, decreased mechanical resistance to distention resulting from depletion of subcutaneous fat in starvation states, may allow edema to become more obvious than it would in an obese or normal subject.

DRUG-INDUCED EDEMA

Drugs that may cause edema of the lower extremities include:

Hormones: Corticosteroids and adrenocorticotrophins
Estrogen
Progesterone
Testosterone
Aldosterone-like substances

The mechanism responsible for edema is sodium retention.

Antihypertensives: Ismelin
Apresoline
Rauwolfia
Monamine oxidase inhibitors
Aldomet
Diazoxide

These agents cause arteriolar dilation, which increases capillary hydrostatic pres-

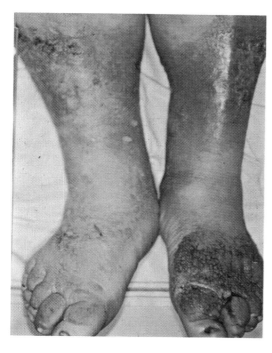

Fig. 13-1. Lymphostasis verruciformis.

Fig. 13-2. Lymphostasis verruciformis. Close-up of lesions on toes.

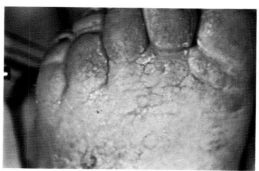

sure and in turn produces the "stretched pore phenomenon"—increased capillary surface area for the transudation of fluid to the tissues.

Anti-inflammatory Drugs: Phenylbutazone

Most drug eruptions with phenylbutazone involve a vascular reaction pattern—edema, seen occasionally, is probably due to alteration of the integrity of the capillary vessels.

Others: Biogastrone
        Monamine oxidase inhibitor-type
        antidepressants

Edema is based on the same mechanism as for the antihypertensive drugs.

ELEPHANTIASIS NOSTRAS VERRUCOSA (LYMPHOSTASIS VERRUCIFORMIS)

Elephantiasis is characterized by enlargement and deformity of the involved area, usualy a limb. These changes are due to hypertrophic fibrosis of the skin and subcutaneous tissues resulting from blocking of the lymphatics.

Elephantiasis is of various types:

1. Congenital (Milroy's disease): congenital and familial form
2. Tropical (filaria, *F. bancrofti*)
3. Nostra of the temperate zone
4. Symptomatic or pseudoelephantiasis secondary to syphilis, frambesia, mycoses, neoplasms, surgery.

Some individuals show a distinct tendency to experience recurrent episodes of erysipelas and cellulitis of the lower leg, ankles, and toes. An elevated temperature and pain in the inguinal region usually accompany an attack. Frequently, insignificant trauma is the precipitating factor. After numerous attacks occurring over a period of time in the same area, permanent, firm brawny edema with hypertrophic warty epidermal changes of the skin appear in the involved portions of the extremity, leading to elephantiasis nostras verrucosa (Figs. 13-1, 13-2).

In lymphostasis verruciformis, chronic low-grade pyoderma is often present, although frequently it is not clinically apparent. Poor hygiene is a contributing factor.

Prophylaxis is the most important aspect of therapy, but when the changes are established, long-term low-dose antibiotic therapy and the wearing of a pressure-gradient stocking are helpful. Forty percent urea lotion or cream will reduce marked hyperkeratotic debris.

LYMPHEDEMA DUE TO MALIGNANCY (NEOPLASTIC INVASION OF NODES AND VESSELS)

Carcinoma of the prostate is the most common cause of this form of secondary lymphedema in the male; lymphoma is the most common cause in the female.

Lymphedema is very common in Kaposi's sarcoma.

TRAUMATIC EDEMA

Anterior Tibial Compartment Syndrome

This syndrome refers to ischemic necrosis of the muscles enclosed in this tight anatomic compartment on the anterior leg due to occlusion of the anterior tibial artery. Signs and symptoms include pain, tenderness, swelling, and induration over the compartment; foot drop and inability to dorsiflex the toes occur due to infarction of the anterior tibial muscle and the long extensors of the toes.

Ruptured Baker's Cyst

The popliteal bursae are found in the popliteal space and are numerous and inconstant. Of these, the gastrocnemio-semimembranosus bursa is of the most clinical importance, as its distention by fluid is the usual cause of a popliteal or Baker's cyst. In other words, this is a bursitis. The popliteal bursae are often connected with the synovial cavity of the knee. When enlarged they stand out as firm, hard swellings when the knee is extended but may disappear when it is flexed. Sudden trauma and strain are important factors in causing symptoms of pain and swelling in the popliteal space and in the calf. The condition can be confused with thrombophlebitis.

Ruptured Gastrocnemius Muscle

This is post-traumatic and is manifested by pain, swelling, and hematoma of the calf. It is usually misdiagnosed as thrombophlebitis. In discussing this condition, one should also mention the syndrome of plantaris tendon rupture as the result of sudden effort or strain; symptoms of pain, swelling, and hematoma also occur. In the latter condition, a tear of the plantaris tendon or muscle fibers is often associated with tear of the sural venous plexus, in which case gravitational ecchymosis of the lower part of the leg and ankle becomes marked. These sural veins are the same culprits involved in high-pressure perforator leaks in the post-phlebitic leg and stasis disease in the gaiter or spat area of the lower leg and ankle, i.e., perforator incompetence.

LIPEDEMA OF THE LEGS

This clinical entity has been aptly called the "painful fat syndrome." Lipedema of the legs was described originally by Allen and Hines in 1940; a subsequent report in 1951 reviewed 119 cases examined during a 9-year period.[1,7] Recent reports have added new data.[3,5]

The characteristic features are (1) symmetrical swelling and aching in the legs, often associated with a weight increase; (2) almost exclusively found in women; (3) minimal to absent pitting edema; and (4) the swelling and aching do not recede at rest. The "stovepipe" lower extremity is a distinctive stigma. There may be a familial history. All pathologic studies are essentially normal except for significant amounts of free fluid fat in biopsy specimens. Roentgenologic studies are of no diagnostic value. Compressive bandages relieve most of the pain and some of the fatty edema temporarily. Elevation of the extremity, low-salt diet, and diuretics are not effective.

PHYSIOLOGIC EDEMA; PUFFY FEET

It must be remembered that dependent edema may be physiologic at times, particularly in people who lead sedentary lives (orthostatic or gravitational edema). It is commonly seen in pregnancy and may also be seen premenstrually.

What about puffy feet and ankles, especially in women, during hot weather? This condition is not uncommon—what is the basis for this complaint? There are many causes that could account for this problem, and Fairbairn has provided some insight: If one can assume that all systemic factors (cardiac, hepatic, and renal) and all local factors (such as lipedema, lymphedema, chronic venous insufficiency, local inflammatory processes) have been excluded as the possible primary causative factor, then one is still left with additional possible causes.[2] These include the use of drugs that may cause edema, such as estrogens, and estrogen-progesterone combinations, certain antihypertensive drugs, and many others. If these factors have been ruled out satisfactorily, then one must consider primarily sodium intake. Fairbairn suggests that many people ingest considerably more salt during the summer months than they do during the winter. Increased sodium intake may then cause mild gravitational edema. If this situation is coupled with any of the systemic or local causes for edema, the process of edema development would be enhanced and worsened.

"IDIOPATHIC" EDEMA

Studies by MacGregor and coworkers offer clarification of this interesting syndrome, "idiopathic" edema.[4] They found that 10 women with so-called "idiopathic" edema had sodium and water retention and a rapid gain in weight when their accustomed intake of diuretics was suddenly stopped. Their findings suggest that the administration of diuretics not only makes the problem worse, but also perpetuates the edema. In addition, the condition in some patients may have been initiated and subsequently aggravated by large fluctuations in sodium and carbohydrate intake. The authors suggest that intermittent edema of unknown cause in most, if not all, otherwise healthy women is due to their use of diuretics, possibly abetted on occasions by self-imposed fluctuations in sodium and carbohydrate intake. In other words, this edema is not idiopathic.

REFERENCES

1. **Allen EV, Hines EA Jr:** Lipedema of the legs: A syndrome characterized by fat legs and orthostatic edema. Mayo Clinic Proc 15:184, 1940
2. **Fairbairn II JF:** In questions and answers. JAMA 230:1201, 1974
3. **Greer KE:** Lipedema of the legs. Cutis 14:98, 1974
4. **MacGregor GA, et al:** Is "idiopathic" edema idiopathic? Lancet 1:397, 1979
5. **Stallworth JM, Hennigar GR, Jonsson HT, et al:** The chronically swollen painful extremity. JAMA 228:1656, 1974
6. **Taylor JS, Young JR:** The swollen limb. Cutaneous clues to diagnosis and treatment. Cutis 21:553, 1978
7. **Wold LE, Hines EA Jr, Allen EV:** Lipedema of the legs: A syndrome characterized by fat legs and edema. Ann Intern Med 34:1243, 1951

14 ULCERS

Although the vast majority of ulcers of the leg are related to venous insufficiency, one must always consider the possibility of other etiologic mechanisms. This is particularly true because differing etiologic factors may produce similar morphologic changes. For our purposes, the following classification according to causal mechanism is relatively simple and reasonably complete.

Classification of Ulcers of the Leg According to Causal Mechanism
I. External
  A. Primary
    1. Trauma
    2. Infections: ecthyma, tropical ulcers
    3. Decubitus (trophic) ulcers
    4. Neurotic excoriations; factitious
  B. Secondary to a Predisposing Lesion
    1. Burns (thermal and chemical)
    2. Radiodermatitis
    3. Neoplasms
II. Internal
  A. Vascular Diseases
    1. Arterial-ischemic
      (a) Arteriosclerotic
      (b) Hypertensive
      (c) Thromboangiitis obliterans
      (d) Livedo reticularis
      (e) Atrophie blanche
    2. Venous
      (a) Stasis
      (b) Thrombophlebitis
  B. Blood Dyscrasias
    1. Anemias (heritable)
      (a) Sickle cell
      (b) Thalassemia
      (c) Congenital hemolytic
    2. Dysproteinemia
      (a) Macroglobulinemia
      (b) Cryoglobulinemia
  C. Neuropathic
  D. Metabolic
    1. Diabetes mellitus
    2. Gout
  E. Autoimmune Diseases
    1. Necrotizing angiitides
    2. Lupus erythematosus
    3. Scleroderma
    4. Rheumatoid arthritis
    5. Polyarteritis nodosa
    6. Pyoderma gangrenosum
  F. Granulomas
    1. Microbiological
      (a) Syphilis
      (b) Erythema induratum
      (c) Atypical mycobacterial
      (d) Leprosy
      (e) Deep fungal infections
    2. Drugs
      (a) Halides
  G. Miscellaneous
    1. Acrodermatitis chronica atrophicans

EXTERNAL CAUSES

Ulcers produced by external causes are self-explanatory; diagnosis depends on the history. Examples of these not uncommon ulcers are presented in Figures 14-1 through 14-6. Some of these ulcers have been described elsewhere in the text; distinctive features of the others are outlined next.

DECUBITUS ULCERS

They occur most commonly in bedridden older patients, but young patients with neurologic disease can be affected. The ulcers localize over bony prominences, the heel region is one of the characteristic sites. They present as deep ulcers with marked peripheral undermining which can extend down to bone. X-ray studies are necessary to rule out osteomyelitis.

FACTITIOUS ULCERS

These ulcers are characterized by their bizarre configurations and are located at sites accessible to self-induced trauma.

ULCERS SECONDARY TO RADIODERMATITIS

The distinctive feature in this type of ulcer is the surrounding area of radiodermatitis: an atrophic skin, loss of hair, mottled hyperpigmentation and hypopigmentation, and telangiectasia.

INTERNAL CAUSES

It is not intended to present this group as final; a degree of overlapping is apparent, particularly in the category of the autoimmune diseases. This group has been discussed under connective tissue disorders. Ulcers complicating vasculitis are discussed in the chapter on vasculitides. Our attention is directed toward the following selected ulcer syndromes.

VASCULAR DISEASES

Arterial—ischemic

Arteriosclerosis Obliterans (Figs. 14-7, 14-8). Leg ulcers of arteriosclerosis are due to infarction following the occlusion of an end artery. Arteriosclerotic ulcers tend to occur on the most distal portions of the extremity and thus are most often seen on the toes or feet. When an ischemic ulcer develops on the leg, it is almost invariably initiated by local trauma (*i.e.*, the patient sustains a break in the skin which does not heal).

Since episodes of trauma may occur anywhere on the leg, there is no typical location for an ischemic ulcer, although many are located on the anterior portion of the limb, the lateral malleolus, and the acral portions of the toes because injuries are somewhat more common in these areas. The base of the ulcer of arteriosclerosis obliterans is necrotic and hemorrhagic with a slight serous discharge. The adjacent skin does not exhibit signs of congestion or stasis changes. Rather, the ulcers are often surrounded by normal-appearing skin or by a rim of blue or purple skin representing infarcted tissue. The ulcers are frequently painful, often severely so, unless diabetic neuropathy is present.

Pedal pulses are often absent, thereby providing confirmatory evidences of arterial disease; they are, however, present in up to 40% of cases. The ulcers usually occur in middle-aged or elderly patients.

Therapy must be individualized; however, there are some general instructions which are applicable. The patient should be warned to avoid physical injury from any source and extremes of temperature. Caution against hot water or ice bags, and against bathing in very hot or very cold water. Interdict the use of tobacco because of nicotine's vasoconstrictor effects. Improve peripheral circulation with vasodilator drugs. Whiskey, 1 or 2 ounces, 4 times daily can also be effective as a mild vasodilator.

If the ulcer results from localized occlusion of small arterial branches, then some will heal solely with bed rest with elevation of the *head* of the bed and cool saline compresses. Others will respond to lumbar sympathectomy combined with complete excision of the ulcer and its surrounding rim of infarcted tissue, followed by a split-thickness skin graft from the abdomen onto the deep fascia. Occasionally, arterial bypass surgery may be warranted. It is of utmost importance to determine that the arterial inflow at the iliac level is adequate before attempting reconstructive arterial surgery on the femoral-popliteal system.

Weismann and Johnson reported the results of therapy in 31 cases of arteriosclerotic ulcers of the leg.[29] Two healed with conservative therapy alone; the remaining 29 patients had a combination of medical and surgical treatment (20 improved and 5 eventually required amputation).

Hypertensive Ulcers of the Leg. These lesions usually occur in women between the ages of 50 and 70 who have been hypertensive for variable, but usually prolonged, periods.[31] Other criteria for establishing the diagnosis are palpable pulses in the legs and an absence of disturbance in the venous circulation. A spontaneously occurring painful red plaque is the initial lesion, most commonly found on the lateral aspect of the ankle, although it may appear low on the posterior and lateral portions of the leg. Within 7 to 10 days, the plaque becomes blue and purpuric. An alternative initial lesion is a simple area of bluish purpuric discoloration of the skin. Soon a hemorrhagic bleb forms on the initial lesion, then breaks down and forms an ulcer which is pale, with little or no granulation tissue, and is very painful. A thick eschar often eventually forms over the ulcer. Generally the lesion develops slowly over a period of months. Some investigators report that the ulcers heal spontaneously in 6 to 9 months if irritating topical medicaments are not applied; in our own and others' experience, these ulcers tend to be extremely chronic and recalcitrant (Fig. 14-9).

Ulcerations in Thromboangiitis Obliterans. Thromboangiitis obliterans or Buerger's disease is a chronic inflammatory disease of the blood vessels with involvement of both arteries and veins occurring in males, particularly Jewish, between 20 and 40 years of age. Recurrent episodes of phlebitis and cellulitis occur, and pain is a prominent symptom. Thrombosis of vessels leads to gangrene, necrosis, and ulceration of the skin of the lower leg and foot.

Therapy is difficult. Tobacco and caffeine,

mechanical and thermal (especially cold) trauma are to be avoided. Sympathectomy and other surgery, including amputation, are often required.

Ulcerations in Livedo Reticularis. Ulcers occasionally occur in areas of skin involved by livedo reticularis. (See Chap. 3 for further discussion.)

Atrophie blanche. Refer to Chapter 3 for discussion of this disorder.

Venous

Stasis Ulcer. The deep venous system of the leg is separated from the superficial veins by the deep fascial layer. This structure provides good support to the deep veins. By contrast, the superficial veins are poorly supported by the subcutaneous tissue and skin. Numerous communicating veins, called perforators, connect the superficial veins to the deep system. The deep venous system contains bicuspid valves to prevent backflow of blood and to facilitate venous return in a cephalad direction. Venous hypertension develops in the veins of the lower legs, resulting in chronic congestion of the tissues. If the perforating veins become incompetent, the pressure in the deep venous system is transmitted directly to the superficial veins.

The medial portions of the ankle and lower leg are the most common sites of stasis ulcers because it is there that the larger perforators occur in greatest numbers (Fig. 14-10).[14] Skin changes resulting from the chronic congestion are edema, pigmentation, induration and ulceration, eczematoid dermatitis, and subacute cellulitis. Often the origin of the ulcer is minor trauma, infection, or occasionally the injudicious use of irritating topical medications.[17] Most ulcers caused by chronic venous insufficiency are rather shallow with irregularly shaped shelving edges and a reddish base with prominent granulation tissue, and are surrounded by the mottled pigmentation of chronic stasis dermatitis. Some patients complain of pain or discomfort in the area of the ulcer, but severe pain is not associated with uncomplicated

Fig. 14-1. Ulcer on heel resulting from shoe trauma.

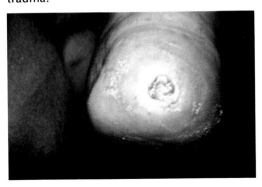

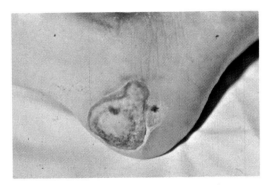

Fig. 14-2. Ulcer caused by pressure from brace.

Fig. 14-4. Factitious ulcer. Patient applied cork soaked in phenol.

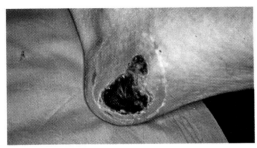

Fig. 14-3. Eschar adherent to ulcer secondary to third-degree burn caused by hot water bag.

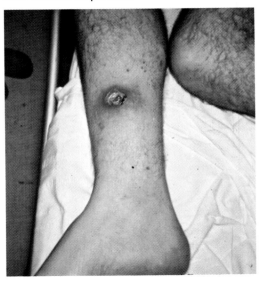

Fig. 14-5. Ulcer following x-ray treatment for epithelioma.

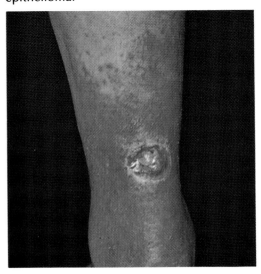

Fig. 14-6. Ulceration in squamous cell carcinoma.

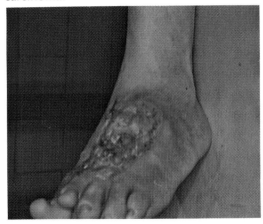

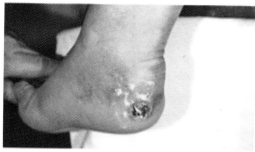

Fig. 14-7. Arteriosclerotic ulcer. Base of the ulcer is necrotic and hemorrhagic (infarcted tissue)

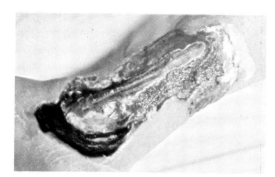

Fig. 14-8. Extensive ulceration in patient with arteriosclerosis and diabetes.

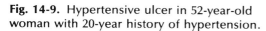

Fig. 14-9. Hypertensive ulcer in 52-year-old woman with 20-year history of hypertension.

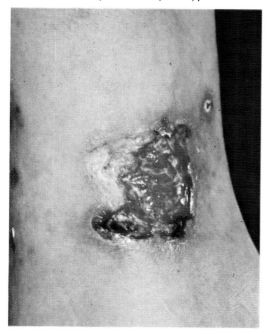

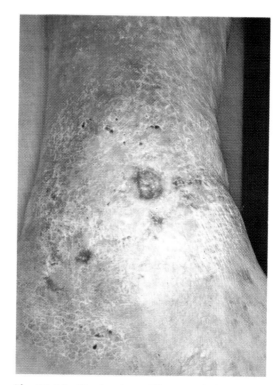

Fig. 14-10. Stasis ulcer. Characteristic localization: "spat" area.

Fig. 14-11. Thrombophlebitic ulcer penetrating to deep fascia.

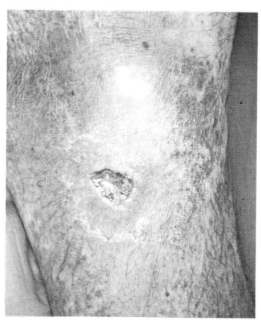

stasis ulcer. (See also stasis dermatitis, Chap. 3.)

The mainstays of therapy consist of bed rest, elevation of the legs (in severe chronic venous insufficiency, elevating the leg to at least 45° is absolutely essential), saline or dilute Burow's compresses, and pressure gradient stockings.[2] Other therapeutic measures which may facilitate healing in selected cases are discussed at the end of the chapter.

Thrombophlebitic Ulcer. In contrast to a varicose ulcer, a postthrombotic ulcer always penetrates the deep fascia. The edges of the ulcer are deep and indurated; the floor is covered with a thick, grayish, firmly adherent crust. Usually the surrounding skin is extensively indurated (Fig. 14-11), and pain is a constant accompaniment.

BLOOD DYSCRASIAS

Anemias

Sickle Cell Anemia. Many patients with sickle cell disease who survive into adolescence or adulthood have chronic leg ulcers or the scars of previous ulcers. These ulcerations may antedate other clinical manifestations of sickle cell disease. The leg lesions themselves (Fig. 14-12) are not distinctive enough to permit a diagnosis clinically, but the ulcer may be the chief complaint and may lead to the detection of sickle cell anemia. The diagnosis is confirmed by laboratory studies showing a normocytic and normochromic anemia with sickling of cells, and by hemaglobin electrophoresis. Oral zinc therapy, discussed at the end of this chapter, has been recommended, but its use is controversial.

Ulcers Associated With Thalassemia. Leg ulcers occur rarely in Mediterranean anemia, only a few cases having been reported in American literature. The ulcers occur around the ankle, may be either unilateral or bilateral, and may involve both the medial and lateral malleolar areas (Fig. 14-13). Leg ulcers appear only in patients with thalassemia minor, since only a rare patient with thalassemia major survives beyond puberty. The pathogenesis of the ulcers is not known. Samitz *et al* postulated that the etiologic factors

giving rise to the ulcers were multiple and nonspecific: trauma, infection, excoriation, hypoxia due to chronic anemia, and peripheral slowing of blood flow.[24] Therapy should be conservative; the ulcers have healed with the application of soaks, rest, elevation, debridement, grafts, Ace bandages, and Unna's boots. Transfusions and splenectomy have not proved beneficial to the healing of the ulcers. High-dose ascorbic acid (3 g daily) has been reported effective in the management of thalassemic leg ulcers; however, further studies are required to confirm this pilot study.[1]

Dysproteinemias

Refer to Chapter 3.

NEUROPATHIC ULCERS

Neuropathic ulcers are secondary to trauma in patients with neurologic disease. Classic examples are those associated with diabetes mellitus, syphilis (tabes dorsalis), leprosy, syringomyelia, and polyneuropathy. The ulcers are sharply marginated and painless. They usually occur on the soles of the feet, especially over bony prominences. See Chapter 5 for the typical neuropathic ulcer as seen in diabetes.

METABOLIC ULCERS

Ulcers in association with diabetes mellitus, necrobiosis lipoidica diabeticorum, and gout are discussed in Chapter 5.

AUTOIMMUNE DISEASES

Ulcers in association with necrotizing angiitides, polyarteritis nodosa, and pyoderma gangrenosum are reviewed in Chapters 3, 4, and 7, respectively.

Systemic Lupus Erythematosus

Although leg ulcers have been reported in lupus erythematosus on several occasions, they do not occur commonly. Tuffanelli and Dubois noted leg ulcers in 5.6% of their series of 520 cases.[27] The ulcers usually occurred over the pretibial or malleolar areas, ranged in diameter from 1 to 10 cm, and had smooth erythematous borders. The ulcers may be associated with livedo reticularis or cryoglobulinemia. Laboratory tests that may be helpful include those used in diagnosing systemic lupus erythematosus, skin biopsy, and immunofluorescent studies. Vasculitis of medium-sized vessels resulting in infarction of the skin and subcutaneous tissues is presumably the cause of the ulceration. Leg ulcers in association with systemic lupus erythematosus heal rapidly with steroid therapy, whereas traumatic ulcers occurring in areas of atrophy heal slowly.

Sclerodermatous Leg Ulcers

In systemic sclerosis, ulcerations of the distal portions of the extremities as well as over the joints are common.[16] On the legs, the ulcers usually occur over the knees and ankles. The lesion may be a shallow erosion or a deep indolent ulceration with deposits of calcium in the crater. The ulcer itself may suggest the diagnosis of scleroderma, but the diagnosis is usually made by finding the cutaneous changes elsewhere and by biopsy.

These ulcers are notoriously recalcitrant to therapy. Herman *et al* reported one case in which skin grafting was successful.[13] Early reports suggested that DMSO might prove efficacious in healing these troublesome lesions; however, further studies are necessary to substantiate this finding.

In general, ulcers due to vasculitis, scleroderma, and dermatomyositis respond poorly, if at all, to pharmacologic agents and need meticulous care given locally.

Ulcers Associated With Rheumatoid Arthritis

Leg ulcers complicating rheumatoid arthritis are described in a separate section in Chapter 7.

Granulomatous Ulcers of the Leg

The ulcerations that may occur on the leg in late syphilis (gummas), erythema induratum, atypical mycobacterial infections, leprosy, and deep fungal infections may frequently be misdiagnosed because the correct etiologic possibility is simply not considered (Figs. 14-14, 14-15). These ulcers are dis-

cussed in Chapter 2 (Microbiological Diseases) and Chapter 4 (in the section on Erythema Induratum). Any ulceration that is clinically atypical, or does not heal with conservative therapy, should be biopsied and appropriate stains should be performed to ascertain whether one of the above causes is present and to rule out the possibility that the ulcer represents an indolent malignancy. Additional studies, such as bacterial and fungal cultures and serologic tests for syphilis, may also be indicated.

Ulcerations Due to Halides

Both bromide and iodide compounds may produce a wide variety of skin eruptions. The most common dermatosis is an acneform or follicular pustular eruption. However, granulomatous fungating or ulcerative lesions of the extremities are also seen; this possibility must be considered in the diagnosis of ulcers that do not respond to the usual modes of therapy, particularly if they have a granulomatous border (Fig. 14-16). Although most drug eruptions fade within two weeks after withdrawal of the offending agent, the lesions produced by the halides characteristically are slow to involute.

MICROBIOLOGY OF LEG ULCERS

Most leg ulcers have a mixed flora of common pathogens. The significance of these organisms is controversial; some authors believe that they exacerbate and worsen the ulcer, while others consider the bacterial flora to be often of little importance. In a study of the bacterial flora of peripheral vascular ulcers, Friedman and Gladstone were unable to show whether the surface infection found in clinically inflamed ulcers is significant and warrants antibacterial therapy.[10] On the other hand, it has been shown that varicose ulcers may act as reservoirs for hospital strains of *S. aureus* and *P. pyocyanea*, and that a high incidence of cross-infection may occur among patients attending a leg ulcer clinic.[19] In another approach, Lookingbill *et al* reported that quantitative bacteriologic measurements can serve as useful tools in evaluating the healing of leg ulcers.[18]

Studies done by English, Smith, and Har-

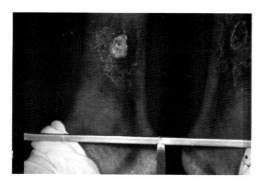

Fig. 14-12. Ulcers with sickle cell anemia.

Fig. 14-13. Ulcer in thalassemia.

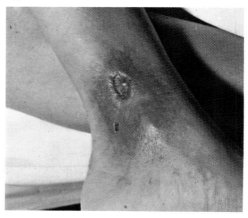

man on the fungal flora of the legs of patients with venous ulcers showed that a Candida species and Fusarium strains were commonly found in the moist skin surrounding the ulcer, rather than in the ulcer itself.[8] Treatment with nystatin did not have any obvious clinical effect on the rate of healing the ulcers.[26] Fusiform bacilli with or without spirochetes have been considered the causal organisms in phagedenic ulcers, which usually occur on the lower leg in children and young adults in hot, humid regions.

DIAGNOSTIC APPROACH TO LEG ULCERS

In the evaluation of a patient with leg ulcers, a careful systematic approach is essential to ensure the greatest probability of arriving at an etiologic diagnosis. The first two steps in this approach are the most important: (1) a careful history; and (2) a complete physical examination.

Following the completion of these steps, a variety of tests may be utilized to establish the diagnosis. In some patients only one or two tests may be necessary, while in others a wide spectrum of studies is essential. Among the procedures indicated are:

1. Complete blood count
2. Blood chemistry profile
3. Serologic test for syphilis
4. Urinalysis
5. Skin biopsy
6. Bacterial smear, anaerobic and aerobic cultures
7. Chest x-ray

8. Fungal KOH preparation and culture, including special culture media when indicated
9. Tuberculin and fungal skin tests
10. Serum or immune electrophoresis, or both
11. LE cell prep, latex fixation, sickle cell prep, and hemoglobin electrophoresis
12. Bone marrow or lymph node biopsy

Additional x-ray, fluorescent antibody, and immunoglobulin studies and other systemic evaluations may also be indicated in specific cases.

The etiologic association between venous disease and leg ulcers has been demonstrated with anatomical, physiologic, and radiologic studies (phlethymography, phlebography) and more recently by Doppler ultrasound. A new quick transcutaneous method using two ultrasound flowmeters can distinguish ischemia due to poor arterial supply from that due to poor venous drainage.[30]

A point worth stressing is that a biopsy should be done in any ulcer which is atypical in appearance, or which does not respond to therapy; in this way unsuspected vasculitis, malignancy, or granulomatous infections may be discovered.

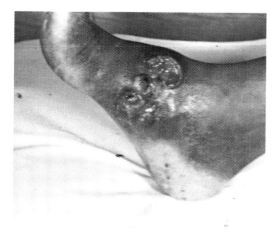

Fig. 14-14. Ulcerative gummas.

Fig. 14-15. Ulcers in maduromycosis.

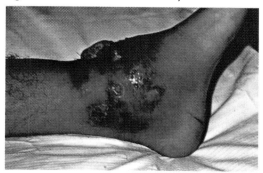

TREATMENT

Treatment depends upon establishing the correct etiologic diagnosis, Then come the basics: posture, topical medications, compression bandages, surgery. We focus here on the stasis ulcer. For ulcers in association with metabolic, autoimmune, and granulomatous disorders, treatment (systemic) is dependent on the underlying disease and is discussed under these diseases; however, local measures are applicable to almost all ulcers.

Bed rest is probably the most effective treatment for an acute leg ulcer.

Hosts of topical preparations have been recommended for local therapy, and this itself suggests that none is entirely satisfactory. Furthermore, one should always keep in mind the possibility of adverse reactions caused by some of these preparations. Topical antibacterial agents and antibiotics, such as nitrofurazone (Furacin) and neomycin, are common offenders. Occasionally, the preservative used in the ointment is responsible. We have observed several cases in which the preservatives, paraben and ethylenediamine, have aggravated eczematization because of sensitization. It is therefore advisable to avoid many of these preparations. In fact, it is a good general rule to avoid any type of ointment, especially on ischemic ulcers. Simple, bland applications are the measures of choice.

Fig. 14-16. Ulcers in granulomas of bromoderma.

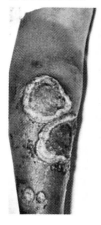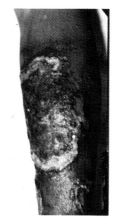

For local infection: As mentioned previously, infection plays a minor role in stasis ulcer, and antibacterial (local or systemic) therapy is not necessary. In ulcers infected with Pseudomonas, Calloway has reported on the use of 1/4% to 1/2% acetic acid.[3] In our experience we have found this highly effective. When ulcers show rapid extension with undermining of the edges, suspicion of an infectious process should be considered. In this situation, aerobic and anaerobic cultures and definition of the organism are important, and specific antibiotic therapy should be instituted.

Enzymatic debridement is useful to clean away detritus but does not otherwise contribute to healing of the ulcer and should be discontinued when the ulcer is clean. The most commonly used are sold under the names of Biozyme, Varidase, Chymar, Elase, and Tryptar. A combination of papain and urea (Panafil) is also useful for enzymatic debridement. Debrisan, a dextran polymer, is a new medication promoted for use in debridement of secreting wounds and ulcers. The product is supplied as dry beads ranging in diameter from 0.1 to 0.3 mm. Debrisan has a powerful hydrophilic action and absorbs serous and purulent exudate from the surface of the ulcers. In a study done by Pace, the beads of dextran were applied to the surface of ulcers in layers 5 mm or more in thickness, covered with plastic film, and held in place with secure bandaging.[22] The exudate-absorbing capacity of the beads was particularly beneficial in ulcers that had uneven surfaces, undercut margins, and sinus tracts. As with other debriding agents, the beads may be used alone until the surface of the ulcer is free of exudate. They should then be used intermittently or discontinued entirely in most cases.

Benzoyl peroxide is one of the most effective agents for debridement and treatment of leg ulcers. The topical application of 20% benzoyl peroxide was developed by Pace, and best results have been obtained in the treatment of stasis ulcers.[21] His regimen consists of the application of a 20% benzoyl peroxide lotion made with pieces of terrycloth toweling cut to fit the size of the ulcer into which it is pressed. The skin surrounding the ulcer is covered with a layer of petrolatum to prevent irritation. Plastic film is applied over the terrycloth dressing and taped to the leg, and a pad is often placed over the dressing to keep the medication in contact with the ulcer. Fresh granulation tissue forms rapidly. Several mechanisms of action have been attributed to benzoyl peroxide: debridement, stimulation of granulation tissue, and an increase of oxygen tension in devitalized tissue.[5]

Whole blood or powdered blood cells have been advocated to stimulate healing of both ischemic and stasis ulcers when applied to the ulcer surface. We prefer packing the ulcer with Gelfoam powder for 24 hours followed by cleansing with fresh hydrogen peroxide. The application of the powder is repeated, and the treated area is covered with a pressure bandage. This regimen can be carried out once a day by the patient himself.

Occlusive agents such as gold leaf, aluminum foil, and polyethylene film have been advanced to promote healing and re-epithelization. Smith *et al*, in a partially controlled study, reported that the response rate (percentage re-epithelization per day) of ulcers treated with gold leaf was no better than the response rate of those treated with a simple dressing.[25] In our experience, aluminum foil has proved helpful in selected cases. We prefer thin aluminum foil. It is inexpensive, readily available, and much easier to apply than gold leaf. The patient can carry out the treatment once a day and can be followed at intervals of one or two weeks. We emphasize that the foil should be cut to measure approximately 1 mm less than the size of the ulcer. The metal is held in place by covering with a gauze pad or an eye-pad dressing.

Occasionally, re-epithelization of an ulcer may be retarded because of excess granulation tissue. Pressure with foam rubber pads, or the application of silver nitrate 0.5% are effective in controlling the problem.

Ambulatory therapy for resistant leg ulcers associated with venous disease and accompanied by persistent edema can be carried out by the use of an Unna's Boot or modification.

The ulcer is cleansed with hydrogen peroxide, packed with Gelfoam powder, and covered with a gauze pressure bandage. An Unna's Boot (Dome-Paste Bandage, Dome Laboratories) is then applied from the base of the toes to just below the knee, with the pressure greatest at the ankles, progressively lessening as one ascends the leg to the knee, and least at the base of the toes. Tubegauz and an elastic stocking or bandage may be worn over the Unna's Boot. The boot is changed every few days depending on the amount of serous drainage from the ulcer and the dermatitis. The Primer and Flexoplast combination,* a modified Unna's Boot, has also proved effective.

*Edward Taylor, Ltd., Tenafly, NJ 07670

For hospitalized patients, topical oxygen therapy can be used to stimulate re-epithelization in indolent ulcers. Elliott described the following simple device: "The affected extremity is placed in a plastic bag and the open end is closed above the ulcer with a rubber band. Oxygen from a tank is allowed to flow through a plastic tube into the deflated bag until it is completely distended. Treatment should last 30 minutes 3 to 4 times daily."[7] Specially constructed devices for hyperbaric oxygenation have been developed that operate much more efficiently.[9,20] Lesions that respond best to this modality are stasis ulcers, decubitus ulcers, and trophic ulcers.

Internal medications, as a rule, have no merit in the management of stasis ulcers, other than a course of systemic antibiotics for secondary pyoderma, if it is present. Husain has reported good results in the healing of chronic leg ulcers with bed rest and topical therapy combined with the use of oral zinc sulfate.[15] Presumably, zinc accelerates wound healing. In his study, the zinc sulfate group of patients seemed clinically to show more rapid epithelization than the control group. The medication was given in capsules containing 220 mg zinc sulfate three times daily, half an hour after meals. In a study done by Halsted and Smith, the mean plasma-zinc value in patients with indolent ulcers was significantly lower than in controls.[12] Upon treatment with zinc sulfate, the plasma-zinc level rose significantly, indicating good absorption. In later studies, others have reported that zinc therapy for venous leg ulcers is ineffective because patients suffering from this disorder are generally not deficient in zinc.[11,28] Ascorbic acid for thalassemic ulcers was discussed previously.

OTHER MODALITIES

Sclerotherapy and two surgical procedures are available: (1) Pinch grafting for ulcers, and (2) operations for varicose veins.

Resistant venous ulcers which do not respond to conservative treatment can be treated by skin grafting using pinch grafts or porcine dermis dressings.[4,23]

TREATMENT OF VARICOSE VEINS

Discussion of this aspect is not within the scope of this text, but an editorial in Lancet very well summarizes the situation: "Sclerotherapy at one time was considered a convenient alternative to surgery but a 'cure' or 'improved' rate of only 35% or so is reported, compared with about 80% for stripping and ligation. Successful operative treatment depends on careful preoperative assessment and marking, on thorough technique, and on the surgeon's willingness to follow the patient and give additional therapy when necessary."[6]

In summary, it is our experience that many physicians approach the problem of leg ulcers, including stasis ulcers, with a sigh of hopelessness. This is, of course, a bad approach. The physician should not force the stasis ulcer patient to a bedridden existence with continuous elevation of the leg, especially a working patient whose occupation may be critical to the livelihood of his family. This is not to say that bed rest with elevation will not encourage healing. Overattention to the bacterial population of the ulcer should also be avoided. Most stasis ulcers will not require an autograft. The great majority of venous ulcers can be managed and cleared up with an ambulatory occlusive and compressive fixed dressing, regardless of the size. Occlusion-induced cutaneous alteration of the microflora, especially an increase in gram-negative organisms, is not a problem insofar as symptomatic infection of skin is concerned. Effective treatment of venous stasis ulcer must be founded on a proper understanding of the basic pathophysiology responsible for the lesion. It is a simple disease; a disease in which too much attention has been directed, and too much importance relegated, to topical therapy and quantitative and qualitative surface bacteriology. Successful treatment of this disease, like many diseases, is equated with one's interest in the disease. Treat the stasis, and the ulcer will heal. Continued elastic support after healing of the ulcer is vital to prevent future manifest stasis disease, a simple point which is too frequently overlooked.

REFERENCES

1. **Afifi AM, Ellis L, Huntsman RG, et al:** High dose ascorbic acid in the management of thalassemia leg ulcers—a pilot study. Brit J Dermatol 92:339, 1975
2. **Beninson J:** Stasis dermatitis and leg ulcers. Postgrad Med 36:524, 1964
3. **Callaway JL:** Chronic leg ulcers. JAMA 186:1080, 1963
4. **Ceilley RI, Rinek MA, Zuehlke RL:** Pinch grafting for chronic ulcers on lower extremities. J Dermatol Surg Oncol 3:303, 1977
5. **Colman GJ, Roenigk HH:** Topical therapy of leg ulcers with 20 percent benzoyl peroxide lotion. Cutis 21:491, 1978
6. **Editorial:** The treatment of varicose veins. Lancet 2:311, 1975
7. **Elliott JA:** Stasis dermatitis and stasis ulcer. In Conn H (ed): Current Therapy, p. 505. Philadelphia, WB Saunders, 1967
8. **English MP, Smith RJ, Harman RRM:** The fungal flora of ulcerated legs. Brit J Dermatol 84:567, 1971
9. **Fischer BH:** Treatment of ulcers on the legs with hyperbaric oxygen. J Dermatol Surg 1:55, 1975
10. **Friedman SA, Gladstone JL:** The bacterial flora of peripheral vascular ulcers. Arch Dermatol 100:29, July 1969
11. **Greaves MW, Ive FA:** Double-blind trial of zinc sulphate in the treatment of chronic venous leg ulceration. Brit J Dermatol 87:632, 1972
12. **Halsted JA, Smith JC Jr:** Plasma-zinc in health and disease. Lancet 1:322, Feb. 14, 1970
13. **Herman BE, et al:** Successful skin graft in patient with generalized scleroderma. JAMA 182:578, 1962
14. **Hines EA Jr:** The differential diagnosis of chronic ulcer of the leg. Circulation 27:989, 1963
15. **Husain SL:** Oral zinc sulphate in leg ulcers. Lancet 1:1069, May 31, 1969
16. **Leinwand I, Duryee AW, Richter MN:** Scleroderma (based on a study of over 150 cases). Ann Intern Med 41:1003, 1954
17. **Lofgren KA:** Stasis ulcer. Mayo Clin Proc 40:564, 1965
18. **Lookingbill DP, Miller SH, Knowles RC:** Bacteriology of chronic leg ulcers. Arch Dermatol 114:1765, 1978
19. **Mitchell AAB, Pettigrew JB, MacGilvray D:** Varicose ulcers are reservoirs of hospital strains of *Staph. aureus* and *Pseudomonas pyocyanea*. Brit J Clin Prac 24:223, 1970
20. **Neubauer RA:** Hyperbaric oxygen and leg ulcers. JAMA 239:1393, 1978
21. **Pace WE:** Treatment of cutaneous ulcers with benzoyl peroxide. Can Med Assoc J 115:1101, 1976
22. **Pace WE:** Beads of a dextran polymer for the local treatment of cutaneous ulcers. J Dermatol Surg Oncol 4:678, 1978
23. **Rundle JSH, Cameron SH, Ruckley CV:** Porcine dermis dressing for varicose and traumatic leg ulcers. Brit Med J 2:216, 1976
24. **Samitz MH, Waldorf DS, Shrager J:** Leg ulcers in Mediterranean anemia. Arch Dermatol, 90:567, 1964
25. **Smith KW, Oden PW, Blaylock WK:** A comparison of gold leaf and other occlusive therapy. Arch Dermatol 96:703, Dec 1967
26. **Smith RJ, English MP, Warin RP:** The pathogenic status of yeasts infecting ulcerated legs. Brit J Dermatol 96:697, 1974
27. **Tuffanelli DL, Dubois EL:** Cutaneous manifestations of systemic lupus erythematosus, Arch Dermatol 90:377, 1964
28. **Weismann K:** What is the use of zinc for wound healing? Int J Dermatol 17:568, 1978
29. **Weismann RE, Johnson M:** Ischemic ulcers of the leg. Surg Clin N Am 43:1263, Oct 1963
30. **Woodcock JP, Alexander S, Durkin M:** Differential diagnosis of ischemic ulceration of the leg using ultrasound. Brit J Dermatol 91:77, 1974
31. **Wooling KR:** Hypertensive-ischemic ulcer. JAMA 187:196, 1964

15 TUMORS

Various tumors show a tendency to occur almost exclusively or regularly on the lower extremities. Is there an explanation for this topographic predilection? Is there a site-specific factor involved?

Tumors of the skin developing on the lower extremities are listed as follows:[37]

Classification of Skin Tumors of the Lower Extremity

BENIGN

Epidermal
   Nevus cell nevus—junctional, compound, intradermal
   Epidermal nevus (including linear form)
   Seborrheic keratoses, stucco keratoses
   Viral—verruca, molluscum contagiosum
   Eccrine poroma
   Clear cell acanthoma

Adnexal
   Pilomatrixoma
   Spiradenoma
   Dermal duct tumor
   Hidradenoma

Dermal and subcutaneous
   Vascular
      Hereditary hemorrhagic telangiectasia
      Nevus flammeus, lymphangioma (circumscriptum and cavernous)
      Hemangioma, cherry angioma
      Klippel-Trenaunay syndrome
      Parkes-Weber syndrome
      Acquired: granuloma pyogenicum, glomus tumor, angiokeratoma
   Neurofibroma—with or without associated Von Recklinghausen's disease

Periungual fibromas with tuberous sclerosis
Blue nevus
Keloid
Plantar fibromatosis
Nodular subepidermal fibrosis—dermatofibroma, histiocytoma, sclerosing hemangioma
Myxoid cyst
Lipoma
Fibroma
Fibrolipoma
Angiofibroma
Radiation fibromatosis
Granular cell schwannoma
Tophi of primary gout
Osteoma cutis
Xanthomatosis
Neurolemmoma
Leiomyoma
Reticulohistiocytoma
Benign subungual exostosis
Warty dyskeratoma

PREMALIGNANT
   Xeroderma pigmentosum
   Actinic keratoses
   Arsenical keratoses
   Bowen's disease
   Chronic stasis ulcer or chronic ulceration of other etiology (tuberculosis, osteomyelitis)
   Chronic radiodermatitis
   Burn scar

MALIGNANT
   Basal cell carcinoma (including basal cell nevus syndrome)
   Squamous cell carcinoma

Epithelioma cuniculatum
Marjolin's ulcer
Malignant fibrous histiocytoma
Melanoma
    Superficial spreading melanoma
    Nodular melanoma
    Melanotic whitlow
    Metastatic melanoma
Kaposi's multicentric idiopathic hemorrhagic sarcomatosis
Lymphoma
    Hodgkin's disease
    Mycosis fungoides
    Lymphocytic and lymphoblastic
    Reticulum cell
    Stem cell
Leukemia cutis
Dermatofibrosarcoma protuberans
Hemangioendothelioma
Hemangiopericytoma
Sarcomas
    Lymphangiosarcoma
    Angiosarcoma
    Leiomyosarcoma
    Fibrosarcoma
    Myxosarcoma
    Liposarcoma
    Neurofibrosarcoma
    Malignant granular cell schwannoma
Intraepidermal epithelioma of Jadassohn
Hidradenocarcinoma
Metastatic
PSEUDOMALIGNANT
    Keratoacanthoma—solitary and eruptive
    Nodular pseudosarcomatous fasciitis
    Masson's pseudoangiosarcoma
    Lymphomatoid papulosis
    Juvenile melanoma
    Atypical fibroxanthoma
    Atypical fibrous histiocytoma
    Pseudoepitheliomatous hyperplasia (borders of chronic ulcers of various etiologies)

Which of these tumors shows a tendency to occur almost exclusively or regularly on the lower extremities? On the basis of our clinical experience augmented by review of the literature, we noted at least 18 types of tumor predisposed to involve the integument and its appendages of the lower extremities (Table 15-1).

Table 15-1. Tumors With Predilection for the Lower Extremities

1. Plantar warts—mosaic and nonmosaic types
2. Eccrine poroma
3. Clear-cell acanthoma
4. Plantar fibromatosis
5. Stucco keratoses
6. Nodular subepidermal fibrosis
7. Periungual fibromas in tuberous sclerosis
8. Benign subungual exostosis
9. Tophaceous gout
10. Arsenical keratoses
11. Kaposi's multicentric idiopathic hemorrhagic sarcomatosis
12. Squamous cell carcinoma on developing chronic stasis ulcer (Marjolin's ulcer) and "toasted skin" syndrome
13. Malignant melanoma on the female lower extremity
    Malignant melanoma on the sole of the Black foot
    Melanotic whitlow
14. Fibrosarcomas
15. Cutaneous liposarcoma
16. Cellular blue nevus
17. Intraepidermal epithelioma of Jadassohn
18. Epithelioma cuniculatum plantare

In this chapter, we discuss distinctive clinical features of tumors with the predilection to occur on the lower extremities as well as some related tumors commonly seen without characteristic selective distribution to the lower extremities.

TUMORS WITH PREDILECTION FOR THE LOWER EXTREMITIES

PLANTAR WARTS

This is the most common tumor on the foot. For detailed discussion, refer to Chapter 2.

ECCRINE POROMA

The eccrine poroma was first described by Pinkus et al in 1956.[37] It is a new growth which is considered by most authors to originate from the distal and intraepidermal portion of the eccrine sweat duct.[15,34,38] This concept evolved from the demonstration by Pinkus in 1939 of evidence of the morphologic and biologic integrity of the intraepidermal portion of the sweat duct.[32] Histochemical and electron microscopic studies by Hashimoto and Lever confirmed this picture of acrosyringium.[16]

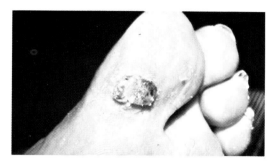

Fig. 15-1. Eccrine poroma. Note sharp demarcation of protruding tumor from surrounding tissue.

Fig. 15-2. Plantar fibromatosis showing characteristic subcutaneous nodular thickening.

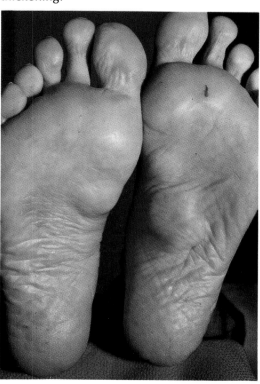

The lesions originally described by Pinkus *et al* were located on the nonhairy surface of the foot.[37] While the sole is apparently the site of predilection, instances of eccrine poroma occurring on the palm, chest, back, and calf have been reported.[11,22,31,40] Poromas are usually single, but Goldner has reported a case in which there were more than 100 such tumors on the palms and soles.[12] Recently Ogino described a patient with multiple eccrine poromas arranged in a linear fashion along the posteromedial aspect of her lower extremity to the right buttock and distally along the lateral aspect of the right foot.[30] Most poromas appear in persons older than the age of 40, and there is no sex predilection.[16,23]

The typical eccrine poroma is a nontender, reddish, soft tumor which protrudes from a shallow cuplike invagination, a feature considered diagnostic (Fig. 15-1). The tumor can be misdiagnosed clinically as a vascular tumor (such as pyogenic granuloma) or as a basal cell epithelioma, but histologically and histochemically the lesion is characteristic.

The clinical course and histologic picture of eccrine poroma emphasize its benign nature, although Darnall and Mopper reported a case in association with Bowen's disease, and Pinkus and Mehregan described a patient with widespread metastatic disease in whom tumor cells shared a symbiotic relationship with epidermal cells within the epidermis, a Paget cell-like relationship.[8,33] According to Shafrir *et al*, only 3 instances of malignant degeneration of the portal epithelium have been reported.[39]

We reported 2 patients with eccrine poroma of the plantar surface of the foot and toe.[29] These cases illustrated the following

aspects of diagnosis and treatment: (1) the clinical appearance of the lesion may be quite specific and permit accurate diagnosis, (2) the lesion may be of long duration, (3) the tumor is benign in behavior, and (4) simple conservative methods of removal are safe and effective.

CLEAR CELL ACANTHOMA

This unique tumor is predisposed to the leg in persons of late middle age. In 1962, Degos described a slow-growing solitary lesion with a characteristic histopathologic picture—malpighian cells which were larger and paler than those of the surrounding epidermis and contained an excess of glycogen.[9] There was almost complete absence of melanin in the basal cell layer of the affected parts. He called the lesion "acanthome a cellules claires" (clear cell acanthoma), and now it bears his name, Degos' acanthoma. It has been described also as pale cell acanthoma.[21,45] Electron microscopic and histochemical studies by other investigators confirmed the finding that clear cell acanthoma is a tumor of surface epidermis involving abnormal glycogen storage in the altered epidermis.[18,21,43,45]

Later studies showed that this tumor was not uncommon.[43,44] With exception of a few cases, the tumors tend to be solitary, ranging from 1.0 cm to 1.5 cm in size. Most lesions have occurred on the leg, especially the calf. Fine and Chernosky emphasized that the tumor has a distinctive clinical as well as pathologic appearance which can be recognized by the clinician with a significant degree of accuracy.[10] The lesion is seen as a slightly elevated dome-shaped papule or nodule, pinkish-gray to reddish-brown in color, and with a tendency to crush or bleed. It appears to be more "stuck on" the skin than infiltrating (in contrast to a seborrheic keratosis), has the vascular look of a pyogenic granuloma, a fine "wafer-like" scale on its periphery, the surface exudation of an eczematous process, and the advancing rounded border of an epithelioma. We have found these features most relevant in making the clinical diagnosis, but biopsy is essential for confirmation. If untreated, the tumor has been known to persist for as long as 25 years. It shows no tendency for spontaneous involution.

Treatment is surgical: shave incision, curettage, or local excision. Recurrences or malignant change have not been observed.

PLANTAR FIBROMATOSIS

The very name of the tumor suggests its preferential distribution. This is fibromatosis of the plantar fascia; it is the fibrous replacement of the plantar aponeurosis, similar pathologically to palmar fibromatosis (Dupytren's contracture), and these two conditions not uncommonly coexist. The disorder is often present but unrecognized in the foot.

Characteristically, plantar fibromatosis presents as a subcutaneous nodular thickening, most frequently occurring in the middle portion of the medial half of the foot (Fig. 15-2). As the fibrous proliferation invades the overlying skin, dermal invaginations occur. Occasionally, constriction of the great toe or second toe produces a hammer-toe deformity. Differential diagnosis is fibrosarcoma. The clinical appearance of the two conditions—a nonencapsulated, slowly growing, diffuse, somewhat asymptomatic nodular enlargement—and the age group in which they occur are similar. Bizarre histologic changes may occur in a region of localized fibromatosis, including the presence of mitotic figures, loss of polarity of the cells, nuclear pyknosis and, at times, atypical mitosis. Accurate histologic diagnosis is mandatory, since there have been instances of needless amputation.

The condition is usually acquired, but there are a few congenital cases that have been reported. In a study of 22 patients done by Aviles et al, no sex predominance was noted.[2] Twelve of the patients had disease in the left foot, 5 in the right, and 5 in both. The bilaterality was synchronous in only 1 patient; in the other 4 patients the second lesion appeared between 2 and 7 years after the first.

The only satisfactory treatment is surgical excision, although surgical excision is probably not indicated for all patients, since many are asymptomatic.

STUCCO KERATOSES

Australian dermatologists have been leaders in the study of these lesions. The term "stucco keratoses" was coined by Kocsard and Ofner to describe the "stuck on" appearance of the lesions on the skin.[24] The stucco keratosis is distinctive in both its features and its localization. The condition occurs on the lower legs; the dorsal and lateral aspects of the feet are the most common sites of involvement, but lesions can be found also on the dorsa of the hands.[42]

The lesions are discrete, grayish-white keratotic papules with flat or convex surfaces.

When viewed with a hand lens, the rough, dry surface is seen; the lesions are more easily seen when viewed with side-lighting.[42] Stucco keratoses are loosely attached ("stuck on" to the skin) and can easily be removed by scratching without causing bleeding, leaving a collarette of scales in the periphery of the lesion.[17] The lesions vary in size from 3 to 10 mm in diameter; in numbers, there is a variation from few to several hundred. The condition is seen with greater frequency after the age of 40, predominantly in males.[14,24] Some of our patients complained of dryness and minimal pruritus; usually the condition was asymptomatic. According to Willoughby and Soter, this often unrecognized acral keratotic disorder probably is more prevalent than the paucity of published reports indicates.[42] Stucco keratoses are common in the US as well as in Australia.

Various agents such as sunlight, dry winter weather, trauma, and tars have been incriminated in the pathogenesis of these lesions, but no specific etiologic factors have been identified. On histologic inspection, the stucco keratosis is that of an epidermal nevus. Some authors consider the lesion a form of seborrheic keratosis.

Therapy consists of a hydration regimen with an emollient which softens the skin, causing the scaly lesions to fall off.

NODULAR SUBEPIDERMAL FIBROSIS

This classification includes histiocytoma, dermatofibroma, sclerosing hemangioma, hemosiderin histiocytoma, and lipoidal histiocytoma.

DERMATOFIBROMA

This benign, asymptomatic fibrous tissue tumor has a predilection for the lower extremities but can occur anywhere. Seen in middle-aged or older patients, it is usually single; rarely, several lesions may be present.

Clinical features: Dermatofibroma presents as a firm, "stony-hard" nodule up to 1 cm in size (rarely even larger), adherent to the skin but freely movable over the underlying tissues. The surface is usually smooth, is rounded or spherical and slightly elevated, and is occasionally surrounded by a furrow-like depression. The color varies from ivory to pinkish, yellow-brown, or bluish-black, depending on the histologic make-up of the tumor, e.g., blood vessels (sclerosing hemangioma), fibrous tissue (nodular fibrosis), and histiocytes containing lipid or hemosiderin, or both.

Dermatofibroma start as a small papule which enlarges to a certain size and then remains stationary. Spontaneous involution occurs only rarely; malignant change almost never occurs.

PERIUNGUAL FIBROMAS IN TUBEROUS SCLEROSIS

Refer to Chapter 16 (Genodermatoses).

BENIGN SUBUNGUAL EXOSTOSIS

The subungual exostosis is the outgrowth of normal bony tissue or calcified cartilaginous remains arising from the terminal phalanx beneath the nail. Subungual exostoses are usually solitary and prefer the great toe, but may be multiple and appear on several toes. The typical lesion initially is a small pinkish nodule, varying in size from a few millimeters to two or more centimeters, that appears beneath the free edge of the nail. The tumor is compressed against the nail plate; the portion of the nail overlying the lesion is lifted and becomes detached—with resultant nail dystrophy (Fig. 15-3).[46] The lesion is indurated and when traumatized is painful, especially when the patient walks. Although seen in all age groups and in both sexes, subungual exostoses develop more frequently during the adolescent years, and occur three times more frequently in women.[25]

The differential diagnosis of subungual exostosis includes: periungual wart, ingrowing toenail, granuloma telangiectaticum, enchondroma, epidermoid cyst, glomus tumor, basal and squamous cell carcinoma, and malignant melanoma.

Radiograph is diagnostic (Fig. 15-4); anteroposterior and lateral firms are advisable. Total surgical excision is the treatment of choice.

TOPHACEOUS GOUT

These tumors represent collections of sodium monourate crystals surrounded by giant cells (foreign body reaction) and encircled by a granulomatous capsule. They vary in size from 1 mm to several centimeters. The lesions occur often in the prepatellar bursae, and in the tendons of the toes, ankles, and heels. Also refer to Chapter 5.

ARSENICAL KERATOSES

These are premalignant lesions which may progress to basal, epidermoid, and squamous cell carcinomas. They characteristically affect the palms and soles. One should look for other evidence of exposure to inorganic arsenic in the remote past. (Ingestion of drugs such as Fowler's solution or Asiatic pills may be responsible, or insecticides. A common source of exposure in Southern United States was Paris Green, which was the conventional poison for the cotton boll-weevil.) Such exposure may produce hypermelanosis and hypomelanosis, the picture of "raindrops on a dusty road" widely over the glabrous skin, Bowen's disease, and basal and squamous

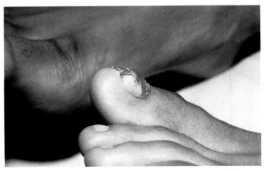

Fig. 15-3. Benign subungual exostosis. The tumor is compressed against the nail plate. (*Courtesy of Dr. S. Lebouitz*)

cell carcinoma, particularly on sites not exposed to sun. The fate of arsenic in the human body has not been well studied. Bettley and O'Shea postulate that carcinoma-prone subjects retain as much as twice the normal, and this, rather than tissue susceptibility to arsenic, may account for their tendency toward arsenical carcinogenesis.[3]

Arsenical keratoses on feet begin as hyperkeratotic yellowish, well-circumscribed papules resembling corns (Fig. 15-5). They enlarge, thicken, increase in number, and frequently coalesce. Differentiation from various types of punctate keratosis and plantar warts is made readily, especially if other skin manifestations of arsenic intoxication are present. Induration, inflammation, and ulceration occur when the lesion becomes malignant.[36]

The multiplicity of the keratoses makes treatment difficult. Paring of the lesions in conjunction with keratolytic ointments or topical retinoic acid and 5-fluorouracil (separately or in combination) is helpful.

KAPOSI'S MULTICENTRIC IDIOPATHIC HEMORRHAGIC SARCOMATOSIS (KS)

The marked predilection of this disease on the basis of race, sex, and anatomic site is probably the most unique of its kind in the entire field of neoplasia. The populations of eastern Europe, northern Italy, and Equa-

Fig. 15-4. Radiograph of Fig. 15-3 showing exostosis of distal phalanx. (*Courtesy of Dr. S. Lebouitz*)

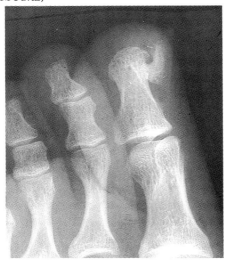

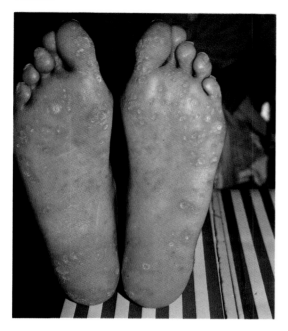

Fig. 15-5. Arsenical keratoses. Patient worked in orchards and used arsenical insecticides. (*Courtesy of Dr. S. Gammer*)

Fig. 15-6. Kaposi's sarcomatosis. Lesions are usually bilateral with a tendency toward symmetry.

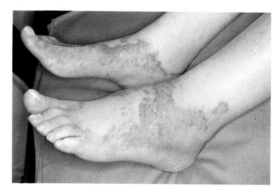

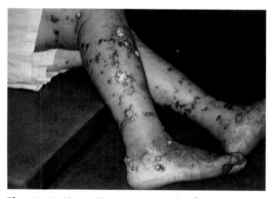

Fig. 15-7. Kaposi's sarcomatosis showing infiltrated lesions of various sizes.

torial and South Africa are more susceptible to this disorder. Ethnic and racial factors have been implicated; predominantly affected are Jews, Italians, and Bantus. The incidence of Kaposi's disease is far more frequent in men than in women; peak frequency is in the fifth to seventh decades of life in Western countries and in the third and fourth decades in Africa.

The cutaneous manifestations are somewhat polymorphus. The eruption is characterized by nodules and plaques that are bluish, bluish red, or reddish brown. It is usually bilateral with a tendency toward symmetry (Fig. 15-6). As a rule, the first lesions occur on the extremities, particularly the legs and feet (a "stocking" distribution). Although there is a distinct predilection for the lower extremities, any part of the body surface may be involved. Kaposi's sarcoma of the skin can be attended by visceral involvement that is often occult and asymptomatic.

The eruption evolves slowly; old lesions may undergo spontaneous involution leaving atrophy and pigmentation. A common clinical picture consists of infiltrated plaques of various sizes on the feet and legs, with scattered or grouped nodules (Fig. 15-7). Unusual features consist of glistening translucent lesions resembling bullae or lymphangioma-like tumors. Indurated plaques are prominent.

Occasionally, petechiae ecchymosis, and widespread purpura may be associated.

Complications of lower extremity involvement include dermal sclerotic changes, and chronic obstructive lymphedema which may lead to lymphedematous keratoderma, lymphostatic verrucosis, and a pyoderma vegetans, particularly between and around the toes. Lesions may also ulcerate.

The histopathology of the disease is characterized by 3 processes: inflammatory, granulomatous, and neoplastic (fibrosarcomatous, predominantly angiosarcomatous, or a mixture). Very often these alterations overlap and produce a mixed picture. The diagnosis of Kaposi's disease is readily made from the clinical features and the histopathology. The disorder cannot be categorized with certainty. At present it must be considered a disease of unknown origin that demonstrates some features of a true neoplasm, an infectious granuloma, an infectious granuloma with neoplastic tendencies, or a reticuloendothelial hyperplasia.

The prognosis for KS is dependent on several factors that include the type of clinical lesion, the histologic pattern, nodal involvement, and immunologic response.[40a] Treatment is directed toward palliation of the disease. Radiotherapy has been the modality of choice; dosage factors are based on the extent, distribution, and depth of lesions. A variety of chemotherapeutic agents such as orally administered nitrogen mustard, vinblastine intravenously, and intralesional vincristine also have been reported as effective measures in various studies.[29a,40a,41a]

MARJOLIN'S ULCER

This special tumor is a squamous cell carcinoma that can develop on chronic stasis ulceration; this can explain its predilection for the lower extremity. It is the most feared complication of chronic stasis disease secondary to chronic deep-venous insufficiency in the postphlebitic leg. Patients with varicose ulcers who also have a history of thermal damage on the same site seem to be predisposed to the development of local malignant change, and possibly both conditions act as stimuli to excess and bizarre cell proliferation leading to cancer. Constant irritation and infection also must play significant roles.

Marjolin's ulcer is characteristically slow-growing. A series of cases reported recently by Liddell serve to describe the syndrome: in 4 patients squamous cell carcinoma developed in chronic venous ulcers; a basal cell carcinoma at the site of chronic varicose ulceration developed in a fifth patient.[26] The first 4 patients had had varicose veins and intermittent ulceration for 30 to 60 years, and the fifth patient for at least 17 years. Those in whom squamous cell carcinoma developed had experienced an enlargement of their indolent ulcers; all had areas of excessive growth of granulation tissue. Three of the first 4 patients had had a burn or scald many years previously.

The accepted treatment for Marjolin's ulcer has been wide local excision and resurfacing the area with split-skin grafts; in Liddell's series, amputation was necessary in 3 of the patients.[5]

Squamous cell carcinoma occurring in *erythema ab igne* is discussed in Chapter 3.

MALIGNANT MELANOMA

This group of tumors is discussed later in this chapter.

FIBROSARCOMA

Fibrosarcoma is essentially a disease of young adults, commonly between the ages of 25 to 45 years. The tumors occur most frequently in the extremities and rarely in the trunk. Initially, these tumors are small, firm, painless nodules which grow slowly for a long time and then develop into large masses. They commonly occur within the muscles, intimately inherent to the fibrous septa. Small satellite nodules are often seen at the tumor periphery, and the surrounding structures may be infiltrated. Adjacent muscles bulge outward; the bone surrounded by the new growth eventually shows compression atrophy.

Definitive diagnosis is established by biopsy. The differential diagnosis should be made from finding of benign tumors, especially fibromatous, and from other types of malignant soft-tissue tumors.

Treatment of fibrosarcoma is wide excision

or a major amputation if the tumor involves an extremity.

CUTANEOUS LIPOSARCOMA

Cutaneous liposarcoma is a malignant tumor composed of undifferentiated sarcoma cells containing fatty elements. The highest incidence of this rare tumor is on the skin of the lower extremity; the upper thigh is the most frequent site. Occasionally it may arise from a preexisting lipoma. Males are affected mostly.

The tumor is a diffuse, nodular infiltration of the soft tissue that undergoes gradual enlargement. Biopsy specimens stained for fat confirm the diagnosis.

Treatment is wide surgical excision.

CELLULAR BLUE NEVUS

Clinically, the cellular blue nevus is a large bluish firm nodule or plaque. The histologic differential diagnosis is a histiocytoma that has bled, i.e., a hemosiderin histiocytoma. Like the common blue nevus, the cellular blue nevus is composed of spindle-shaped cells; these are dermal melanocytes. In both, the melanin tends to be aggregated about adnexal structures. In the cellular type of blue nevus, one also sees variously sized islands of densely packed, rather large, rounded or spindle-shaped cells. They show variously shaped nuclei and abundant, pale, vacuolated cytoplasm.

In the hemosiderin histiocytoma, the pigment tends to increase perivascularly, whereas in a blue nevus it tends to increase periappendigeally. An iron stain will differentiate the two; the dermal melanocytes are dopa-positive.

Another differentiating point between these two pigmented lesions is the epidermis; the epidermis overlying the blue nevus is normal or thin ("ironed out"), whereas the epidermas over the histiocytoma is hyperkeratotic, hyperplastic, and also hyperpigmented.

On low-power microscopic examination, one must consider a metastatic melanoma when looking at a blue nevus; these are about the only two lesions that will produce this much melanin so deep in the skin. The epidermis is normal in both a metastatic melanoma and a blue nevus.

INTRAEPIDERMAL EPITHELIOMA OF JADASSOHN

This is an intraepidermal squamous cell epithelioma, i.e., squamous cell carcinoma in situ. It is characterized by nests of intraepidermal tumor cells; these nests of cells distinguish it from Bowen's disease, in which there are a vast variety of tumor cells involving full-thickness anaplasia of the epidermis.

Clinically, this is a sharply marginated plaque, slightly erythematous or tan, and resembles superficial seborrheic keratosis. Most occur on the leg.

EPITHELIOMA CUNICULATUM PLANTARE

Epithelioma cuniculatum, a rare and unusual tumor peculiar to the foot, was described by Aird et al in 1954 and was first reported in the American literature in 1976.[1,6] Recently, Brownstein and Shapiro described 8 such cases and termed the tumor "epithelioma cuniculatum plantare."[7] The point emphasized in all reports is that the tumor is a true malignancy—a variant of squanmous cell carcinoma.

All the patients were middle-aged, and the tumor had usually been present on the sole for many years. The tumors varied from 1-cm wart-like lesions to larger, fungating boggy masses (Fig. 15-8). Papillomatosis is the most prominent feature; secondary changes include inflammation, fibrosis, and accumulation of debris in sinuses and crypts.[6] (The crypts resemble the burrows of rabbits, hence the name "cuniculatum.") These sinuses, filled with decomposed keratin, have a characteristic foul smell. Most lesions were initially considered to be plantar warts that had been treated with a variety of modalities. Aird et al and Thompson consider the tumor as a variety of squamous cell carcinoma that produced abundant keratin which, on repeated pressure, forced portions of the tumor deep into soft tissue of the foot.[1,41]

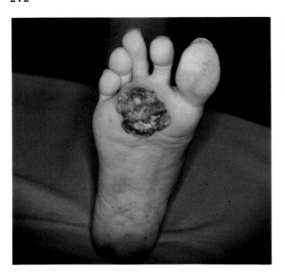

Fig. 15-8. Epithelioma cuniculatum plantare. This lesion had been present for several years and was initially treated for a plantar wart with various modalities. A biopsy showed a variant of squamous cell carcinoma.

Fig. 15-9. Granuloma telangiectaticum on sole.

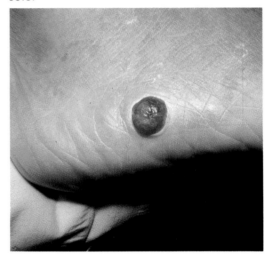

On histologic examination, the surface was markedly papillomatous; well-differentiated sheets of pale-staining keratinocytes extend into the dermis, surrounded by a moderate inflammatory infiltrate.[7] There is a similarity between this lesion and certain papillary squamous tumors that occur in other sites and are termed verrucous carcinoma, florid papillomatosis, or giant condyloma.[6]

Wide local excision of the entire lesion is the only satisfactory method of treatment. Because of the location and size of the lesion, good function on the weight-bearing surface can produce problems after treatment. When extensive growth has caused deformity of the foot, amputation should be considered.[35]

SKIN TUMORS COMMONLY SEEN WITHOUT SELECTIVE DISTRIBUTION TO THE LOWER EXTREMITIES

GRANULOMA PYOGENICUM (TELANGIECTATICUM)

Its cause is not definitely known. Granuloma pyogenicum can arise *de novo* from normal skin, but often follows trauma or infection or both, and is rapidly growing. Seen in both sexes at all ages it has predilection for hands, feet, lip, cheeks, chin, back, and umbilicus.

The tumors are sessile or pedunculated, often showing a characteristic constricting

epithelial collar at skin level (Fig. 15-9). They vary from pea-sized to cherry-sized, are very vascular, and bleed easily. Their color varies from light pink to bluish-red. The surface may be smooth; more often it shows areas of necrosis and ulceration and is bathed in a malodorous seropurulent secretion which may dry to form a loosely adherent crust.

On the lower extremity, the plantar surface of toes and the sole are commonly involved, and the moist eroded type of lesion predominates with frequent troublesome bleeding and pain on walking. Differentiation from a melanoma and Kaposi's sarcoma is of paramount importance.

KELOIDS

This is a neoplasm of the dermis following trauma, infection, or inflammation; common

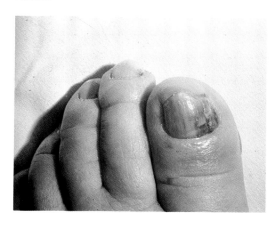

Fig. 15-10. Glomus tumor. (*Courtesy of Dr. S. Lebouitz*)

factors are burns and surgical incisions. So-called spontaneous keloids probably arise owing to inapparent trauma. They occur as single or multiple elevations, irregular in shape, smooth or corrugated, whitish to pink in color, and resembling a thickened hypertropic scar. They are dense elastic tumors arising from the corium which project above the skin surface and are firmly attached to it. A great variety of shapes and sizes are encountered. Often, there is a central mass or "body," with flatter, less distinct extensions or "claws."

Pruritus is the most common complaint, less often a hypersensitivity to pressure and heat. Occasionally, depending on the location, a sense of constriction with limitation of motion of the area is encountered. After reaching a maximum size, few changes occur unless additional trauma is inflicted, especially surgical intervention, when further growth can be anticipated.

"Hypertrophic scar" is a term applied to a keloid-like scar occurring at the site of trauma which does not surpass the limits of the original lesion.

GLOMUS TUMOR (GLOMANGIOMA)

The glomus tumor is an uncommon benign hamartomatous lesion. These tumors originate from vascular glomus bodies which are located predominantly on the extremities, especially subungual areas (Fig. 15-10). The solitary type is more common than the ge-

netically determined multiple glomus tumors. It appears as a soft or firm, blue-red papule, is tender, and gives rise to severe paroxysms of pain initiated by trauma, pressure, or exposure to cold. Treatment consists of surgical excision.

SEBORRHEIC KERATOSES

This benign epidermal hyperplasia ordinarily develops as a small yellowish or tan, well-demarcated, slightly elevated superficial lesion covered by a thin greasy scale and having a "stuck on" appearance. Multiple lesions are the rule with progressive increase in size and number of lesions and a darkening to brown or black color as they become more elevated, thicker, and friable. Many have a pitted or granular surface because of keratinous plugs. The surface is readily curetted away, often without bleeding, in contrast to the actinic keratosis. Seborrheic keratoses continue to enlarge as new lesions appear so that there is a mixture of lesions varying in size, shape, color, and thickness, present at any one time. Onset is in middle age (40 to 45 years)—earlier and more profuse in those with a familial predisposition.

Sites of predilection are the trunk, face, scalp, neck, and extremities, in that order. The lower extremities are commonly involved and the lesions may become irritated with a subsequent change in clinical appearance. Their differentiation from pigmented nevi, pigmented basal cell carcinoma, and intraepidermal epithelioma of Jadassohn is important. The latter lesion is often located on the legs and invariably is in association with lesions of seborrheic keratoses.

KERATOACANTHOMA—SOLITARY TYPE

Keratoacanthoma (KA) is a benign self-healing tumor closely resembling a squamous cell carcinoma. Sunlight is probably the primary provocative agent, since they usually develop on sun-exposed areas. Ninety percent of lesions involve the face, neck, hand, and forearms. The lower extremity is occasionally involved when actinically damaged skin is evidenced, similar to that from which squamous cell and basal cell carcinoma arise.

The classical picture of the solitary keratoacanthoma is that of a firm round nodule with a keratin-filled crater in its center. Fine telangiectasias may be seen on its surface; generally, there is no induration or inflammation at the base, unless it is irritated. The lesion is characterized initially by rapid growth; it remains almost unchanged in appearance for two to eight weeks, and then spontaneously begins to involute slowly. This whole cycle takes two to eight months, resulting finally in a slightly depressed scar. The remarkable rapid growth and the property of self-healing distinguish the lesion clinically from squamous cell carcinoma. An adequate eliptical biopsy through the center of the lesion is critical. The histologic findings are fairly characteristic, and together with the clinical picture the diagnosis can be made with confidence. It is important that the patient be followed until complete involution has occurred for only then can the diagnosis be confirmed.

PRECANCEROSES

In common usage, the term precanceroses is limited to Bowen's disease, actinic keratosis, keratoses from arsenic, irradiation, and tars, and leukoplakia. All but leukoplakia can occur on the lower extremities.

Bowen's disease is a variant of cutaneous intraepidermal squamous cell carcinoma with a specific clinicopathologic picture. The lesions can be single or multiple, varying from 1 to 10 cm in size. They are sharply demarcated, rounded to polycyclic in shape, reddish or brownish in color; crusted, fissured or hyperkeratotic. When the scale or crust is removed, a flat, red, moist granular base is revealed. The evolution of a lesion is one of slow, centrifugal growth. Nodule formation and ulceration often mark the development of invasive cancer, a complication occurring in 5% to 10% of patients. Bowen's

disease can occur on exposed as well as non-exposed areas of the body.

Differential diagnosis from psoriasis, numular eczema, actinic keratosis, and superficial basal carcinoma may be difficult, but biopsy readily confirms the diagnosis.

Some investigators have postulated a correlation between arsenic exposure and Bowen's disease, but a history of specific exposure is often not obtained. Other studies have shown that Bowen's disease predisposes to other premalignant and malignant skin lesions and to the simultaneous or subsequent development of noncutaneous cancer.

The lesions seen on the lower extremities occur both on sun-exposed (damaged) and nonexposed areas. In the former, the concomitant findings of actinic keratoses as well as telangiectases, freckling, and whitish sclerotic areas is not unusual.

Liquid nitrogen, 5-fluorouracil with occlusion, surgical excision, and curettage and electrocoagulation are effective therapeutic measures. Long-term followup is advisable to determine possible development of noncutaneous cancer.

Actinic keratosis (senile keratosis, solar keratosis) is the most common precancerous disease causing skin cancer. The lesions are caused by the cumulative effects of solar radiation.

Clinically, the lesions occur on sun-exposed areas predominantly in middle-aged and elderly patients who are fair complexioned and have had a greater than average amount of sun exposure. These patients usually present a characteristic skin picture that is dry and wrinkled, with brownish spots, telangiectases, and white sclerotic lesions. Actinic keratoses occur in both sexes.

The keratoses are usually multiple. The lesions are round or irregular in shape and are barely elevated; they vary in color from gray to a yellowish brown or dull red. There is a thickening of the horny layer with the formation of adherent scales in the early stage of their development, and the lesion can best be detected by palpation. The continued adherence of the scales may result in a piling up to produce a warty or hornlike surface. Malignant change is suspected when there is a palpable infiltration of the base of the lesion with an erythematous halo. This change is to squamous cell cancer, often low grade with infrequent metastasis (0.1% or less). Basal cell carcinoma occurs frequently in actinic skin, but it arises without a preceding keratosis.

The keratoses usually occur on the face, dorsum of the hands, forearms and neck, but with new trends in sunbathing, more actinic keratoses are being seen on the lower extremities.

Topical (1% to 2%) 5-fluorouracil, curettage and desiccation, cryotherapy and surgical excision are acceptable methods of treatment.

Aresenical Keratosis. Discussed earlier in this chapter.

Chronic radiodermatitis results from exposure to ionizing radiation. It may arise from an earlier acute reaction to an intensive exposure or from repeated smaller doses, each in themselves incapable of eliciting an acute reaction.

Early x-ray sequelae consist of well-demarcated areas of telangiectasis, hyperpigmentation and whitish discoloration, and atrophy. The skin changes may occur months to many years following irradiation and may be the sole manifestations for many years before keratoses, ulcerations and later, neoplastic changes occur. The malignancies can be basal cell or squamous cell carcinoma and rarely, malignant melanoma.

On the lower extremities, the sequelae are most often seen in patients who had been radiated for plantar warts, dyshidrotic eczema, or hyperhidrosis.

BASAL CELL AND SQUAMOUS CELL CARCINOMAS

Basal cell carcinoma and squamous cell carcinoma are the most common skin cancers that occur in Caucasians.

The *basal cell carcinoma* is derived from epidermal and adnexal basal cells. It frequently presents as a slow-growing shiny nodule with surface telangiectasia; it is com-

posed of masses of cells with darkly staining nuclei that simulate epidermal basal cells. The clinical configuration, however, can assume variations such as papulonodular, cystic, ulcerative, cicatricial, and pigmented types. Basal cell carcinomas invade locally, but rarely metastasize. The tumors are found primarily on the head and neck, that is, in sun-exposed areas, and sunlight is the chief predisposing factor.

Basal cell epitheliomas on the foot are rare. Recent case reports with reviews of the literature emphasized this finding.[4,28]

Actinic basal and squamous cell carcinomas on the legs are uncommon, but not rare, especially in the southern "cotton belt." One would speculate that the cotton chopping (hoeing) and handpicking of yesteryear would account for this, secondary to a chronic cumulative actinic insult from long hours in the fields. In our experience, these epitheliomas are much more common in women, probably because they wear dresses rather than trousers, and hence have more direct sun exposure. Exposure to Paris Green and its inorganic arsenic may explain some of these cases. It is also interesting to note that actinic keratoses are not rare on the legs, ankles, and dorsal feet in elderly women in the rural South: We have not seen any on the lower extremities of men. Many of these women also commonly worked barefoot in the fields.

In a series treated by one of us (Dr. John E. Lewis) over a 3-year period, there were 22 patients with 34 leg tumors (23 basal cell carcinomas, 6 Bowen's, and 5 squamous cell carcinomas): 18% of the patients were men, 82% were women; 12% of the tumors occurred in men, 88% in women; 14% of these patients presented with one or more chronic leg ulcers, and all were women; average age of the male patient was 55, average age of the female patient was 75.

The nevoid basal cell carcinoma syndrome has an interesting association with the foot. The syndrome is an autosomal dominantly inherited disease complex affecting primarily the skin, endocrine, skeletal, and nervous systems.[13] Dyskeratosis of the palms and soles, manifested by 1- to 2-mm pits in the stratum corneum, is a very frequent finding and is the result of a focal defect in keratinization.[20] Seventy percent of patients present with pits; on a rare occurrence, a microscopically typical basal cell epithelioma has been observed in a pit.

Squamous cell carcinoma is the second most common skin cancer in Caucasians and is found more often than basal cell epithelioma in the pigmented races. The tumor is a relatively slow-growing lesion composed of masses of cells that simulate epidermal cells and tend to form keratin. However, the individual cells frequently show bizarre forms and shapes as well as malignant dyskeratosis. Squamous cell carcinomas do metastasize at times.

The evidence for the participation of sunlight in producing squamous cell carcinomas in Caucasians, albinos (personal experience in Tanzania), and patients with xeroderma pigmentosum is even more convincing than it is for producing basal cell epitheliomas; chronic irritation and injury, rather than solar damage, play important roles on the lower extremities, as seen in squamous cell carcinomas secondary to Marjolin ulcers, "toasted skin" syndrome, and epithelioma cuniculatum plantare.[27]

Intraepidermal epithelioma of Jadassohn and Bowen's disease are both squamous cell carcinomas *in situ*, and both become invasive if neglected.

Similarly, an arsenical keratosis on the sole may be the progenitor of an invasive squamous cell cancer.

MALIGNANT MELANOMA

Malignant melanoma is the most serious skin neoplasm.

Melanoma is a cancer of the pigment-producing cells of the skin, eyes, and mucous membranes. Untreated, this disease usually spreads widely within the body and is fatal. Melanoma may develop from a mole that becomes malignant, or it may arise from pigment cells in normal-appearing skin. The recognition of melanoma during its early stages is fateful because a patient may be cured if the tumor is eradicated completely before the cells have spread throughout the body.[12]

Melanoma constitutes 1% of the cancers in the United States. The cause of melanoma, like that of other cancers, is unknown; exposure to ultraviolet light may contribute to its development.

Clark has opened new avenues in elucidating the evolution of cutaneous malignant melanoma. In his studies of the histokinetics and biological behavior of melanomas, specific histologic patterns characterize the development of the tumor and help to determine the inherent malignancy and the degree of containment that can be achieved by the host's immunoinflammatory systems.[4,7] In a more recent publication, clinical features are correlated with histogenic concepts.[14]

Mihm *et al* complement this clinical study with a color atlas in which it is often possible—through inspection of the color of the lesions, with particular attention to shades of blue—to recognize malignant melanoma in its early stage.[16] Thus, melanomas undergo predictable sequential changes that permit precise clinical diagnosis. In essence, according to Clark "There are different forms of cutaneous malignant melanoma and that the clinical appearance of each of the forms is quite distinctive—distinctive enough to presume that the diagnostic accuracy of malignant melanoma should exceed 90%, and the index of suspicion should be beyond 100%."[5] Such levels of diagnostic accuracy were not achieved 10 to 20 years ago.[11]

Three types of malignant melanoma have been distinguished: lentigo-maligna melanoma, superficial-spreading melanoma, and nodular melanoma. Biopsy readily confirms the clinical diagnosis; definitive histologic criteria establish guidelines for the most effective therapy.

The regional evaluation of malignant melanoma has clinical advantages in the recognition of their biological activity. The following forms of malignant melanoma are seen on the lower extremity: lentigo-maligna melanoma, superficial-spreading melanoma, nodular melanoma, melanotic whitlow, and metastatic melanoma. It is beyond the scope of this review to decribe all the clinical characteristics of these lesions (Figs. 15-11, 15-12, 15-13 portray some of the features) and their histologic counterparts—the aforemen-

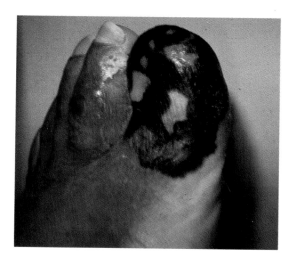

Fig. 15-11. Melanotic whitlow.

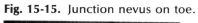

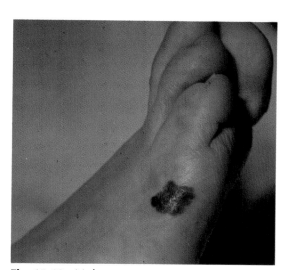

Fig. 15-12. Melanoma.

Fig. 15-14. Junction nevus on sole.

Fig. 15-15. Junction nevus on toe.

Fig. 15-13. Melanoma on leg.

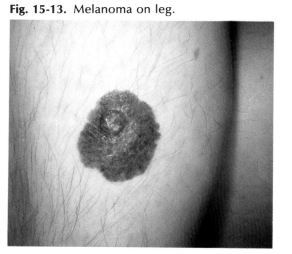

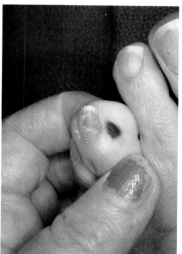

tioned publications are requisite and preferable.

The incidence of cutaneous malignant melanoma on the lower extremity is formidable. The lower limb was (and continues to be) the most frequent site of melanoma in the survey done by Cosman *et al*, who reviewed statistics from the Columbia-Presbyterian Medical Center and from five other centers in the United States and abroad.[8] Lower limb distribution ranged from 26.1% to 39.6%. In the study done by Beardmore and Davis from Australia, primary cutaneous melanomas appeared most frequently on the trunk, next most frequently on the head and neck in males, and on the lower limbs in females (48%).[3] In a comparison of the clinical behavior of melanoma of the hands and feet in 283 patients, Keyhani reported that 228 patients had malignant melanoma of the feet and 55 had melanoma of the hands, roughly a 4:1 ratio; in the hands, 45.4% of melanomas occurred subungually, while in the feet 50% occurred on the sole.[10] According to Fitzpatrick, there was a striking increase in melanomas on the legs of females, especially the left (four times greater than on the left leg of males).[9] He attributes this to their spending more time outdoors and wearing less clothing, especially since nylon stockings have replaced light-opaque stockings or long dresses. Clark *et al* reported that malignant melanoma of the superficial-spreading type is about three times as common on the thigh (15:6) and on the leg (22:6) in females as in males.[6]

Malignant melanoma of the lentigo-maligna type occurs occasionally on the thigh or leg. Acral lentiginous melanoma is a recently described subgroup of melanomas that appears on the palms and soles and may mimic plantar wart.[1,2,13,15,18]

Nodular melanoma occurs twice as commonly in men as in women. The preponderance of these tumors in men occur on the back and on the head and neck; elsewhere on the body, nodular melanoma occurs in approximately equal frequency in both sexes. The data of Clark *et al* also show that although Blacks do not commonly develop malignant melanoma, they do develop them with some frequency on the foot.[6] Sole, heel, and nail bed (melanotic whitlow) are the preferred

sites. Initially, on the sole, melanomas appear as a brown-black, irregular pigmented "stain" which may or may not be related to a pre-existing nevus.[5] The possibility that pigment-deficient areas may represent the target organ for sunlight-induced melanomas in Blacks and dark-skinned subjects is suggested in the report by Pantoja *et al*.[17] The clinical features of 57 melanomas of the lower extremity occurring in native Puerto Ricans were studied. The melanomas had a distribution similar to that reported in Blacks, whereas most melanomas of the lower extremity among Caucasians occur above the ankle.

THE VEXING PROBLEM OF THE PIGMENTED NEVUS ON THE FOOT

The most common tumors of the skin appear during childhood or adult life as pigmented nevi.

The most immature lesions appear as macular, tan to brownish areas in children which on histologic study show primarily junctional (basal layer) activity. In an adult, such a lesion represents a lentigo, while junctional activity is revealed by a spreckling of pigment and a hazy irregular border. As these lesions mature, they become progressively elevated to produce a whole spectrum of varying shapes, sizes, surfaces, and shades of color, from tan to dark brown. The surface changes produce verrucoid, polypoid, sessile, and dune-shaped forms. These more mature forms present fewer junctional and more intradermal locations of the nevus cells. The end stages of this evolution are represented clinically by fibrous papules or pigmented papillomas.

Most pigmented nevi never become clinically suspicious, and other than for nevi that are constantly irritated, such as those occurring at the beltline or under a bra strap, removal is not necessary. For some as yet inexplicable reason, nevi on the palms, soles, and genitalia remain junctional in type. Since the majority of nevi that undergo malignant transformation are of the junctional type, the excision of all nevi on the palms and soles has been advocated because of the high incidence of malignant melanoma at these sites. (Malignant melanoma of the plantar surfaces occurs more frequently than on the palms and genitalia. Can we hypothesize that a site-specific factor is involved or that some additional provocative, perhaps the repeated trauma of weight-bearing, is required?)

MANAGEMENT OF PIGMENTED NEVI

In children, except where a serious cosmetic problem exists, decision regarding removal of pigmented nevi may be safely deferred until late childhood or puberty. The "juvenile melanoma of Spitz" is a compound cellular nevus and is benign. It usually occurs on the face as a smooth, pink papular lesion but may occur on the trunk and be varying shades of brown in color. Its importance lies in the possibility of misdiagnosis histologically by a pathologist unfamiliar with this entity.

In adults, treatment of pigmented nevi on the soles is controversial. Can we make a case for the routine removal of all nevi on the feet? This is more theoretical than realistic; one cannot be certain of the pathology of any nevus without its surgical removal and histologic examination. The actual incidence of malignant melanomas in these areas is remarkably low in comparison to the high incidence of pigmented nevi, and the excision of every such nevus certainly does not appear to be warranted.

Attacking the Problem

Individuals who might have this lesion on the sole should be alerted to the significance of any change in the mole (Fig. 15-14). Suspect any lesion in which there is a change in color and its distribution, with the shape of its margin producing a notching effect. Recent pigment leakage to form a tan or brown halo, and the development of localized areas of infiltration or nodules are evidence of malignant change. Bleeding, oozing, and ulceration, when traumatic factors can be eliminated, are late signs of malignant melanoma. Reasonable criteria for removal are (1) any junction nevus undergoing any unusual change (2) if the patient is extremely frightened concerning the possibility of malignancy (preoccupation with a cancerophobia

with his nevus), perhaps because of a family history of melanoma (3) junction nevi greater than 0.5 cm (This would give the clinician an empiric criterion to "hang his hat on," and would avoid removal of all these lesions on the sole.)

Removal of Lesions

Excisional biopsy should be employed for all suspicious smaller lesions. The method of removal of the small junction nevus on the sole could be subsection with a razor blade to avoid the consequence of a painful scar which might occur after scalpel surgery. When a nevus is very large, an incisional biopsy may provide adequate tissue for diagnosis; however, an excisional biopsy of the entire nevus should be performed whenever possible. The biopsy should include a small margin of skin surrounding the nevus. Needless mutilating surgical removals where plastic revisions may be required should be avoided unless one first knows the procedure is medically indicated, *e.g.*, a benign lesion aggressively removed would require grafting after total excision. Lesions on intertoe areas tend to be junctional in character (Fig. 15-15), but unless they are subject to trauma they should be evaluated on the basis of the criteria just listed. Subungual pigmented lesions cannot be properly evaluated or followed and should be excised prophylactically.

REFERENCES

TUMORS

1. **Aird I, Johnson DH, Lennox B, et al:** Epithelioma cuniculatum: a variety of squamous carcinoma peculiar to the foot. Brit J Surg 42:245, 1954
2. **Aviles E, Arlen M, Miller T:** Plantar fibromatosis. Surgery 69:117, 1971
3. **Bettley FR, O'Shea JA:** The absorption of arsenic and its relation to carcinoma. Brit J Dermatol 93:563, 1975
4. **Black CI:** Basal cell epithelioma on the sole. Cutis 14:74, 1974
5. **Bostwick J, Pendergast WJ Jr, Vasconez LO:** Marjolin's ulcer: an immunologically privileged tumor? Plast Reconstr Surg 57:66, 1976

6. **Brown SM, Freeman RG:** Epithelioma cunniculatum. Arch Dermatol 112:1295, 1976

7. **Brownstein MH, Shapiro L:** Verrucous carcinoma of the skin: epithelioma cuniculatum plantare. Cancer 38:1710, 1976

8. **Darnall TW, Mopper C:** Eccrine poroma associated with Bowen's disease. Arch Dermatol 82:548, 1960

9. **Degos R, et al:** Tumeur epidermique d'aspect particulier: Acanthome a cellules claires. Ann Dermatol Syph 89:361, 1962

10. **Fine RM, Chemosky ME:** Clinical recognition of clear cell acanthoma (Degos'). Arch Dermatol 100:559, 1969

11. **German AL:** Eccrine poroma. Arch Dermatol 89:382, 1964

12. **Goldner R:** Eccrine poromatosis. Arch Dermatol 101:606, 1970

13. **Gorlin RJ, Vickers RA, Kellin E, et al:** The multiple basal cell nevi syndrome: An analysis of a syndrome consisting of multiple nevoid basal cell carcinoma, jaw cysts, skeletal anomalies, meduloblastoma, and hyporesponsiveness to parathormone. Cancer 18:89, 1965

14. **Green A:** Verruca dorsi manus et pedis. Aust J Dermatol 5:10, 1959

15. **Hashimoto K, Lever WF:** Eccrine poroma. J Inv Dermatol 43:237, 1964

16. **Hashimoto K, Lever WF:** Appendage Tumors of the Skin. Springfield, Ill, Charles C Thomas, 1968

17. **Helm, F, McEvoy BF, Milgrom H:** Stucco keratoses. Cutis 15:669, 1975

18. **Hollmann K.H, Civatte J:** Electron microscopic study of clear cell acanthoma. Ann Dermatol Syph 95:139, 1968

19. **Holubar K, Wolff K:** Intra-epidermal eccrine poroma. Cancer 23:626, 1969

20. **Howell JB, Mehregan AH:** Pursuit of the pits in the nevoid basal cell carcinoma syndrome. Arch Dermatol 102:586, 1970

21. **Hu F, Sisson JK:** Ultrastructure of pale cell acanthoma. J Inv Dermatol 52:185, 1969

22. **Hunter GA, Hellier, FF:** Tumors of the palm and sole resembling basal cell epithelioma. Brit J Dermatol 72:283, 1960

23. **Hyman AB, Brownstein MH:** Eccrine poroma. Dermatologica 138:29, 1969

24. **Kocsard E, Ofner F:** Keratoelastoidosis verrucosa of the extremities (stucco keratoses of the extremities). Dermatologica 133:225, 1966

25. **Lebouitz SS, Miller DF, Dickey RF:** Subungual exostosis. Cutis 13:426, 1974

26. **Liddell K:** Malignant change in chronic varicose ulceration. Practitioner 215:335, 1975

27. **Malignant and benign neoplasms of the skin.** In Analysis of Research Needs and Priorities in Dermatology, Chap IV. J Inv Dermatol 73:433, 1979

28. **Montgomery RM:** Two basal cell epitheliomas on the sole. Cutis 12:739, 1973

29. **Morris J, Wood MG, Samitz MH:** Eccrine poroma. Arch Dermatol 98:162, 1968

29a. **Odom RB, Goette DK:** Treatment of cutaneous Kaposi's sarcoma with intralesional vincristine. Arch Dermatol 114:1693, 1978

30. **Ogino A:** Linear eccrine poroma. Arch Dermatol 112:841, 1976

31. **Okun MR, Ansell HB:** Eccrine poroma. Arch Dermatol 88:561, 1963

32. **Pinkus H:** The wall of the intra-epidermal part of the sweat duct. J Inv Dermatol 2:175, 1939

33. **Pinkus H, Mehregan AH:** Epidermotropic eccrine carcinoma. Arch Dermatol 88:597, 1963

34. **Pinkus H, Rogin JR, Goldman P:** Eccrine poroma. Arch Dermatol Syph 74:511, 1956

35. **Reingold IM, Smith BR, Graham JH:** Epithelioma cuniculatum pedis, variant of squamous cell carcinoma.

36. **Rook A, Wilkinson DC, Ebling FJG:** Textbook of Dermatology, p 1711. Philadelphia, FA Davis Company, 1968

37. **Samitz MH, Lewis JE:** Skin tumors of the lower extremities. Int J Dermatol 17:558, 1978

38. **Sanderson KV, Ryan EA:** The histochemistry of eccrine poroma. Brit J Dermatol 75:86, 1963

39. **Shafrir A, Lichtig C, Hirshowitz B, Mahler D:** Eccrine poroma. Isr J Med Sci, 10:1133, 1974

40. **Stritzler C, Stritzler R:** Eccrine poroma on the calf of a leg. Arch Dermatol 94:370, 1966

40a. **Templeton AC, Bhana D:** Prognosis in Kaposi's sarcoma. J Natl Cancer Instit 55:1301, 1975

41. **Thompson SG:** Epithelioma cuniculatum. An unusual tumor of the foot. Brit J Plast Surg 18:214, 1965

41a. **Tucker SB, Winkelmann RK:** Treatment of Kaposi's sarcoma with vinblastine. Arch Dermatol 112:958, 1976

42. **Willoughby C, Soter NA:** Stucco keratosis. Arch Dermatol 105:859, 1972

43. **Wilson-Jones E, Wells GC:** Degos' acanthoma (Acanthome a cellules claires). Arch Dermatol 94:286, 1966.

44. **Wilson-Jones E, Wells GC:** Degos' acanthoma (Acanthome a cellules claires). Brit J Dermatol 79:249, 1967

45. **Zak FG, Martinez M, Statsinger AL:** Pale cell acanthoma. Arch Dermatol 93:674, 1966
46. **Zimmerman EH:** Subungual exostosis. Cutis 19:185, 1977

MELANOMA

1. **Arrington JH, Reed RJ, Ichinose H, Krementz ET:** Plantar lentiginous melanoma: A distinctive variant of human cutaneous malignant melanoma. Ann J Surg Pathol 1:131, 1977
2. **Bart RS, Kopf AW:** A darkly pigmented lesion of a great toe (acral lentiginous melanoma). J Dermatol Surg Oncol 3:158, 1977
3. **Beardmore GI, Davis NC:** Multiple primary cutaneous melanomas. Arch Dermatol 111:603, 1975
4. **Clark WH Jr:** A classification of malignant melanoma in man correlated with histogenesis and biological behavior. In Montagna W, Hu F (eds): Advances in Biology of Skin, Vol. 8, The Pigmentary System, pp 621–647. Oxford, Pergamon Press, 1967
5. **Clark WH Jr:** Clinical diagnosis of cutaneous malignant melanoma. JAMA 236:484, 1976
6. **Clark WH Jr, Ainsworth AM, Bernardino EA, et al:** The development biology of primary human malignant melanomas. Sem Onco 2:83, 1975
7. **Clark WH Jr, From L, Bernardino EA, et al:** The histogenesis and biological behavior of primary human malignant melanoma of the skin. Cancer Res 29:705, 1969
8. **Cosman B, Heddle SB, Crikelair GF:** The increasing incidence of melanoma. Plast Reconstruct Surg 57:50, 1976
9. **Fitzpatrick TB:** SST, aerosols increase risk of skin cancer. Skin and Allergy News 6:1, 1975
10. **Keyhanl A:** Comparison of clinical behavior of melanoma of hands and feet: 283 patients. Cancer 40:3168, 1977
11. **Kopf AW, Mintzis M, Bart RS:** Diagnostic accuracy in malignant melanoma. Arch Dermatol 111:1291, 1975
12. Malignant melanoma and vitiligo. In Analysis of Research Needs and Priorities in Dermatology, Chap IX. J Inv Dermatol 73:491, 1979
13. **McBurney EI, Herron CB:** Melanoma mimicking plantar wart. J Am Acad Dermatol 1:144, 1979
14. **Mihm MC Jr, Clark WH Jr, From L:** The clinical diagnosis, classification and histogenic concepts of the early stages of cutaneous malignant melanomas. N Engl J Med 284:1078, 1971
15. **Mihm MC Jr, Clark WH Jr, Reed RJ:** The clinical diagnosis of malignant melanoma. Sem Oncol 2:105, 1975
16. **Mihm MC Jr, Fitzpatrick TB, Lane Brown MB, et al:** Early detection of primary cutaneous melanoma: A color atlas. N Engl J Med 289:989, 1973
17. **Pantoja E, Llobet RE, Roswit B:** Melanomas of the lower extremity among native Puerto Ricans. Cancer 38:1420, 1976
18. **Reed RJ:** Acral lentiginous melanoma. In New Concepts in Surgical Pathology of the Skin, pp 89–90. New York, John Wiley & Sons, Inc., 1976

16 GENODERMATOSES

Genodermatoses are hereditary skin diseases or malformations due to pathologic units of heredity which are transmitted through the germ cells from one generation to the next. Transmission from generation to generation follows certain genetic mendelian rules. The nature of the responsible gene may be autosomal or sex-linked, complete or incomplete, dominant or recessive, and incompletely or fully penetrant. Expressivity may be variable or invariable (a "forme-fruste" syndrome would connote variable expressivity).

The classification of genodermatoses is according to dominant or recessive, autosomal or sex-linked. The number of sex-linked diseases is smaller, for we are dealing with genes located on only one pair of sex chromosomes, in contrast to autosomal genes, which are located on 23 pairs. (Chromosomal disorders were alluded to in the section on Dermatoglyphics.)

Autosomal dominant dermatoses are much more frequent and also more easily recognized. It is probable that many disorders in medicine that are not considered to be hereditary are due to recessive genes.

Recessive diseases tend to have an earlier age of onset, in fact, they are frequently congenital (manifest at birth). However, there are many recessive genes that become manifest later in life—a good example is pseudoxanthoma elasticum, in which the skin changes may become manifest in the first or second decade, and the cardiovascular involvement later in life.

Dominant diseases tend to be less severe and are compatible with life, while recessive ones are more disabling, and sometimes incompatible with life. This fact is exemplified by genodermatoses that resemble each other clinically, but that differ in their mode of inheritance and in their degree of severity. Such dermatoses are: ichthyosis vulgaris and congenita, epidermolysis bullosa simplex and dystrophica, angiokeratoma of Mibelli and angiokeratoma corporis diffusum, partial and complete albinism, minor (hidrotic) and major (anhidrotic) ectodermal dysplasia, and dyskeratosis congenita.

An important factor is that in recessive inheritance, the phenotypic abnormality is characterized by horizontal spread (in one or more members of the same generation), but the genotypic abnormality may be transmitted in vertical spread (from one generation to the next). Mutations caused by excessive radiation are usually of a recessive nature.

Some genodermatoses have been known for centuries. The number of disorders that are considered genetic continues to grow, and it is only in recent years that we have learned to investigate gene expression. With the constant advances in genetic diagnosis and the recognition of these disorders by the physician, followed by appropriate family studies and preventive counseling, the frequency of these disorders can be reduced.

GENODERMATOSES (WHICH MAY HAVE CLINICAL EXPRESSIVITY ON THE LOWER EXTREMITIES)

AUTOSOMAL DOMINANT:

Atopic dermatitis—eczema and nail plate dystrophy if eczema on dorsal toes

Psoriasis—nail changes, skin lesions including plantar keratoderma

Tuberous sclerosis—Koenen's periungual fibromas

Albinism and piebaldism

Angiokeratoma of Mibelli—lesions may be present on dorsal toes

Hidrotic ectodermal dysplasia—nail dystrophy, plantar keratoderma

Ehlers-Danlos syndrome—pseudoscars on knees, hyperextensible joints

Epidermolysis bullosa simplex—blisters; may be mild dystrophic changes with the dominant dystrophic type

Milroy's lymphedema—lymphedema may be mild, moderate, or severe

Ichthyosis vulgaris—increased sole markings, hyperkeratosis over knees, scales on extensor legs

Darier's disease—nail changes; plantar keratoderma may be present

Palmoplantar keratoderma—several types

Neurofibromatosis—neurofibromas, café au lait spots

Porokeratosis (of Mibelli)—especially on feet

Xanthomas—especially Type II familial hyperlipoproteinemia with tuberous and tendon xanthomas

Nail patella syndrome—nail dystrophy

Pityriasis rubra pilaris (some cases)—keratodermic sandal; typical salmon-colored eruption with islands of spared skin; follicular papules

Marfan's syndrome—arachnodactyly

Peutz-Jehger's syndrome—nail changes may be present on the toes

Familial Mediterranean fever—erysipelas-like lesions on lower legs

Lipoid proteinosis—papules on knees

Primary gout—tophi; most common on metatarsophalangeal joint of great toe

Pachyonychia congenita—pachyonychia (thickened nails and thickness increases distally); plantar keratoderma

Follicular atrophoderma (Bazex)—dimple-like depressions of follicular orifices on dorsal feet and toes

Cowden's disease (multiple hamartoma syndrome)—small keratoses on soles and plantar surfaces of toes

Multiple glomus tumors

Leukonychia

Anonychia

Periodic shedding of nails

Diabetes mellitus—infections, neuropathic lesions, arteriosclerosis obliterans, tinea pedis, onychomycosis, erythrasma

Hereditary angioedema—angioedema soles

Erythrokeratoderma variabilis—geographic hyperkeratotic patches, may have plantar keratoderma

Basal cell nevus syndrome—pits on soles, basal cell cancers

Osler-Weber-Rendu disease (hereditary hemorrhagic telangiectasia)—mat telangiectases on soles and in nail beds

B-K mole syndrome—origin of familial malignant melanomas from heritable melanocytic lesions

Koilonychia

Onychauxis

Connective tissue diseases (? ? ? ? ?)

Arteriosclerosis obliterans (? ? ? ? ?)

Cortical hyperhidrosis—is familial and probably autosomal dominant, and this is emotional hyperhidrosis which includes sweating on the soles

AUTOSOMAL RECESSIVE:

Acrodermatitis enteropathica—acral dermatitis

Epidermolysis bullosa dystrophica—severe dystrophy including nails

Lamellar ichthyosis

Werner's syndrome—signs and symptoms of arteriosclerotic occlusive disease and premature aging of skin

Xeroderma pigmentosum—freckling, epitheliomas, increased incidence of melanoma

Rothmund-Thompson syndrome—telangiectasia and mottled pigmentation on the lower legs; keratoses on feet which may become squamous cell cancers; atrophy of skin

Albinism

Erythropoietic porphyria—dystrophic changes

Conradi's syndrome—soles may be thickened

Ataxia telangiectasia—telangiectasia in the popliteal fossae

Familial chronic mucocutaneous candidiasis—nail involvement including granulomas around nails

SEX-LINKED:

Anhidrotic ectodermal dysplasia—minimal or absent nail changes

Osteoarthropathy—seen in males

Sex-linked ichthyosis—seen in males

Fabry's disease—angiokeratomas, may have symptomatic (burning and tingling) flushing of feet and legs

Incontinentia pigmenti—female

Dyskeratosis congenita—constant and severe nail changes

Chronic granulomatous disease—nails and periungual tissue

Ichthyosis vulgaris (some cases)

As gleaned from the preceding list, an extraordinary variety of heritable syndromes upon occasion may involve the skin or nails of the feet. However, as we have done in other sections of this text, we have selected certain of the disorders to present here; some were reviewed in the chapter on toenails, and several disorders were discussed in the chapter on pediatric-dermalogic problems.

PALMOPLANTAR KERATODERMAS

The palmoplantar keratodermas are a group of hereditary disorders characterized by diffuse or focal thickening of the soles and palms, or occasionally, of only one of these sites.

The six following syndromes are all characterized by an autosomal dominant inheritance pattern:

1. **Diffuse Palmoplantar Keratoderma (Tylosis; Thost-Unna syndrome).** In this disorder, a diffuse thickening of the palms and soles is noted in early infancy and is often fully developed by the age of 6 months. The hyperkeratosis is smooth, uniform, and sharply demarcated from normal skin by an erythematous border. Hyperhidrosis and painful fissuring may occur, but some patients are asymptomatic. The nails may be normal or thickened.

   An association between esophageal carcinoma and palmoplantar keratoderma has been reported in several families. In these cases, the hyperkeratosis did not appear in infancy but rather between the ages of 5 and 15 years.

   Tylosis is an autosomal dominant form of keratosis palmaris et plantaris of late onset which has been reported in several families. In association with the skin lesions is an abnormality of the lower esophagus. At this site can occur peptic ulceration, followed by stricture in which squamous cell carcinoma develops. In these cases, the hyperkeratosis did not appear in infancy but rather between the ages of 5 and 15 years. In patients with tylosis, abnormalities of the oral mucosa, either preleukoplakia or leukoplakia, also have been recorded.

2. **Mutilating Keratoderma (Vohwinkel syndrome).** In this disorder, the keratoderma of the palms and soles appears in infancy and shows a surface honeycombed with small depressions. Linear keratoses and starfish-shaped keratoses have been noted on the knees, elbows, and the dorsal as-

Fig. 16-1. Typical punctate keratoderm.

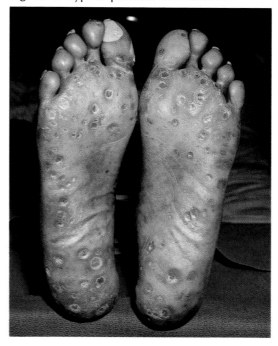

pects of the hands and feet. At any time after age 5, constrictive bands develop around the smaller digits and progress to auto-amputation of the affected digits.

3. **Progressive Palmoplantar Keratoderma (Greither's syndrome).** This rare syndrome also begins in infancy, but unlike tylosis is characterized by slow progression over a variable number of years, sometimes until the fourth decade. The sides and dorsa of the feet and hands as well as irregular patches on the legs and arms may be affected with patchy hyperkeratotic lesions.

4. **Punctate Keratoderma.** This genodermatosis is marked by punctate, round to oval, hard keratotic lesions on the palms and soles (Fig. 16-1), and develops between 15 and 30 years of age. The keratotic plugs may be removed by trauma and leave a depression surrounded by a horny wall. Onychogryphosis, longitudinal fissuring of the nails, and other nail dystrophies may ocur in association. Arsenical keratoses may simulate this keratoderma.

5. **Striate Keratoderma.** In this syndrome, linear keratoses involving the soles or palms may extend onto the digits.

6. **Disseminated Palmoplantar Keratoderma With Corneal Dystrophy.** This hyperkeratotic syndrome is manifested by diffuse, punctate, or linear keratoderma which may be associated with corneal dystrophy or comma-shaped, punctate, or dendritic opacities. The keratoderma does not develop until the second decade of life.

The following three disorders are characterized by an autosomal recessive inheritance pattern:

1. **Mal de Meleda.** This rare syndrome, named after the Dalmatian island of Meleda (Mljet), is primarily due to inbreeding. Redness of the palms and soles in early infancy is followed by scaling and thickening which is more often diffuse than focal. The sides and dorsa of the feet and hands are covered in part by the hyperkeratotic lesions. Hyperhidrosis with secondary eczematization is common. Circumscribed areas on the knuckles, knees, and elbows may be affected as well. A sharp erythematous border surrounds the lesions. The area of involvement tends to increase with age.

2. **Palmoplantar Keratoderma with Periodontosis (Papillon-Lefevre syndrome).** This rare syndrome exhibits redness and thickening of the palms and soles beginning at ages 1 to 5 years and extending along the Achilles tendon and the sides of the hands and feet. Hyperhidrosis and periodontosis are present. The latter causes loss of deciduous and permanent teeth early in life.

3. **Circumscribed Palmoplantar Keratoderma.** This keratoderma develops as tender callosities at pressure points on the soles and palms. Mental deficiency, leukoplakia of the buccal mucous membrane, and corneal dystrophies may be associated.

ICHTHYOSIFORM DERMATOSES

The classification adapted for this group of disorders is largely that of Frost and Van Scott, based upon epidermal proliferation rates, histopathologic findings, and clinical characteristics.[2]

1. **Ichthyosis Vulgaris.** This dermatosis is inherited as an autosomal dominant disorder, possibly with incomplete penetrance. It is not present at birth but begins between the ages of 1 and 4 years and becomes more severe over the next several years. Small, fine scales occur on the trunk and arms with larger scales noted on the legs. The antecubital and popliteal fossae are relatively spared. The turnover rate of the skin is less than normal, that is, the horny layer is abnormally retained. The rate of keratinization is not increased.

2. **Lamellar Ichthyosis.** This disorder is inherited as an autosomal recessive trait, although spontaneous mutations probably occur. Universal erythema and scaling from birth to adulthood is usual. The flexures are not spared. In an untreated case, the scales are large, thin, gray-brown in color, centrally adherent with an elevated margin. Ectropion and corneal scarring with vascularization occasionally occur.

3. **Epidermolytic Hyperkeratosis.** Present at birth as a thick scaly mantle, the skin is shed almost immediately to leave a raw body surface. Thick gray-brown, often verrucous, scales then form over most of the body, particularly in the flexural creases such as the antecubital and popliteal fossae. Flaccid bullae due to bacterial infection of the skin may occur. The inheritance is autosomal dominant.

4. **X-Linked Ichthyosis.**[3] Generalized dry skin and scaling, particularly of the legs, arms, trunk, and neck, occur in very early infancy in this sex-linked dermatosis. The characteristic scales are large and yellow, brown, or black in color. Palms and soles are uninvolved. Deep corneal opacities are noted not only in affected individuals, but also in the carriers of this trait. They are of no clinical significance but are useful in determining the type of ichthyosis. An association with mental retardation, skeletal anomalies, and pituitary hypogonadism has been reported.

5. **Psoriasiform Erythroderma.** These patients show generalized erythema and scaling, often from infancy. The scales are micaceous and desquamate in large quantities. On clinical and histologic study, the disorder is identical to generalized psoriasis. This disorder is not an ichthyosis but is included here, since it is often confused clinically with the ichthyotic states.

Histologic studies are helpful in differentiating the clinical types of ichthyosis.

Therapy for all types of ichthyosis consists of hydration baths followed by the application of hydrophilic ointment, aqua and aquaphor or petrolatum or by applying 40% urea in Keri lotion; 3% salicylic acid added to the emollients may also be helpful. Antibacterial soaps and systemic antibiotics will heal the bullae and eradicate the odor of epidermolytic hyperkeratosis.

EPIDERMOLYSIS BULLOSA

This is a group of genetically determined syndromes characterized by bulla formation as a response to trauma.

1. **Epidermolysis Bullosa Simplex.** This is an autosomal dominant disorder usually first manifested, when the infant begins to crawl or walk, by clear tense bullae on the palms, soles, and knees or other areas of frequent trauma. The lesions heal without scarring. Some patients may improve at puberty, but in any case, longevity is not impaired.

2. **Cockayne Syndrome or Recurrent Bullous Eruption of the Feet.** This disorder, also referred to as the "march syndrome," is variously considered as a mild variant of the simplex form of epidermolysis bullosa or as a separate entity. Bullae develop on the feet subsequent to friction as in prolonged marches in the army, or subsequent to normal trauma of walking, especially during the summer months (Fig. 16-2). Affected individuals seldom have blisters on parts other than their feet.

3. **Hyperplastic Epidermolysis Bullosa.** In this autosomal dominant disorder, bullae develop on the knees and feet, forehead, and hands as well as on other sites of trauma either in infancy or not until puberty or later. they heal with atrophic scars and milia or at times keloids. Ichthyosis, keratosis pilaris, and palmoplantar keratoderma with hyperhidrosis and thickened dystrophic nails are common. Leukoplakia of the buccal mucosa may develop following repeated erosions at the site.

4. **Polydysplastic Epidermolysis Bullosa.** This form of epidermolysis bullosa is inherited as an autosomal recessive trait. Bullae appear at birth or in early infancy. Bullae develop on the feet and legs as well as in any traumatized area of the body. The bullae are large and flaccid and may be hemorrhagic. Scarring with pseudo-webbing of the digits is common following repeated injury. Squamous cell carcinoma may develop on the legs in scarred atrophic skin. Scarring of the conjunctiva, mucous membranes, and esophagus may also occur. Leukoplakia of the buccal mucosa with subsequent carcinoma formation, and stricture of the esophagus leading to aspiration pneumonitis and occasionally to carcinoma of the esophagus have been reported.

5. **Epidermolysis Bullosa Letalis.** This au-

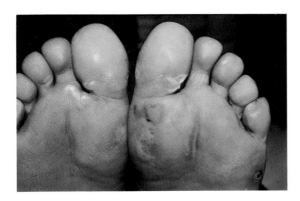

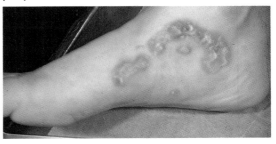

Fig. 16-2. Cockayne syndrome. A variant of the simplex form of epidermolysis bullosa.

Fig. 16-3. Porokeratosis of Mibelli. The original lesion was a horny papule that gradually enlarged to form a circinate plaque.

tosomal recessive disorder is usually incompatible with life. Bullae develop within hours after birth, leading to the shedding of sheets of skin. The mucous membranes are extensively involved. The entire picture presents an insuperable nursing problem, and most children do not survive 3 months.

POROKERATOSIS

1. **Porokeratosis of Mibelli.** This is a benign disorder of keratinization characterized by extending plaques of hyperkeratosis followed by atrophy. The original lesion, a horny papule, gradually enlarges to form a plaque of circinate or irregular contour (Fig. 16-3). The periphery of the plaques is raised, and from this raised area, a thin crest of keratin emerges. The central zone of the plaque may be normal or atrophic. The feet, hands, face, and upper trunk are often affected. Most cases begin in childhood. A dominant inheritance pattern is occasionally manifested, but many random cases occur.
2. **Disseminated Superficial Actinic Porokeratosis.** In this autosomal dominant disorder described by Chernosky and Freeman, follicular keratotic papules which evolve to annular keratotic lesions occur primarily on sun-exposed sites such as the face, legs, and arms.[1] The lesions tend to enlarge slowly in an irregular circinate fashion. The eruption tends to regress during the winter months and exacerbate in the summer. Symptomatic complaints such as pruritus are minimal. Clinically, the lesions differ from those of porokera-

tosis of Mibelli, but the histologic picture is the same though the findings are minimal.

ANHIDROTIC ECTODERMAL DYSPLASIA

This disorder is recessive in inheritance, and 90% of the cases are males. Partial or complete absence of sweat glands and other epidermal appendages results in absent or reduced sweating, hypotrichosis, and total or partial anodontia. The manifestations of the syndrome are widely variable. In the complete form, there is a characteristic facies with prominent chin and frontal ridges, saddle nose, thick everted lips, large ears, and sparse hair. The skin is dry and smooth, with fine wrinkles leading to an appearance of premature aging. When the ability to produce sweat is markedly reduced, exertion or a hot environment may cause the individual to become very uncomfortable.

There is no available satisfactory therapy.

DYSKERATOSIS CONGENITA (DKC)

This syndrome consists of nail dystrophy, atrophy and pigmentation of the skin, and leukoplakia. It is inherited as a partially sex-

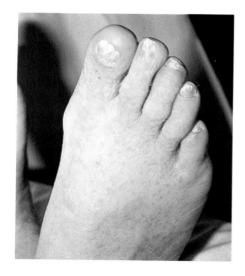

Fig. 16-4. Darier's disease. The follicular lesions resemble flat warts or acrokeratosis verruciformis.

present at birth or may occur progressively over the first 5 years of life. Repeated infection and swelling of the nail folds and repeated shedding of the nails often occur. Subungual hyperkeratosis may be severe.

Keratoderma and hyperhidrosis of the palms and soles become apparent during childhood.

Leukoplakia of the tongue, buccal mucosa, and larynx is very common during the teenage years and may undergo malignant changes.

No treatment is available.

linked recessive disorder with almost all cases occuring in males. DKC is a disorder of DNA repair.

The nail changes usually appear first with the nails becoming dystrophic and being shed between the ages of 5 and 13 years.

Reticulated brownish pigmentation along with some atrophy and telangiectasia results in a poikilodermatous appearance of the skin. These changes usually begin 2 or 3 years after the nail changes and reach their maximum within 5 years. The changes are most prominent on the neck and thighs but also involve large areas of the trunk.

The skin over the dorsa of the hands and feet is atrophic, shiny, and transparent. Thickening and hyperhidrosis of the palms and soles may also occur.

The mucous membrane involvement consists of leukoplakia and is significant because of a high risk of carcinoma occurring in the areas of leukoplakia.

A high proportion of DKC patients show features of Fanconi's anemia, which is also a disorder of DNA instability.

The prognosis is rather poor with a fatal outcome due to either a carcinoma or the blood dyscrasia.

PACHYONYCHIA CONGENITA

In this autosomal-dominantly inherited disorder, the finger- and toe-nails develop a yellow thickening and curvature which may be

DARIER'S DISEASE (KERATOSIS FOLLICULARIS)

Darier's disease, a disease of unknown cause, is inherited as an autosomal dominant, but most pedigrees do not extend beyond two generations because the marriage rate and fertility are low.

The distinctive lesion is a greasy crusted papule which may be flesh-colored or yellow-brown. Warty or papillomatous masses result from the coalescence of lesions and may be malodorous. The lesions most commonly occur on the chest, upper back and shoulders, lumbosacral and buttocks areas, scalp, face, and the flexures. When the papules occur on the dorsal surfaces of the hands or feet, they resemble flat warts or acrokeratosis verruciformis (Fig. 16-4). Punctate keratoses or

Fig. 16-5. Tuberous sclerosis. The tumors protruding from under the nail folds are characteristic.

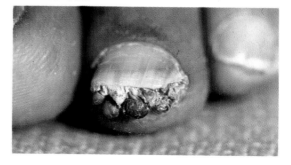

minute pits are seen on the palms and soles. Keratoderma of the palms and soles is seen in approximately 10% of cases.

TUBEROUS SCLEROSIS

The characteristic features of this syndrome are epilepsy, mental retardation, and skin lesions.

Epilepsy develops in about 80% of the cases and usually appears in infancy or early childhood, thus often antedating the appearance of the skin lesions by years.

Mental deficiency is noted in about 70% of cases and may be progressive.

The characteristic skin manifestations are: (1) adenoma sebaceum of Pringle, which are yellowish or telangiectatic firm papules occurring on the nasolabial folds, cheeks, and chin; (2) the shagreen patch, which is a thickened plaque located in the lumbosacral area; and (3) the periungual fibromata occurring on either the finger- or toenails at or after puberty. The fibromas appear as firm, smooth, flesh-colored tumors protruding from under the nail folds (Fig. 16-5).

REFERENCES

1. **Chernosky ME, Freeman RG:** Disseminated superficial actinic porokeratosis (DSAP). Arch Dermatol 96:611, 1967
2. **Frost P, Van Scott EJ:** Ichthyosiform dermatoses. Arch Dermatol 94:113, 1966
3. **Wells RS, Kerr CB:** Clinical features of autosomal dominant and sex-linked ichthyosis in an English population. Brit Med J 1:947, Apr 16, 1966

17 SWEAT DISORDERS

Many mammals possess eccrine sweat glands on their foot pads, presumably to moisten the skin surface and thereby improve their grip. Eccrine sweat glands are widely distributed, numerous, and highly developed in some of the higher primates where they serve a thermoregulatory function. In man, eccrine glands reach the maximum degree of development. They are located on all areas of the body surface except the lips and mucous membrane portion of the genitalia and are most concentrated on the soles, palms, and in the axillae. The eccrine sweat glands are the only skin appendages on the soles.

The first appearance of the forerunner of eccrine glands is a specialized downgrowth of the epidermis in the fourth fetal month. The sweat glands begin to develop first in the palms and soles and then elsewhere over the skin of the body. No additional sweat glands are formed after birth. Many sweat glands that are histologically normal are nonfunctioning. By 2½ years of age, all eccrine sweat glands which are to be functional in the adult have become active.

The eccrine sweat gland is the most dynamic structure in the skin as far as immediacy of action—it turns off and on rapidly in response to many types of stimuli.

Thermal sweating is regulated by a hypothalamic center that responds to changes in the temperature of the blood perfusing it. This type of sweating is rather generalized, occurring most prominently on the upper trunk and face. The eccrine glands of the palms and soles respond only weakly to thermal stimuli.

Mental, emotional, or psychic sweating is most striking on the palms and soles, analagous to the action of sweat glands on the friction surfaces of lower animals that prepare mammals to cope with danger by running away. Centers for psychic sweating are located in the frontal region of the brain, but the precise position and pathways are not known.

The eccrine sweat glands depend upon an intact sympathetic nerve supply to function. This sympathetic innervation is unusual in that it is cholinergic. Sweat is usually hypotonic and contains sodium, chloride, potassium, urea, and lactate as its most significant constituents.

HYPERHIDROSIS

Hyperhidrosis is an abnormal increase in the amount of sweat produced; on the feet it may be part of a generalized hyperhidrosis, or it may be local.

Generalized hyperhidrosis may be due to such factors as a hot humid environment, increased internal heat production from work or exercise, febrile illnesses, hypothalamic disorders, or endocrine disorders.

Although hyperhidrosis of the feet is often due to emotional stimuli, there are also numerous individuals in whom there is no apparent primary emotional disorder. Rather, there would seem to exist some facilitation of the neural pathways causing physiologic psychic sweating. In these persons, hyperhidrosis may be virtually constant. Other causes may be poor foot mechanics, faulty footwear, neural changes (neuritis, syringomyelia, tabes, paresis), and certain skin lesions (trench foot, frostbite).

In most cases of hyperhidrosis of the feet, moisture may be seen; however, in many instances the moisture can only be felt. The feet feel wet and soggy. The skin is whitish and may be macerated. Between the toes especially there is maceration, and there may be splitting of the skin. The skin may be thickened and may even appear worm-eaten (Figs. 17-1, 17-2). Either sex may be affected,

and the onset is usually in childhood or around puberty. The hyperhidrosis may persist many years; however, it tends to lessen spontaneously after the age of 25 years. The disorder may show a familial tendency.

Many of these cases may be mistaken for fungal infections. Hyperhidrosis may predispose to and prepare a favorable soil for fungal infection. The paradox, however, is seen in children. Hyperhidrosis of the feet is particularly common in children; yet fungal infection is relatively rare before puberty. Hyperhidrosis may also be a predisposing factor for contact dermatitis and dyshidrotic eczema.

In an entity known as *symmetric lividity of the soles* there is a hyperkeratotic reaction of the sole to hyperhidrosis. The condition is characterized by cyanotic color changes reflecting the vasomotor activity seen in association with hypersympathotonia and presents as bluish-red plaques of thickened, soggy hyperkeratosis (Fig. 17-3). The disorder is often seen in young foot soldiers.

TREATMENT

Systemic and topical therapy are by no means satisfactory.

Systemic therapy with anticholinergic drugs (*e.g.*, propantheline bromide [Pro-banthine], atropine, belladonna, and glycopyrrolate) to block the action of acetylcholine on the sweat glands often produces side effects such as dryness of the mouth, blurring of vision, dizziness, palpitation, and urinary retention, which are more trouble-

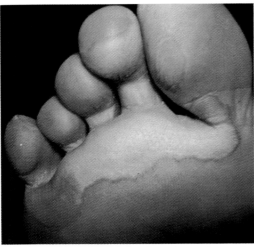

Fig. 17-1. Hyperhidrosis of undersurface of toes.

Fig. 17-2. Hyperhidrosis of soles.

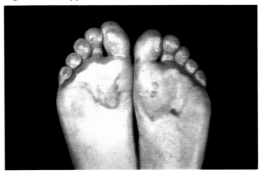

Fig. 17-3. Symmetrical erythema of soles.

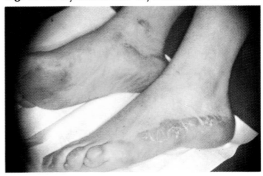

some than the hyperhidrosis itself. In cases in which there is an obvious emotional factor, tranquilizers or antihistaminics (*e.g.*, diphenhydramine hydrochloride [Benadryl], hydroxyzine hydrochloride [Atarax], and hydroxyzine pamoate [Vistaril]), for their sedative properties, may occasionally be of some help, but their tendency to produce drowsiness limits their use. In general, systemic therapy for hyperhidrosis is disappointing.

Topical therapy may consist of simple foot soaks with tap water, saline, or Burow's solution. Soaking for 20 to 30 minutes will usually inhibit sweating locally up to several hours. The use of noncaking dusting powder will help reduce perspiration. These powders should be of a simple absorbent type (*e.g.*, Zeasorb powder, Stieffel) and those containing numerous "medications" incorporated into the powder should be avoided, since at times irritant or allergic reactions may occur.

In our experience, the following set of directions has proved helpful in controlling mild to moderate hyperhidrosis:

1. Soak feet in Burow's solution (1:20), morning and evening.
2. Dry feet well.
3. Dust powder freely into shoes and hosiery.
4. Cotton hose or peds are preferable. Change twice daily, morning and evening.
5. Change shoes twice daily, morning and evening.

In patients with excessive plantar sweating, measures such as the following can be tried:

1. Formalin soaks (5% to 10% aqueous formalin solution) are helpful but may cause overdrying with fissuring and sensitization.
2. Topical 5% methanamine, available in a gel stick formulation, decreases palmar and plantar sweating.[1] Its action depends on a slow release of formaldehyde.
3. Glutaraldehyde solutions can substantially inhibit sweating but produce an objectionable discoloration.[3] It is used as a 10% solution with distilled water or can be buffered with sodium bicarbonate to get pH of 7.3.[2] The 10% solution is applied to the soles three times a week for two weeks; after the sweating is diminished, the patient tapers the applications to once weekly or when needed.

4. Alcoholic solutions of aluminum chloride are more effective in controlling axillary sweating than sweating on the palms and soles. In this category is Drysol* a 20% solution, used with an occlusive technique overnight on the feet (Saran wrap secured in place with a sock).

Local radiation therapy for hyperhidrosis should not be used because of the danger of late radiodermatitis. In extreme cases, when all other measures have failed, one may consider sympathectomy. The second, third, and fourth lumbar ganglia are resected.

DYSHIDROSIS

Dyshidrosis, also called pompholyx, is a recurrent eruption of numerous deep-seated vesicles occurring singly and in groups on the palms and soles with minimal inflammatory signs. Hyperhidrosis frequently is also present. The name, dyshidrosis, is unfortunate since studies have failed to show that the primary lesion of dyshidrosis is a sweat retention vesicle. Rather, dyshidrosis is an eczematous reaction pattern of the skin, unique by virtue of the anatomy of the affected sites. Secondary sweat retention may occur in the vesicles, with resulting exacerbation of the dyshidrosis.

Therapy for dyshidrosis is similar to that described for hyperhidrosis. In addition, topical steroids and systemic broad-spectrum antibiotics are often useful therapeutic modalities.

BROMHIDROSIS

Bromhidrosis or foul-smelling sweat frequently occurs on the feet. Eccrine sweat itself, as secreted, is odorless. However, sweat promotes bacterial growth, and the odor associated with sweating is the result of bacterial decomposition of surface protein debris. (See Foot Odor, Chapter 20).

*Person & Covey, Inc., Glendale, California 91201

Therapy should be directed toward the hyperhidrosis, as discussed previously, against the bacterial flora of the skin by the use of antibacterial soaps, and against the proteinaceous debris by frequent washing. As a temporary measure, dusting the feet once or twice daily with equal parts of baking soda and talc is helpful in reducing the foot odor syndrome.

ANHIDROSIS

Anhidrosis is the inability of the body to produce and/or deliver sweat to the skin surface. Anhidrosis of the feet may be part of a generalized anhidrosis or may be local. Causes of generalized anhidrosis are: damage to the hypothalamus such as in heatstroke, neurosurgical procedures, tumors, and mechanical trauma; hysteria; anticholinergic drugs; congenital ectodermal defect; Atabrine dermatitis; skin conditions such as atopic dermatitis, contact dermatitis, pemphigus, exfoliative dermatitis; hormonal disturbances such as Addison's disease, myxedema, diabetes mellitus, and diabetes insipidus; poisoning as by arsenic, fluorine,

formaldehyde, lead, morphine, and thallium; fluid imbalance; malignancy; glomerulonephritis; and cirrhosis.

Causes of anhidrosis localized in the feet may be cord lesions as with poliomyelitis, multiple sclerosis, syringomyelia, and tumors; alcoholic polyneuritis; leprosy; nerve tumors; diabetes mellitus; gout; orthostatic hypotension; localized congenital absence of sweat glands; atrophy of glands due to senile skin, radiodermatitis, lymphedema, acrodermatitis chronica atrophicans, and so forth; antiperspirants; interference with blood supply in skin, as by continuous pressure of a cast; and skin diseases such as lichen planus and psoriasis.

Therapy must be directed toward the responsible etiologic agent.

REFERENCES

1. **Cullen SI:** Topical methanamine therapy for hyperhidrosis. Arch Dermatol 111:1158, 1975
2. **Gordon BI:** "No Sweat." Cutis 15:401, 1975
3. **Juhlin L, Hansson H:** Topical glutaraldehyde for plantar hyperhidrosis. Arch Dermatol 97:327, 1968

18 TOENAIL DISORDERS

The most common disorders of toenails encountered by the practitioner might be listed as follows.

1. Onychomycosis—95% caused by *Trichophyton rubrum.*
2. Dystrophies due to impaired circulation, with arteriosclerosis obliterans and diabetes mellitus being the salient underlying diseases.
3. Changes due to physical trauma—with ingrown toenails involving the great toe heading the list.
4. Psoriasis, lichen planus, alopecia areata.
5. Dystrophy of the nailplates due to dermatitis of the dorsal surface of the toes.
6. Miscellaneous.

In view of the magnitude of this subject, this chapter is restricted to general considerations, but includes a more detailed description on nail biopsies, ingrown toenails, pincer nails, and avulsion of nails.

Following is a categorization of nail disorders using a basic etiologic classification of disease, with the realization that it is not possible to "pigeonhole" all diseases into one category to the exclusion of others. Most of the problems are self-explanatory.

CONGENITAL-HEREDITARY:

Hereditary osteoarthropathy—sex-linked, seen in males
Periungual fibromas of tuberous sclerosis (Koenen's tumors)

Psoriasis
Nail-patella syndrome—hypoplasia or anonychia of nails, hypoplastic or absent patellae, iliac horns
Leukonychia totalia—and some cases of partial leukonychia
Congenital great toenail dystrophy
Epidermolysis bullosa—simple and dystrophic types may have nail involvement from thinning to dystrophy to anonychia
Koilonychia—there is a rare familial variety
Anonychia
Darier's disease—longitudinal striations; maybe onychauxis
Pachyonychia congenita—hypertrophic nails
Hidrotic ectodermal dysplasia—usually thickened toenails (nail changes are an insignificant feature of the anhidrotic type)
Wilson's disease—azure blue lunulae
Marfan's syndrome—enlarged toes
Porokeratosis of Mibelli—may involve nail matrix with secondary dystrophy of the nailplate

Peutz-Jehger's syndrome—bands of brown melanin pigmentation or diffuse melanin pigmentation of nails may occur
Chronic mucocutaneous candidiasis—with candidiasis of nailplates
Onychogryphosis
Onychauxis
Dyskeratosis congenita—a rare syndrome which may have nail dystrophy or onychomadesis
Congenital lymphedema (Milroy's)—yellow nails may be present
Incontinentia pigmenti

TRAUMATIC:

Onychauxia—trauma is the most common cause (thickened nails)

Onychogryphosis (thickened claw-like nails)—usually due to trauma and most common in the elderly

Splinter hemorrhages—trauma is the most common cause

Subungual hematoma—most common cause of blackening of part of a nail (Fig. 18-1)

Ingrown toenail—trauma is the most common cause

Pincer and trumpet nail—attributable to the wearing of ill-fitting shoes

Acquired digital fibrokeratoma—trauma to granulation tissue accompanying an ingrown toenail

Koilonychia—occupational, trauma-induced

Post-traumatic shedding (onychomadesis)

Post-traumatic onycholysis

Post-traumatic leukonychia—trauma is the most common cause of the striate variety

Periungual or subungual chilblains (thermal trauma)—with secondary changes in nailplate

Onychoschizia—most common cause of this horizontal splitting of the nailplate is frequent immersion in warm water, especially if the water is soapy

Post-traumatic atrophy and anonychia

INFLAMMATORY:

Psoriasis—pits, onycholysis, gross dystrophy (usually hypertrophy), onychomadesis, subungual debris, chromonychia

Pustular psoriasis—nail dystrophy or anonychia

Acrodermatitis continua—nail dystrophy or anonychia

Pityriasis rubra pilaris—nail dystrophy (usually hypertrophy)

Alopecia areata—atrophic nails

Pseudomonas and proteus infections—the former characterized by green chromonychia and the latter by black chromonychia

Leprosy—neurotrophic changes

Norwegian scabies—dystrophy

Acute paronychia—a primary pyoderma (S. aureus)

Chronic paronychia—occasionally seen on the toes

Viral warts—periungual and subungual warts occasionally seen on the toes

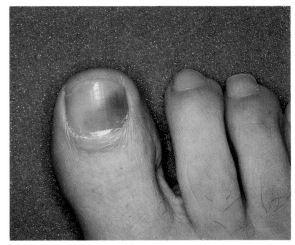

Fig. 18-1. Subungual hematoma. Most common cause of blackening of part of nail. It can be confused with melanoma.

Dermatophyte—*Trichophyton rubrum* most common pathogen—usually yellow chromonychia, may be splinter hemorrhages, onycholysis, hypertrophy, dystrophy

Aspergillus and Scopulariopsis—these fungi are occasionally found, usually in the great toeplates, which have been damaged from another cause

Eczematous conditions with secondary dystrophy of the nailplates—eczema on the dorsal surfaces of the toes with involvement of the skin of the posterior nailfold produces inflammation of the underlying matrix, leading to "washboard nails"

Lichen planus—especially with bullous and ulcerative lichen planus of toes, which may result in anonychia or dystrophy. Ordinary lichen planus produces atrophy of the nailplate, and occasionally pterygium

Reiter's disease—nail changes like the gross changes in psoriasis

CONNECTIVE TISSUE DISEASES:

Lupus erythematosus—chilblain lupus (Hutchinson) lesions, especially on the toes—said to occur in patients with generalized discoid L.E.

Rheumatoid arthritis—atrophic nails may occur; Bywater's lesions are microinfarcts involving the nailfolds

Scleroderma—atrophy of nails is most common; may also see pterygium inversum unguis as a result of soft tissue atrophy and scarring of the pulp

Hybrid connective tissue diseases

Sarcoidosis—may have nail changes due to involvement of the underlying distal phalanx

Chronic mucocutaneous candidiasis—gross dystrophy

Trichinosis—it is said that transverse splinter hemorrhages occurring in all nails simultaneously is pathognomonic

Fixed drug eruption—if it occurs in the nailbed it may impart a dark color to the nail

NEOPLASTIC—BENIGN:

Granuloma telangiectaticum—is an impetiginized pyogenic granuloma and is seen particularly secondary to ingrown great toe plates as an exophytic lesion arising from the lateral nailfold

Enchondroma—of distal phalanx

Subungual exostosis—prefers the great toe

Glomus tumor—painful benign tumor of the glomus (arteriovenous) shunt

Myxoid cyst—involvement of the matrix usually produces a linear canaliform dystrophy of the nailplate

Melanocytic nevi—in the nailbed or matrix

Keratoacanthoma—in the nailbed

NEOPLASTIC—MALIGNANT:

Melanotic whitlow

Hutchinson's freckle—has been reported to occur in the nailbed

Kaposi's sarcoma—lesions frequent around and under the toenails; the acquired lymphedema seen with this disease may also produce yellow nails

Bowen's disease—may occur in the nailbed

Squamous cell carcinoma—may occur in the nailbed

Remember that metastases have been reported on the toes

ENDOCRINE:

Onycholysis—may occur with hyperthyroidism (Plummer's nail) or with hypothyroidism

Thyroid acropachy—clubbing occurring in a patient with Graves'disease

Addison's disease—diffuse black-brown discoloration of all nails, or multiple pigment streaks may occur. Addison's disease may also be seen in patients with chronic subcutaneous candidiasis who may have Candida granulomas of the nails

Acromegaly—enlarged toes

Broad short toes with en raquette-like nails—may be seen in pseudohypoparathyroidism ane pseudo-pseudohypoparathyroidism

Onychomycosis—common in diabetes mellitus, and patients with Cushing's syndrome

Pallor of nails—in Simmonds' and Sheehan's syndromes

METABOLIC:

Acquired clubbing (osteoarthropathy) secondary to chronic ulcerative colitis, chronic hepatitis, Crohn's disease, subacute bacterial endocarditis, cystic fibrosis, and cyanotic congenital or acquired heart disease—clubbing is due to local connective tissue changes

Diabetes mellitus—trophic nail changes secondary to ischemia or neuropathy

Terry's nail—ivory white color in some patients with advanced liver disease who usually have ascites and edema.

Hypoalbuminemia (less than 2 g/%)—two parallel transverse white bands in nailbed which do not move with nail growth—disappear with IV albumin—these are Muerhcke's lines

Mee's lines—transverse white lines in nails of patients surviving acute renal failure

½–½ nail—in chronic renal failure and uremic patients—proximal nail is dull white and distal nail is brown

NUTRITIONAL:

Hypoalbuminemia—white nails, maybe in bands (Muerhcke's lines) Iron-deficiency anemia—brittle nails and koilonychia have been described

Scurvy—splinter hemorrhages may occur

Beau's lines—these lines are an atrophy of the plate indicating a recent illness, and due to temporary interference with nail growth. When Beau's lines appear on isolated nails, the cause is unlikely to be any general disturbance, but local causes such as prolonged spasm of a proper digital vessel in Raynaud's syndrome are more likely

TOXIC:

Methemoglobinemia—cyanotic nails

Photo-onycholysis—especially with demethyl-chlortetra-cycline (Declomycin)

Arsenical keratoses—may be subungual or periungual

Dark longitudinal bands of discoloration—may occur in chronic arsenic poisoning

Blue lunulae—may be seen in argyria

Cherry red nails—of carbon monoxide poisoning

NEUROLOGIC:

Trophic nail changes—in neuropathic diseases

VASCULAR:

Polycythemia—dark red nails

Anemia—pallor

Brittle nails—from impaired peripheral circulation

Onycholysis—from impaired peripheral circulation

Onychomadesia—from impaired peripheral circulation

Pterygium—from impaired peripheral circulation

Atrophy of nails—from impaired peripheral circulation

Chilblains—may be periungual or subungual

Pallor of nails—Raynaud's disease or syndrome

Cyanosis—from pulmonary insufficiency or cyanotic heart disease

Yellow nail syndrome—lymphedema, pleural effusion and nephrotic syndrome—nail changes are permanent and untreatable. Yellow nails may be seen with congenital or acquired lymphedema

IDIOPATHIC:

Many types of nail changes are idiopathic

Trachyonychia—rough nails—disorder seen more often in children

Acanthosis nigricans—may be associated with variable nail changes

Pachydermoperiostosis

Clawlike little toenails

Leukonychia

Thinning

Pterygium

Onycholysis

Onychauxis

Koilonychia

Clubbing

Pitting

Ridging

Rippling

Black streaks are very common in Blacks owing to active melanocytes in the matrix; this may indicate a junction nevus in the matrix in a Caucasian

IATROGENIC—DRUG PIGMENTATIONS:

Common ones are gold, silver, phenothiazines, any antimalarial, cytotoxic drugs

Onycholysis—PUVA photo-onycholysis, tetracyclines (especially Declomycin)

Cytotoxic drugs may cause onychomadesis

Changes in the structure of the nailplate, nailfolds, nailbed, or matrix secondary to local surgical procedures

Chemicals applied locally, *e.g.,* onycholysis from nail lacquer, may also produce discoloration and dystrophy; golden brown color of nail plate from glutaraldehyde; variable shades of brown on the nail plate surface due to formaldehyde, tincture benzoin, anthralin, and potassium permanganate; variable colors on nail plate surface from shoe polish.

NAIL BIOPSIES

Although most nail disorders are readily diagnosed from the history and the altered features in the nail, in some instances a biopsy may be needed to confirm a clinical impression. For example, psoriasis, lichen planus, and alopecia areata of the nails can be difficult to diagnose clinically, especially when the disease is confined to the nails, but they do show characteristic histopathologic pictures. Tumors of the nail unit always require biopsy for exact diagnosis. Many practitioners tend to veer away from nail biopsies, but they are no more difficult to do than skin biopsies.

BIOPSY OF UNGUAL TISSUE[10]

1. Primary indications for matrix or nailbed biopsy are the diagnosis of tumors and research into nail disorders.

2. Biopsy of matrix and margin of the pos-

terior nailfold is likely to produce permanent deformity.

3. X-ray studies of firm deforming lesions should be done before biopsy.

4. Use 1% lidocaine (Xylocaine) without epinephrine.

5. Use 2-mm biopsy punch for posterior nailfold, matrix, and proximal nailbed lesions.

6. When nail is intact, reduce thickness of nailplate before performing biopsy on matrix and proximal nailbed lesions.

7. Less deformity results if remaining nail is left intact to prevent contraction.

8. Distal nailbed lesions—remove overlying nailplate and biopsy lesion.

9. Specimens with attached nail should be fixed in 10% formalin with 5% trichloroacetic acid. This softens nailplate.

INGROWN TOENAILS

This painful disorder is a troublesome problem, especially among the aged. It is not uncommon in athletes, caused by footgear worn during certain sport activities, and in people who wear pointed-toe and high-heeled shoes. According to Lathrop, the chief factor is the incurving of the medial side of the distal phalanx of the toe; pressure forces exert a lateral shift.[6] This squeezes the nailplate, which turns downward and digs in. Once the nail has penetrated or damaged the cuticle fold, inflammation, erosion, granulation tissue, swelling, pain, and disability quickly follow.

In the simple incurved nail, the lateral aspects of the nail are markedly curved inward resulting in tenderness and pain. Therapy consists of packing cotton or lamb's wool under the advancing edge of the curved nail, thereby forcing it upward sufficiently to allow the nail to grow over the skin of the toe rather than into it. The packing is kept in place for the several months required. Prophylactic therapy consists of cutting the nails straight across and not too short.

In a true ingrown toenail, a pointed spicule of nail that remains attached to the lateral portion of the nail following improper trimming penetrates into the soft tissues of the toe as the nailplate grows forward (Fig. 18-2). This results in exquisite pain and, often, secondary infection.

Therapy consists of locating the nail sliver and removing it by cutting it away with a straight-edge nail-cutting forceps, followed by treating the infection with warm soaks and antibiotics, topical and systemic. When the infection has cleared, packing is placed under the nail as described previously for the incurved nail, and the nail plate is allowed to grow out over it.

In McGlamry's experience, conservative treatment can be completely satisfactory in instances in which packing and debridement of nail grooves is followed by a change to properly spacious shoes and stockings.[7] If subsequent ingrowing epiodes occur, surgical intervention may be necessary. Surgical techniques have been described by various authors.[5,6,7]

PINCER AND TRUMPET NAILS

This nail dystrophy is probably the result of an anomaly of developmental origin. The dystrophy is characterized by a transverse overcurvature that increases along the longitudinal axis of the nail and reaches its greatest proportion at the distal part.[8] At this point, a particular type of ingrown nail is seen: The lateral borders tighten around the soft tissues and pinch them without necessarily breaking through the epidermis.[2] The soft tissue may actually disappear and can even be accompanied by resorption of the underlying bone.[3] The lateral borders of the nail maintain a permanent constriction of the deformed nail, forming tunnels or claw-like forms. Pressure from ill-fitting shoes can be a factor in this. The great toe is the usual site of involvement; the condition occurs predominantly in women. Pincer toes can be extremely painful; avulsion of the nail or destruction of the nail matrix are the only measures providing relief.

AVULSION OF NAILS

Nail avulsion may be the only effective treatment for nail dystrophies such as ingrown toenails and pincer nails. Avulsion also can

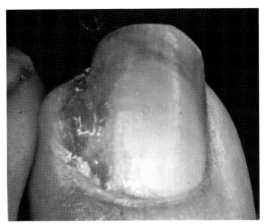

Fig. 18-2. Ingrown toenail.

be used in conjunction with griseofulvin for the treatment of onychomycosis (see Chap. 2) and as a method for treating psoriatic nails (see Chap. 11)

For a single affected nail, surgical avulsion is the modality of choice; when multiple nails are involved as in onychomycosis and psoriasis, nonsurgical avulsion is suggested.

SURGICAL AVULSION

Albom described a simple procedure that has proved effective:[1]

1. Complete anesthesia (digital block) of the affected digit is induced.
2. A spatula tip (#24A dental spatula) is first pushed under the posterior and posterolateral nail folds, and the nail plate is separated on its dorsal surface.
3. The spatula is then placed under the distal tip of the nail plate and advanced between the nail plate and the nail bed. The top of the instrument is passed forward along the ventral surface of the nail plate until the entire ventral surface of the plate is separated from the bed.
4. With a straight hemostat or needle holder, the nail plate is easily pulled off from its bed.
5. A Telfa dressing with Ilotycin or Polysporin ointment is applied and Surgitube is rolled into the digit, making an excellent nonbulky covering.

NONSURGICAL AVULSION

Farber and South have advocated nail avulsion with urea ointment.[4,9] Their formulation and technique consist of the following:

Formulation

urea	40%	120 g
white beeswax (or paraffin)	5%	15 g
anhydrous lanolin	20%	60 g
white petrolatum	25%	75 g
silica gel type A	10%	30 g
	100%	300 g

Technique

1. Cloth adhesive tape is used to cover the surrounding paronychial surfaces after pretreatment with tincture benzoin, or other medical adhesive.
2. The urea ointment is then generously applied directly to the diseased nail surface and covered with a piece of plastic film wrap, which is anchored proximally with more adhesive tape.
3. The entire digit is then covered with a "finger" cut from a plastic or vinyl glove, and then held in place with more adhesive tape. (Manufactured "finger cots" should never be used for this purpose, as they are too tight and will not expand adequately with edema, thus risking the vascular integrity of the digit.)
4. The patients are instructed to keep the dressings completely dry. Plastic booties are used for this purpose.
5. The patients then return in 7 days. At that time, the treated nails are removed (without anesthesia). This is done by lifting the entire nail from the nail bed with a periosteal elevator and trimming it just under the proximal nail fold with a nail clipper.
6. Pinpoint bleeding is easily controlled by compression.
7. The nail bed hardens in 12 to 36 hours when left open to the air, and patients can resume their normal activities immediately.

The authors recommend this technique in treating hypertrophic nail dystrophies that cause discomfort in shoes and in the chronic podiatric care of structural nail dystrophies such onychrogryphosis. (For this condition, this procedure must be repeated on a biannual basis.) Dermatophyte nail disease constitutes the major condition for which patients seek this treatment and is combined with oral griseofulvin or topical miconazole, or both.

REFERENCES

1. **Albom MJ:** Avulsion of a nail plate. J Dermatol Surg Oncol 3:34, 1977
2. **Baran R:** Pincer and trumpet nails. Arch Dermatol 110:639, 1974
3. **Cornelius CD, Shelley WB:** Pincer nail syndrome. Arch Surg 96:321, 1968
4. **Farber EM, South DA:** Urea ointment in the nonsurgical avulsion of nail dystrophies. Cutis 22:689, 1978
5. **Gibbs RC:** Treatment of the uncomplicated ingrown toenail. J Dermatol Surg Oncol 4:438, 1978
6. **Lathrop RG:** Ingrowing toenails: causes and treatment. Cutis 20:119, 1977
7. **McGlamry ED:** Management of painful toes from distorted toenails. J Dermatol Surg Oncol 5:554, 1979
8. **Samman PR:** The nails. In Rook A, Wilkinson DS, and Ebling FJG (eds): Textbook of Dermatology, pp 1663–1664. Oxford, Blackwell Scientific Publication, 1972
9. **South DA, Farber EM:** Urea ointment in the nonsurgical avulsion of nail dystrophies—A reappraisal. CUTIS 25:609, 1980
10. **Stone OJ, Barr RJ:** Biopsy of nail area. Cutis 21:257, 1978

19 SKIN DISORDERS IN ASSOCIATION WITH SPORTS

These syndromes received comparatively little mention in medical literature prior to 1970. Heretofore these unique syndromes were restricted to a trained minority of athletes, professional and amateur, for whom athletics was a means or way of life. In this decade, the sports explosion ignited a rash of these syndromes when an untrained or poorly trained majority began participating in recreational activities. We are living in an era of fun, fads, slim figures, and preoccupation with health—thus this tremendous fervor to jog, hike, and bike, with their toll of a variety of skin disorders. Of all the skin areas on the athlete, the foot is probably the most susceptible to skin problems.

Various exposure factors, depending on the sport, account for cutaneous problems that can occur on the lower extremities. Table 19-1 lists clinical syndromes observed by us or reported in the literature—this provides but a general perspective; it is by no means a catalog of all the skin problems caused by sports activities with predilection for the feet and legs. Athlete's foot, one of the most common problems encountered in athletes, was not included in this classification because it is not restricted to sports participants and can occur as readily in any individual. Athlete's foot syndrome is discussed in Chapter 2.

The very name of some of the syndromes (tennis toe, surfers' nodules, jogger's toe, skiers' shins) usually defines the causal relationship. The etiologic agents or appliances vary according to age, sex, geographic loca-

Table 19-1. Skin Disorders of the Lower Extremities In Association With Sports

Sport	Skin Disorders
Football (Soccer) and Basketball	Black heel
Basketball	Pitted keratolysis (PK)
Tennis	Calcaneal petechiae (tennis heel)
	PK
	"Tennis toe"
Hunting	Hunting phenomenon Acute pernio, frostbite
Hiking	Corns, calluses, warts, and blisters
Jogging	Jogger's toe, friction blisters, "runner's bumps"
Skiing	Skiers' shins
Surfing	Surfers' nodules
Any sport requiring special footwear (training shoes)	Allergic contact dermatitis

tion, season of the year, and the sport played. What is highly pertinent and often overlooked is to ask the leading question of the patient: "What sport do you indulge in?" Effective treatment and measures to prevent recurrence are dependent on the practitioner's understanding of this cause-effect picture.

BLACK HEEL

Black heel, also called calcaneal petechiae, is a traumatic lesion found in football (soccer) and basketball players.[9,12,13] It occurs most commonly as a consequence of pressure affecting the back or posterolateral aspect of the heel. It is seen almost exclusively in adolescents or young adults engaged in active sports, notably football and basketball, but also lacrosse, tennis, rodeo events, and so forth. The lesion is disposed horizontally at the upper edge of the calcaneal fat-pad and consists of grouped punctate hemorrhages. The black color is due to pigment derived from blood.

The lesion is caused by a shearing or pinching stress resulting from abrupt contact of the foot with a floor or hard ground.[13] The condition is symptomless; it may be observed only by chance and is self-healing. In England, Verbov's cases were related to rubbing or pinching of the heel where the reinforced heel piece of the players' football boots was stitched to the inner part of the boot.[12] The lesion was treated successfully with use of a slight heel raise with felt. The condition usually occurred early in the season; hardening of the skin as the season progressed seemed to protect it from this lesion.

PITTED KERATOLYSIS

The condition is seen primarily in basketball and tennis players. Occlusive footwear and

Fig. 19-1. Pitted keratolysis in a basketball player.

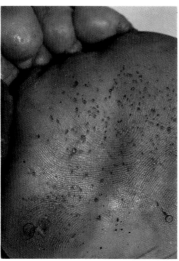

hyperhidrosis favor the corynebacterium infection; the combination is responsible for pitted keratolysis. The lesions, small shallow pits, develop in the stratum corneum of the sole over the weight-bearing surfaces, particularly the heels, balls of the feet, and toe pads. The pits range from 1 to 3 mm in diameter and 1 to 2 mm in depth. Some of the pits have a dirty brown to black pigmentation of the crater floor and walls (Fig. 19-1). The lesions are asymptomatic; they clear rapidly with the elimination of local moisture, but when this is not accomplished, topical 5% formalin or oral erythromycin can be used.[6]

For an overall description of pitted keratolysis, the reader is referred to Chapter 12.

TENNIS TOE

Tennis (or sportsman's) toe is merely a subungual hemorrhage caused by special stresses on the great toes.[2,8] Gibbs described this entity as pain associated with the appearance of hemorrhage beneath the toenails. The toe affected is that which extends furthest. According to Gibbs, in approximately 25% of normal people this is the second toe; in a similar percentage it is the hallux; and in roughly half the population, both the first and second toes extend the same distance. In tennis, the damage occurs because the player is frequently stopping abruptly and the forward motion of the body propels the toes into the box toe and tip of the sneakers. The hemorrhage under the nail shows a characteristic blue-black color. If the pain is severe, the nail should be cut to release the fluid underneath.[8] The shoe is also cut away above the affected nail to relieve the pressure.

Other problems due to tennis are friction blisters and tennis heel (calcaneal petechiae). Friction blisters, as would be expected, are the most common problem in tennis players. Tennis heel is relatively uncommon and is caused by friction. It presents as a pinpoint discoloration due to extravasated capillary blood on the posterior heels (see black heel). The condition is painless and usually disappears if active tennis is discontinued.

JOGGER'S TOE

This entity was described by Scher: Jogger's toe tends to involve the toe on the lateral surface of the foot.[10] The third, fourth, and fifth toes are most commonly involved. Rather than sudden changes in motion, which cause tennis toe, the jogger's toe appears to be due to the constant pounding of the foot on the running surface. Inappropriate or poorly fitting footgear also contribute to the pathogenesis of this condition. The process usually appears with erythema, edema, and separation of the toe nail from the nail bed; with less severe injury, subungual hemorrhage is the feature. Throbbing pain often accompanies the skin changes. Secondary infection resulting in cellulitis is an occasional complication. Temporary discontinuation of jogging and use of appropriate footgear are helpful in alleviating the condition.

"Runner's bumps" present as scaly and hyperkeratotic patches caused by rubbing of parts of the heels against shoes, especially in runners. Persons afflicted with so-called rearfoot varus are more prone to this problem in their attempt to compensate for the anatomic aberration.[3] Insert supports (wedges) in the running shoes help to alleviate the abnormal biomechanics caused by the foot fault.

SKIERS' SHINS

The appellation is the stigma of the skier: an abrasion or even ulceration of the skin over the mid-tibia is a specific skin sign of skiing. Ski enthusiasts are constantly attempting to "unbend" their knees, and this lesion results from forward leaning in a rigid boot.[11]

SURFERS' NODULES

The popularity of surfboarding, especially on the beaches of southern California, introduced a hazard that presents with typical surfers' nodules. The lesions are movable, subcutaneous, nontender masses, 1 to 6 cm in diameter localized to the knees and the middle of the top of the feet.[1] The earliest lesion may be a small red papule or pustule found at sites of pressure when riders kneel on their surfboards. Trauma is responsible for the lesions; they are caused by the friction of particles of sand that adhere to the wax on the surfaces of the board. This irritant reaction progresses into superficial erosions and ulcerations. The ulcers appear within 2 to 21 days of the primary lesion, varying in size from 0.5 to 3 cm. The ulcers are painful, become covered by a brownish hemorrhagic crust, and later form deep crateriform pockets with undermining indurated borders. Continued immersion during a prolonged surfing day alters the ulcer to a boggy, oozing, edematous mass.[1] On histopathologic examination, the surface nodule shows the picture of a hyperplastic granuloma.

The nodules usually involve spontaneously with abstinence from surfing. For prevention, paddling in the prone position and the wearing of elastic knee and ankle supports with sponge-rubber reinforcements are advisable. Ulcerations respond to local antiseptics, systemic antibiotics, and surgical debridement.

EFFECTS OF COLD

The hunting phenomenon discussed in Chapters 1 and 3 and acute pernio due to water-

Fig. 19-2. Callus from friction of boot and abnormal foot biomechanics in a hiker.

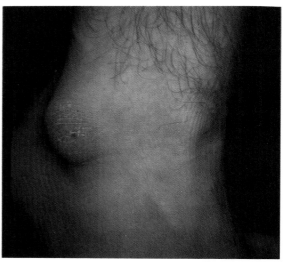

proof shoe boots described previously (Chap. 10) are minor problems that can be triggered by cold. Persons with Raynaud's disease or Raynaud's phenomenon associated with other disorders can find winter sports devastating and should be instructed to protect their hands and feet during these activities.[6]

Frostbite is a more serious problem. Although not encountered during planned winter sports, frostbite can occur in hunters, skiers, and others exposed to prolonged subfreezing temperatures. Tissue injury is believed to be the direct result of freezing. Upon exposure to intense cold, dermal vasoconstriction occurs, followed by a sensation of warmth and burning. As the tissues freeze, a white, waxy color and complete anesthesia supervene. Gradual thawing seems to give satisfactory results in superficial frostbite. Rapid rewarming of the frostbitten area in a 40° to 44°C water bath offers greatest tissue salvage. Excessive heat—temperatures greater than 115°F—gives disastrous results. Application of ice or snow as well as friction massage is contraindicated because this results in further tissue destruction.

HIKERS' HAZARDS

These common problems are the hiker's bane and are produced as a result of pressure-trauma-friction to the feet.[4] They include blisters, corns, and calluses (Fig. 19-2). Pressure can play an important role in causing plantar warts (see section on verrucae). If the amount of friction and pressure is increased beyond a certain point, traumatic blisters are induced. (The pathogenesis of friction blisters is discussed in Chap. 1.) In the genetic disorder, Cockayne syndrome, bullae develop on the feet subsequent to friction, as in prolonged marching (see Chap. 16). Corns and calluses have been discussed throughout the text, and particularly in Chapter 20.

Dusting the feet and socks with talc is the simplest and probably the most practical measure for reducing skin friction.

ALLERGIC CONTACT DERMATITIS

This disorder, discussed in Chapter 10, is not an uncommon problem among athletes. Re-

cently, Hanifin reported a new and apparently highly potent source of contact allergy that threatened many of those individuals caught up in the jogging craze.[5] Several individuals were highly allergic to an insole component used in Nike athletic shoes. This component is easily identified by its bright blue nylon covering, which overlies a black neoprene foam pad and covers the entire inner sole area of the shoes. Hanifer traced this allergy to the adhesive that bound the nylon to the neoprene. Testing with the other components of the shoes caused no reactions.

The patients showed a diffuse plantar dermatitis; testing with the cured adhesive produced a considerable flare reaction, not only on the feet but also on other areas of the body.

For treatment, refer to Chapter 10.

MISCELLANEOUS SPORTS HAZARDS

These can range from common problems such as insect bites and rhus dermatitis on the legs of sports enthusiasts walking around in shorts, for example, golfers, to an unusual subungual exostosis due to a bicyclist's toe clip, which caused trauma to the hallux.[7,14]

REFERENCES

1. **Erickson JG, Von Gemmingen GR:** Surfer's nodules and other complications of surfboarding. JAMA 201:148, 1967
2. **Gibbs RC:** "Tennis toe." Arch Dermatol 107:918, 1973
3. **Gibbs RC, Boxer MC:** The biomechanics of locomotion: Applicability to dermatologic and orthopedic conditions of the foot. J Dermatol Surg Oncol 6:252, 1980
4. **Glickman FS:** Hikers' hazards. Cutis 19:497, 1977
5. **Hanifin JM:** Nike training shoe dermatitis. Arch Dermatol 114:289, 1978
6. **Houston SD, Knox JM:** Skin problems related to sports and recreational activities. Cutis 19:487, 1977
7. **Mattikow MS:** The ubiquitous golfer. Cutis 19:471, 1977
8. **Montgomery RM:** Tennis and its skin problems. Cutis 19:480, 1977
9. **Nabai H, Mehregan AH:** Black heel. Cutis 6:751, 1970

10. **Scher RK:** Jogger's toe. Int J Dermatol 17:719, 1978
11. **Spoor HJ:** Sports identification marks. Cutis 19:453, 1977
12. **Verbov J:** Calcaneal petechiae. Arch Dermatol 107:918, 1973
13. **Wilkinson DS:** Black heel: A minor hazard of sport. Cutis 20:393, 1977

20 MISCELLANEOUS FOOT DISORDERS

Plantar Keratotic Lesions
Burning Feet
Erythromelalgia (Erythermalgia, Erythralgia)
Foot Odor
Piezogenic Papules
Lichen Aureus
Annular Lipoatrophy of the Ankles

PLANTAR KERATOTIC LESIONS

Corns and calluses—the most frequently encountered foot complaints—plantar warts, and porokeratosis plantaris discreta are plantar keratotic lesions seen by the podiatrist, dermatologist, and orthopedic surgeon. Pathomechanical faults cause corns and calluses; they play an important role in plantar warts. Although each lesion has its own distinctive features, the conditions are often confused and because of this can be wrongly treated.

Plantar warts are discussed in Chapter 2.

The *plantar corn* appears as a hard, horny papule with a core of impacted keratin. Corns develop over abnormal pressure points, usually under the second and third metatarsal heads (Fig. 20-1). Invariably, there are external pressure and friction acting in concert with the underlying bony prominence to cause vise-like constriction and irritation of the affected skin.[4] On paring, one exposes a hard central compressed mass, several millimeters in diameter. There is no pinpoint bleeding; it occurs only if excess paring is done (Fig. 20-2). Corns are painful and ex-

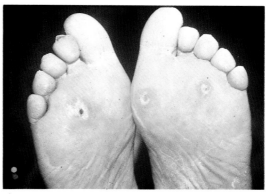

Fig. 20-1. Corns. Note how they develop over abnormal pressure points.

Fig. 20-2. Appearance of corn site after paring; there is no pinpoint bleeding.

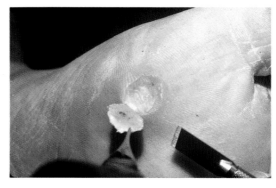

quisitely tender on vertical pressure. Treatment of plantar corns requires relieving pressure at the affected areas. Temporary relief may be achieved with salicylic acid plasters and paring.[2] Conservative measures can often provide relief of symptoms; they focus on comfortable and corrective shoes. The addition of metatarsal bars that are affixed to the outside of the shoes and that mechanically rearrange the weight-bearing characteristics of the foot more toward the heel are useful in relieving pressure from the metatarsal head.[3] Treatment of corns with injectable silicone was effective in a report done by Balkin.[1] In more intractable cases, an operative procedure may be required, either removal of an underlying bony prominence or a redirection of its weight-bearing role. The pros and cons of surgical treatment should be weighed very carefully before deciding to operate. It is cheaper and safer to get corrective shoes.

Calluses occur on the soles or edges of the feet where there is excessive pressure; an acute excess will produce a blister, while chronic friction produces a callus.[2] Clinically, the callus appears as a hard, dry plaque-like lesion. Care of calluses requires softening by hydration, salicylic acid gel under plastic wrap overnight or salicylic acid plasters for keratolysis, and avoidance of the causal irritation. Occasionally, a corn can be present within a callus. In our experience, surgical debridement of callus tissue and corns, special pads, and shoes are handled best by the podiatrist.

Porokeratosis plantaris discreta is an uncommon plantar hyperkeratosis that can be mistaken for a plantar wart. The condition has become better known following the extensive histologic study done by Taub and Steinberg: a horny plug microscopically comparable to the cornoid lamella of porokeratosis.[7] They theorized that pressure over a sweat pore causes hyperkeratosis of the duct, obstructing the orifice and causing a cystic dilation of the deeper portion.

Clinically, the lesion occurs singly or in a group. It presents as a keratin plug 1 to 2 mm in diameter, but groups of lesions may reach 1 cm or more. The plugs are sharply marginated and conical in shape; they press into the stratum malpighii, which is the base of the lesion, to a depth of 4 or 5 mm.[6] The plugs are connected loosely to the surrounding skin and can be separated easily by using a small curet or by paring. Montgomery advises that the base should be lightly electrodesiccated or the lesion will recur.[6]

KERATODERMA PLANTARIS (ACQUIRED)

Keratoderma plantaris may be acquired as well as hereditary. Numerous inflammatory disorders, such as psoriasis, lichen planus, syphilis, chronic arsenic intoxication, and Reiter's disease, may give rise to hyperkeratosis of the soles. Palmar and plantar keratoderma have been described in association with systemic cancers; however, this relationship has not been established with certainty. Occasionally, patients are seen who have striking plantar hyperkeratosis for which no cause is established and whose family history is negative for similar conditions.

Acquired hyperkeratosis of the soles has, in the past, been treated with macerating soaks or keratolytic agents such as salicylic acid—forms of treatment that have been messy, inconvenient, and rather unsatisfactory.

Heiss and Gross reported excellent success with the application of 0.3% vitamin A acid ointment twice daily with plastic occlusion during the night.[5] This would appear to be an effective and relatively simple therapeutic approach to a previously difficult problem (Figs. 20-3, 20-4).

BURNING FEET

Burning of the soles would rarely be a primary skin disease, and if so, other skin lesions would be observed, for example, the burning pain in association with erosion injury (see Chap. 12).

Does this condition represent a banal problem, *e.g.*, muscle cramping from awkward positioning, or does it imply impaired peripheral circulation or neuropathy (as in diabetes) or possibly a nutritional deficiency of niacin, pyrodoxine, or thiamine as seen in pernicious anemia and pellagra? The presenting symptoms should alert the physician to search for an etiologic diagnosis, but explanations for the localized variation in the sensitivity of this limited region are elusive.

The symptom complex is not uncommon in elderly patients with nutritional deficiencies and in alcoholics with malabsorption. Relief is often obtained when the dietary deficiencies are corrected.

Painful burning of the feet has been reported in patients with graft-versus-host disease (GVHD) after allogeneic marrow transplantation.[1] In children, the syndrome appeared as red, painful burning and scaly feet; the burning sensation persisted after the scales cleared. (Uberti MO, observations in Children's Hospital, Philadelphia, Nov 80, personal communication.) This distressing symptom could be a manifestation of the neuralgia characteristic of GVHD and appears to be a consequence of inflammation and fibrosis occurring around and within small dermal and subcutaneous nerves.

Another unusual example is the burning of the soles with flushing and pellagrous complication seen in carcinoid. An increase in bradykinin excretion is responsible for the flushing, which in turn provokes the burning sensation. Increased prostaglandin excretion has been suggested as the provocative factor for this burning sensation in erythromelalgia. This disorder is one of the most distinctive expressions of burning feet. Erythromelalgia is described next.

ERYTHROMELALGIA (ERYTHERMALGIA, ERYTHRALGIA)

Erythromelalgia is a rare distinctive syndrome characterized by three components: burning pain, local redness, and heat in the distal portions of the extremities. Symptoms of erythromelalgia occur intermittently, and the attacks are usually provoked by elevation of the skin temperature of the affected parts—from the internal heat of exercise or from external heat—and are diminished by cold.[3,4] The condition occurs in two forms, a primary (idiopathic) and a secondary type related to hematologic, nervous, peripheral vascular, or other diseases.[1,2,4,5] Little is known about the pathogenesis, and it is also unknown whether the pathogenesis of the

secondary type of erythromelalgia is similar to that of the primary type.[3]

Erythromelalgia is often an extremely uncomfortable condition: Burning and stinging pain mainly affecting the sole is at times intolerable. The erythematous areas are warmer than the surrounding skin and tender. Elevation of the legs and cooling of the feet (cool compresses or cool air from an electric fan or air conditioner) usually provide relief. More significantly, prompt relief of symptoms has been obtained with aspirin. One of the actions of aspirin is to inhibit prostaglandin synthesis. This therapeutic response suggests the possibility that prostaglandins may be involved in the pathogenesis of erythromelalgia because the redness and burning of the skin could be attributed to increased prostaglandin synthesis.

FOOT ODOR*

Bromidrosis or sweat odors commonly result from the interaction of skin secretions, including eccrine, sebaceous, and apocrine secretions, with resident skin microorganisms. Foot odors, in particular, most likely arise from microbial action on eccrine sweat and epidermal lipid. Characterization of isovalerianic acid as the "sweaty foot odorant" suggests that this chemical along with other short-chain acids might contribute to the observed odor. However, no studies have been directed toward *in vivo* sampling and characterization of the odors or correlating specific microorganisms or substrates with odor production.

In contrast, recent studies of axillary and scalp odors have shown that organisms residing in these skin areas can produce the observed odors *in vitro*. Thus, the yeast *Pityrosporum ovale*, the major scalp resident, produces unique fruity odorants (γ-lactones) when incubated on lipid substrates (lecithin, triglycerides). This same organism imparts a scalp-like odor to cultures that contain sebum as the primary substrate. These odors are probably formed on the scalp from a cooperative effort of *Propionibacterium acnes*, which acts to hydrolyze triglycerides

---

* Contributed by John N. Labows, Ph.D.

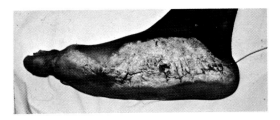

Fig. 20-3. Keratoderma plantaris (before treatment).

Fig. 20-4. Keratoderma plantaris after treating it with 0.3% vitamin A acid under occlusion.

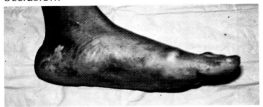

in hair follicle, and *P. ovale*, which metabolizes the resultant fatty acids or glycerol, or both. Similarly, axillary odors arise from the action of two bacterial species on apocrine secretion. Apocrine secretion provides a unique substrate which includes androgen steroids, cholesterol, protein, and lipid. Incubation of micrococci with apocrine secretion gives a sweaty odor, which has been characterized as that of isovalerianic acid. Diphtheroid (corynebacteria) bacteria produce a heavy musk/urine-like odor when incubated with the secretion. Moisture has been shown to effect the relative proportion of these two bacteria, with more humid conditions favoring the diphtheroids. Controlling of odor has been directed at (1) reducing eccrine secretion with antiperspirants (drying agents); (2) masking of the odors with deodorants; and (3) reduction of the bacterial population with antibacterial agents.

The interdigital spacings of the foot provide a similar area for colonization by both bacteria and fungi. Eccrine secretion provides various salts and amino acids as well as lactic acid and urea, and with epidermal lipid can serve as a substrate for microbial growth. The foot does not provide as rich a substrate as the scalp or axillae. However, the daily occlusion of the foot area serves to concentrate the available substrate and promote microbial growth. Dermatophyte fungi can generally be demonstrated in situations with low-grade peeling or scaling (dermatophytosis simplex), but no strong or unusual odors are present. However, the combination of an overgrowth of aerobic diphtheroid bacteria in an area already damaged by dermatophytes (dermatophytosis complex) can result in skin maceration, itching, and malodor. The Corynebacteria found on the foot differ from those isolated from the axillae in their ability to produce the odorous methanethiol. Taxonomically, they are similar to the Brevibacteria and to dairy isolates, which produce methanethiol an important flavor component of cheddar cheese aroma, although some confusion exists as to the complete classification of the skin diphtheroids. Diphtheroids have been isolated from the skin in cases of pitted keratolysis and may be responsible for the foot odor observed in this condition.

More serious cases of foot infection may involve the gram-negative organisms such as Pseudomonas and Proteus. Various Pseudomonas species are efficient producers of odorous sulfur metabolites (dimethyl disulfide—cabbage, and methyl mercaptan—cheddar cheese aroma). Several amine compounds (fishy odors) as well as sulfur metabolites have been identified in cultures of Proteus species. Whether any of these bacteria produce the same odorous metabolites from the natural substrates present on the foot has not been determined. However, research is in progress to determine if these metabolites are unique to the given bacteria and can be used for their detection in a mixed bacterial growth such as might be found on the foot. Such an approach might also be useful in distinguishing a fungal from bacterial colonization.

Treatment of foot odors should involve reductions in moisture and bacterial population. Antibacterials can be applied to eliminate bacterial growth; however, continued exposure to antibacterials could destroy the bacterial ecology of the foot. A better approach involves the use of drying agents for moisture removal, or aeration of the affected area to enhance the evaporation of moisture. This approach of modifying the environmental conditions in order to restore the natural ecology is preferable.

PIEZOGENIC PAPULES

This disorder is not uncommon, although it is often unrecognized. Herniation of fatty subcutaneous tissue through a defect of the connective tissue into the dermis produces lesions that are not noted when the patient is recumbent but which become apparent when the upright position is assumed.[1,2,5,6] The most common site is the posterior part of the medial sides of the heels. The patient is asymptomatic when reclining; although in one reported case the papules were exquisitely painful even when lying in bed.[3] The herniations may remain asymptomatic or may become painful when the patient stands. A detailed histologic study done by Schlappner et al confirmed the pathogenesis of the disorder.[4]

Palliative measures, such as supportive devices in the shoes and a change from a standing occupation to one of a more sedentary nature, are helpful. In some instances, surgical correction, excision of the fatty tissue protrusion at its base, may be indicated.

LICHEN AUREUS

Lichen aureus presents a distinct clinical picture and in its early stage may resemble an atypical progressive pigmentary dermatosis. This rare disease can occur anywhere on the body; in the report by Waisman and Waisman, the lesions were distributed symmetrically on the legs.[1] The eruption presented as discolored patches composed of closely aggregated or confluent follicular, superficial, rust-colored flat papules with a thin adherent scale. The histologic picture was that of a nonspecific angiodermatitis, distinguished from the pigmented purpuric eruptions by its lack of epidermal changes and exocytosis.

ANNULAR LIPOATROPHY OF THE ANKLES

This unusual clinical entity represents a form of partial lipodystrophy; basically, it involves mainly the subcutis, while the overlying skin is intact.[3] The condition is characterized by its clinical features and localization. The skin lesion is striking: a band of atrophy encircling the ankles. The atrophy was preceded by a short period of symptomless, noninflammatory subcutaneous swelling of the ankle regions.

Pathogenesis is obscure. Some authors classify the conditions as an idiopathic localized lipoatrophy; Shelley and Izumi consider the atrophy to be a cutaneous symptom of systemic disease—endocrinologic, neurologic, or metabolic, with the possibility of latent diabetes.[1-3] The patients described by Jablonska et al had no neurologic disorders and were in good health.[2] The disease causes neither contractures nor difficulty in walking.

REFERENCES

KERATOTIC LESIONS

1. **Balkin SW:** Treatment of corns by injectable silicone. Arch Dermatol 111:1143, 1975
2. **Carney RG:** Confusing keratotic lesions of the sole. Cutis 7:32, 1971
3. **Engler GL, Gibbs RC:** Common plantar hyperkeratoses. J Dermatol Surg 1:59, 1975
4. **Gibbs RC:** Foot notes: variations on a corny theme. J Dermatol Surg Oncol 4:289, 1978
5. **Heiss HB, Gross PR:** Keratosis palmaris and plantaris treatment with topically applied vitamin A acid. Arch Dermatol 101:100, 1970
6. **Montgomery RM:** Porokeratosis plantaris discreta. Cutis 20:7111, 1977
7. **Taub J, Steinberg M:** Porokeratosis plantaris discreta, a previously unrecognized dermatological entity. Int J Dermatol 9:83, 1970

BURNING FEET

1. **Shulman HM, Sale GE, Lerner KG, et al:** Chronic cutaneous graft-versus-host disease in man. Am J Path 91:545, 1978

ERYTHROMELALGIA

1. **Alarcon-Segovia D, Babb RP, Fairbairn JF II, et al:** Erythermalgia. Arch Intern Med 117:511, 1966

2. **Alarcon-Segovia D, Diaz-Jovanen E:** Erythermalgia in systemic lupus erythematosus. Am J Med Sci 266:149, 1966
3. **Jorgensen HP, Sondergaard J:** Pathogenesis of erythromelalgia. Arch Dermatol 114:112, 1978
4. **Redding KG:** Thrombocythemia as a cause of erythermalgia. Arch Dermatol 113:468, 1977
5. **Smith LA, Allen EV:** Erythermalgia (erythromelalgia) of the extremities: A syndrome characterized by redness, heat and pain. Am Heart J 16:175, 1938

PIEZOGENIC PAPULES

1. **Cohen HJ, Gibbs RC, Minkin W, Frank SB:** Painful piezogenic pedal papules. Arch Dermatol 101:112, 1970
2. **Galinski AW:** Cutaneous herniations. A case report. J Am Pod Assoc 60:128, 1970
3. **Harman RRM, Matthews CNA:** Painful piezogenic pedal papules. Brit J Dermatol 90:573, 1974
4. **Schlappner OLA, Wood MG, Gerstein W, Gross**
PR: Painful and non-painful piezogenic pedal papules. Arch Dermatol 106:729, 1972
5. **Shelley WB, Rawnsley HM:** Painful feet due to herniation of fat. JAMA 205:308, 1968
6. **Woerdeman JJ, Van Dijk E:** Piezogenic papules of the feet. Acta Dermatovener (Stockholm) 52:411, 1972

LICHEN AUREUS

1. **Waisman M, Waisman M:** Lichen aureus. Arch Dermatol 112:696, 1976

ANNULAR LIPOATROPHY OF ANKLES

1. **Geschwandter WR, Munzberger H:** Lipoatrophia semicircularis. Hautarzt 25:222, 1974
2. **Jablonska S, Szczepanski A, Gorkiewicz A:** Lipo-atrophy of the ankles and its relation to other lipo-atrophies. Acta Dermatovener (Stockholm) 55:135, 1975
3. **Shelley WB, Izumi A:** Annular atrophy of the ankles. Arch Dermatol 102:326, 1970

INDEX

Numerals in *italics* indicate color illustrations